Step by Step

Tubo-uterine Factors in Infertility

System requirement:

- **Windows XP or above**
- **Power DVD player (Software)**
- **Windows Media Player version 10.0 or above**
- **Quick time player version 6.5 or above**

Accompanying DVD Rom is playable only in Computer and not in DVD player.

Kindly wait for few seconds for DVD to autorun. If it does not autorun then please do the following:

- Click on my computer
- Click the **drive labelled ANSHAN** and after opening the drive, kindly double click the file **Anshan**

DVD CONTENTS

1. Laparoscopic Myomectomy

2. Hysteroscopic Removal of Submucous Myoma

3. Hysteroscopic Excision of Intrauterine Adhesions

4. Laparoscopic Adhesiolysis

5. Fimbrioplasty—Laparoscopic Approach

6. Laparoscopic Removal of Ovarian Endometrioma

7. Ectopic Pregnancy—Laparoscopic Salpingectomy

Step by Step
Tubo-uterine Factors in Infertility

Surveen Ghumman MD

Specialist
Department of Obstetrics and Gynecology
Vardhman Mahavir Medical College and Safdarjung Hospital
New Delhi

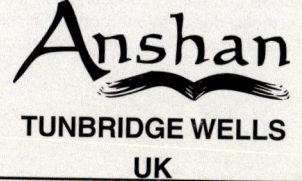

TUNBRIDGE WELLS
UK

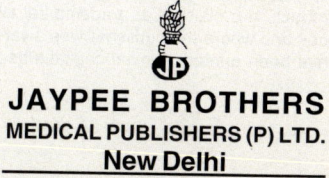

JAYPEE BROTHERS
MEDICAL PUBLISHERS (P) LTD.
New Delhi

First published in the UK by

Anshan Ltd
in **2008**
6 Newlands Road
Tunbridge Wells
Kent TN4 9AT, UK

Tel: +44 (0)1892 557767
Fax: +44 (0)1892 530358
E-mail: info@anshan.co.uk
www.anshan.co.uk

ISBN 13 978-1-905740-81-9

British Library Cataloguing in Publication Data
A catalogue record for this book is available from the British Library

Printed in India by Paras Offset Pvt.Ltd.,C-176, Naraina Phase-1,New Delhi -28

Contributors

Neena Singh Kumar
Consultant Endoscopic Surgeon
Department of Obstetrics and Gynecology
Batra Hospital and Research Center, New Delhi

Punita Bhardwaj
Consultant
Gynae Endoscopic Unit
Sir Ganga Ram Hospital, New Delhi

Reeti Sahni
Senior Consultant
Radiology and Imaging Sciences
Indraprastha Apollo Hospital, New Delhi

Sudha Salhan
Professor and Head
Department of Obstetrics and Gynecology
Vardhman Mahavir Medical College
and Safdarjung Hospital, New Delhi

Surveen Ghumman
Specialist
Department of Obstetrics and Gynecology
Vardhman Mahavir Medical College
and Safdarjung Hospital, New Delhi

Shweta Mittal
Consultant
Centre of IVF and Human Reproduction
Sir Ganga Ram Hospital, New Delhi

Foreword

In the past decade, developments in the field of ART have intensified the hopes and wishes of infertile people to resolve their infertility and have resulted in an increasing demand for such services in both developed and developing countries. The increasing effort and determination on the part of researchers, clinicians and surgeons alike to overpower and eliminate the crippling stigma of infertility and the 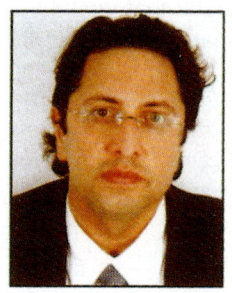 promise to help every infertile couple experience the reality of parenthood has led to aggressive research and a plethora of information in the fields of reproductive endocrinology and infertility. The growing challenge of providing a therapy for every cause of infertility is obviously accompanied with efforts to obviate the complications that beset these therapies.

This remarkably concise and clear book deals with the many issues relating to uterotubal factor in infertility, including evaluation of the uterine cavity and the laparoscopic and hysteroscopic management of the condition. Not all problems are alike, and this book will satisfy different needs of different people by touching upon a diverse range of problems, from fibroids to intrauterine adhesions to endometriosis. It holds a treasure of information for all interested in helping infertile patients. I am sure that any practicing physician who treats infertile patients will greatly benefit from reading this well written book.

I would like to congratulate the contributors and the editor Dr. Surveen Ghumman of the book for their valuable effort and time in creating an interesting and scientifically stimulating book that would be hard to put down.

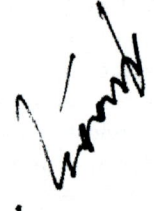

Gautam N Allahbadia MD DNB FNAMS
Consultant Fertility Physician
Dr LH Hiranandani Center for Human Reproduction
Dr LH Hiranandani Hospital, Powai, Mumbai

Scientific Director
Prince Aly Khan Hospital IVF Center and the Aesculap
Academy – Asia Pacific Center for Minimally Invasive
Surgery, Training and Research, Mazagaon, Mumbai

Medical Director
Rotunda – The Center for Human Reproduction
Bandra, Mumbai

Preface

Fertility therapy continues to expand most rapidly into superspecialized areas of assisted reproductive techniques. While the scientists have been busy making successful advances in these areas the clinical approach and therapy has also taken a great step forward to minimize the time taken to reach a diagnosis and direct a couple to appropriate therapy.

Tubo-uterine causes of infertility have been gradually increasing in importance in the field of infertility management. Their incidence is between 25 to 40% in the infertile patient. Keeping these factors in mind this book has been written to enable a practicing clinician to have a concise road map in dealing with such patients.

Evaluation of the uterine cavity, tubal structure and function along with their imaging forms the basis on which the diagnosis depends are dealt in detail. The various conditions like fibroids, ectopic pregnancy and other intrauterine, tubal and peritubal pathologies have been discussed in the various chapters with special reference to their diagnosis and management. Medical and surgical management have been explained with flow charts, diagrams and photographs. Keeping in view the theme of the book the chapter on endometriosis deals extensively with the postsurgical management of the infertile woman. With the advent of endoscopes, early diagnosis and minimal tissue handling during surgical procedures has led to successful treatment of a vast number of cases. Separate chapters on the minimal invasive surgical management have been incorporated. This includes photographs of instrumentation and of the actual procedure. Along with this the videos in the DVD-ROM of the techniques have been presented with the aim of reinforcing the surgical steps. Postoperative adhesions in the abdominal cavity are an important cause of infertility and a separate chapter deals with its prevention.

This book has been written as a practical guide with the aim of placing the modern approach to the management of infertility in the context of sound theory, evidence based therapy and recent advances. A comprehensive classification, investigation and management of all tubouterine factors causing infertility have been presented in the book and the accompanying DVD-ROM.

In this day of information overload this book is an attempt to integrate information into a practice management protocol that is rational, logical and rewarding for the reader.

I hope this book is stimulating enough to help every practising infertility specialist to solve dilemmas in dealing with tubouterine pathologies in their patients enabling them to achieve the desired goal—A successful pregnancy in all patients.

Surveen Ghumman

Acknowledgements

I am indebted to Dr R.N. Salhan, Medical Superintendent of Safdarjung Hospital and Vardhman Mahavir Medical College for his encouragement and support. I sincerely thank Dr Sudha Salhan, Professor and Head of Department of Obstetrics and Gynecology at Safdarjung Hospital for encouraging me in this academic pursuit.

I thank all the contributors for their well researched chapters and for sparing their invaluable time and intellectual skills. I have thoroughly enjoyed interacting with all the authors during this academic venture.

I would also like to acknowledge the invaluable contribution of the team and artists at my publishers, M/s Jaypee Brothers Medical Publishers (P) Ltd. for making this volume in its present form.

I would like to extend my gratitude to my family for bearing with me for the time I have invested in this project rather than spend with them. The constant support, help and encouragement I received from my husband went a long way in bringing this book together. A special thanks to my daughters who helped in many ways. I would also like to thank my parents for guiding me to reach this day.

Although this book has my name on it but it is a combined effort of all above without which it would not have its present form.

Contents

1. **Evaluation of Uterine Cavity and Endometrium** **1**
   Surveen Ghumman

2. **Tests for Evaluation of Tubal Structure and Function** **29**
   Surveen Ghumman

3. **Fibroid** **53**
   Surveen Ghumman

4. **Endoscopic Management of Fibroid** **101**
   Neena Singh Kumar, Surveen Ghumman

5. **Uterine Anomalies** **135**
   Surveen Ghumman

6. **Intrauterine Adhesions** **187**
   Surveen Ghumman

7. **Hysteroscopic Infertility Surgery** **207**
   Punita Bhardwaj

8. **Tubal Reconstructive Surgery** **225**
   Surveen Ghumman

9. **Laparoscopic Surgery for Tubal and Peritubal Pathology in Infertility** **269**
   Punita Bhardwaj

10. **Laparoscopic Tubal Anastomosis** **291**
    Neena Singh Kumar, Surveen Ghumman

11. **Pelvic Inflammatory Disease** **303**
    Surveen Ghumman

12. Endometriosis 321
    Surveen Ghumman

13. Ovarian Endometriosis—Laparoscopic
    Management 361
    Neena Singh Kumar, Surveen Ghumman

14. Ectopic Pregnancy... 369
    Sudha Salhan, Surveen Ghumman

15. Prevention of Postoperative Adhesions 405
    Surveen Ghumman

16. IVF and Tubo-uterine Factors in Infertility 427
    Shweta Mittal

17. Imaging Techniques in
    Tubo-uterine Pathology 435
    Reeti Sahni

    Index 459

CHAPTER 1

Evaluation of the Uterine Cavity and Endometrium

Surveen Ghumman

Uterine anatomical defects are common in women with infertility and recurrent pregnancy loss. Therefore, it is essential that fertility work-up includes an evaluation for structural uterine abnormalities (Table 1.1).

Table 1.1: Tests for assessing the uterine cavity structural abnormalities and endometrial receptivity

I. Tests for assessing uterine cavity and structural abnormalities:
  1. Hysterosalpingography
  2. Hysterosalpingosonography
  3. Magnetic resonance hysterography
  4. Hysteroscopy
  5. Endometrial biopsy
  6. Ultrasonography
  7. MRI
 II. Tests for assessing endometrial receptivity:
  1. Tests that assess endometrial changes
   • Endometrial biopsy
   • Ultrasound and Doppler
   • Hormonal levels
  2. Markers of the embryo-endometrial dialogue

I. *Tests for Assessing Uterine Cavity and Structural Abnormalities*

HYSTEROSALPINGOGRAPHY

Hysterosalpingography (HSG) is the radiographic visualization of the endocervical canal, the endometrial cavity and the lumina of the fallopian tube after instilling a radiographic contrast media through the cervix.

In infertility unless specific information points towards a uterotubal disease, a hysterosalpingogram should be performed after completion of ovulation assessment and semen analysis. Likelihood of tubal disease would lead to an HSG, early in investigation of infertility.

The risk factors for tubouterine disease are:
1. History of salpingitis
2. A positive clamydia IgG titer ($>$1:32)
3. Postpartum dilatation and curettage
4. Previous ectopic pregnancy or pelvic surgery
5. Exposure to diethylstilbestrol
6. Recurrent pregnancy loss
7. Previous abnormal HSG
8. Menstrual problems.

Although this examination does not define the extent of certain conditions such as endometriosis and periadenexal adhesions, it does reveal the shape of the uterine cavity and characteristics of the tubal lumina and their patency. Despite advances in endoscopy. HSG retains a special place in investigating the infertile women because it is a simple, painless and non-surgical screening procedure.

Contraindications

1. Infection
2. Pregnancy
3. Bleeding—Active uterine bleeding is a contraindication because there is:
   - Increased chance of intravasation
   - Obscuring of uterine pathology by blood clots
   - Potential for retrograde menstruation and induction of endometriosis.

Time

It is usually done in follicular phase when the endometrium is thin. If an incompetent OS is to be diagnosed it should be done premenstrually when physiological contraction of the lower uterine segment is greatest.

Interpretation of Abnormal Hysterosalpingogram

Abnormalities Involving the Endometrial Cavity

The various abnormalities of endometrial cavity seen are:

1. Outpouching
2. Filling defect
3. Abnormal shape or size of cavity.

   1. **Outpouching:** It is seen in
      i. *Cesarean or myomectomy scar:* Outpouching is seen at site of scar.
      ii. *Adenomyosis:* It is seen as spicules of contrast medium with varying length of 1 to 2 cm extending perpendicularly from the endometrial cavity into the uterine wall and frequently terminating in a small sac 2 to 4 mm in diameter. It can also appear as small sacculations and branching channels which may extend into outer uterine wall (Fig. 1.1).
      iii. *Previous interstitial segment ectopic pregnancy:* It results in saccular outpouching at the cornua.

   2. **Filling defects**
      i. *Submucous polyp or myoma:* They produce smooth round sometimes pedunculated filling defects (Fig. 1.2)
      ii. *Nabothian cyst:* It can produce filling defects in the cervical canal.
      iii. *Intrauterine adhesions:* They are seen as linear or irregular filling defects which are sharply defined. Large adhesions will constrict and deform the endometrial cavity. Extensive adhesions may obliterate the cavity completely, obstructing the tube and causing vascular intravasation (Figs 1.3 and 1.4).
      iv. *Endometrial hyperplasia:* This causes irregular filling defects along the contour of the endometrial cavity.
      v. *Blood clots or retained products of conception:* They will produce tubular or serpiginous filling defects. An early pregnancy will cause a round filling defect in the upper uterine cavity like a myoma.

   3. **Abnormal size or shape of cavity**
      i. *Anomalies of the müllarian duct:*
         • *Unicornuate uterus:* Oblong cavity displaced, to one side with a single fallopian tube. It should be

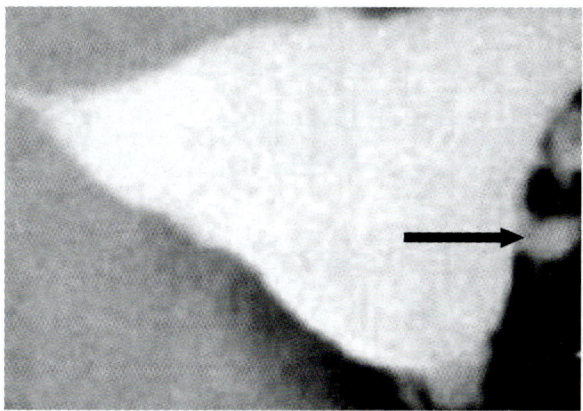

Fig. 1.1: Sacculations seen in adenomyosis on HSG

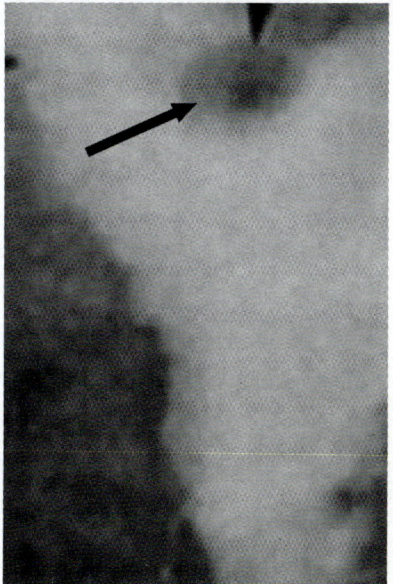

Fig. 1.2: Endometrial polyp on HSG

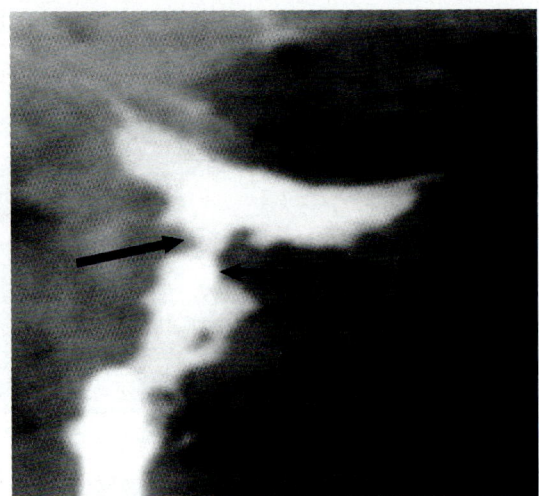

Fig. 1.3: Intrauterine adhesions seen on HSG

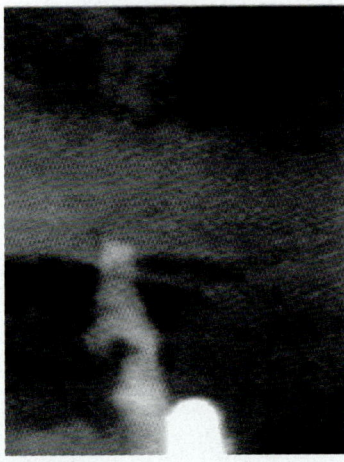

Fig. 1.4: Contracted uterine cavity
due to adhesions seen on HSG

differentiated from an incompletely filled cavity, an intense spasm of one horn and blockage by dense synechiae preventing access to opposite horn. A lateral film and uterine manipulation may help to differentiate it from these condition.

- *Bicornuate uterus:* Bicornuate uterus will show a V shaped endometrial cavity (Fig. 1.5)
- *Uterus didelphus:* Duplicated endocervical canal and oblong endometrial cavities are seen. In these cases Foley's catheter is inserted on one side since the vagina may not be able to accommodate 2 sets of instruments (Fig. 1.6)
- *Septate uterus:* Endometrial cavity in septate uterus appears as in bicornuate uterus (Fig. 1.7)
- *Arcuate uterus:* It is a minor malformation in which the fundus appears concave although the depth of depression is less than 1.5 cm.

ii. *Antenatal diethylstilbsterol exposure:*
- Symmetric or asymmetric deformity of the endometrial cavity with a reduced size of the cavity. The uterus appears T shaped and hypoplastic, with indentations on its lateral border.

iii. *Large submucous myoma:*
- If it is large it will produce an elongation of the uterine cavity. A large intramural myoma may produce enlargement of a portion of the cavity.

iv. *Intrauterine adhesion:*
- Moderate to large intrauterine adhesions can deform endometrial cavity.

Media

All media used for HCG contains iodine. A water contrast medium is recommended for optimum delineation of the uterine tubal mucosa. This is particularly important for evaluating tubal disease as preservation of mucosal folds in the ampulla is a determinant of success of the reconstructive

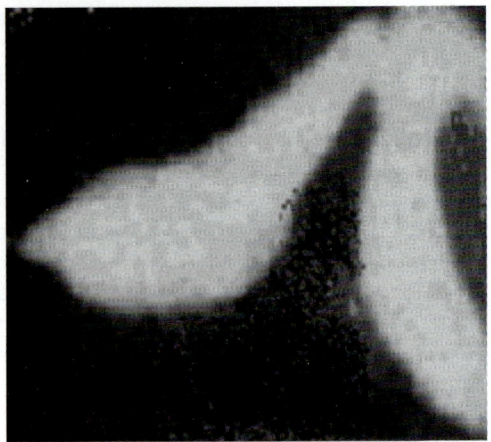

Fig. 1.5: Bicornuate uterus on HSG

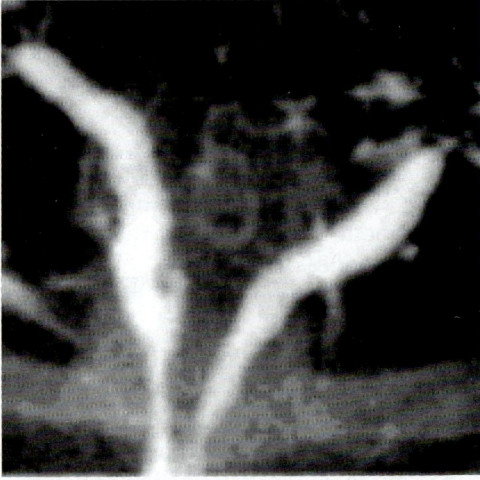

Fig. 1.6: Uterus didelphus on HSG

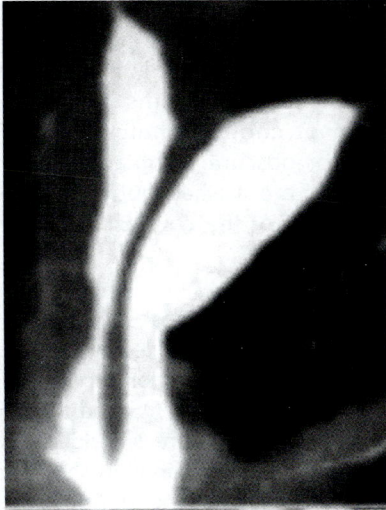

Fig. 1.7: Intrauterine septum on HSG

surgery. When an oil based contrast is used the mucosa is obscured but a more clear radiographic image with sharper borders and more contrast is achieved in comparison to water based contrast medium. There are new media which have a low osmolality (assumed to cause less pain from peritoneal irritation) or contain iodine in non-ionic form (less likely to result in allergic reaction to iodine).[1]

Fallacy

1. On introducing contrast air bubbles are inadvertently introduced and appear as mobile round filling defects which can mimic a small polyp. Differentiation can be made by moving the patient from supine to prone position causing bubbles to migrate. Occasionally the bubble may lodge in the cornua and prevent contrast from passing into the fallopian tube. This can be corrected by placing the patient

in a lateral decubitus position which allows the bubble to rise from the cornua. It can be avoided by initially filling the cannula with contrast medium before its placement.

2. Sometimes a plexus of veins can be visualized by intravasation of contrast material. This may mimic adenomyosis or obscure fallopian tubes. However, the venous channels are washed out by nonopacified blood once the injection of the contrast medium is stopped.

Technique

The cannula is filled with contrast material to flush out the air. Posterior vaginal wall is retracted with a Sims speculum. A tenaculum is fixed on the anterior cervical lip, the cannula inserted into the external cervical OS and the two instruments are held together. Some pressure should be maintained on the fluid filled syringe. The examination should be carried out using image intensifier fluoroscopy, which allows appropriate amount of contrast material to be injected. Two spot radiographs are needed. First one is taken with early filling of endometrial cavity as a submucous polyp may become obscure once endometrial cavity is fully distended with contrast. The second is taken before intraperitoneal spill is seen so as to optimally visualize the tubal details.

The typical examination requires 10 seconds of fluoroscopic time. Radiographs in anteroposterior and lateral positions should be taken. A follow-up film should be taken 30 minutes later for water-soluble material and after 24 hours for oil-soluble material.

Fluoroscopy with image intensification gives the best results. Insufficient dye injection will give an incomplete study. Too much dye injection, especially under pressure, might cause extravasation of the dye into the vascular system or conceal the fimbrial ends of the tubes.[2]

Endocervical canal: It has serrated borders that are caused by normal anatomic plicae palmatae. The normal lower uterine segment has parallel borders that are usually regular. This segment if wider than 1 cm suggests an incompetent OS.

Uterine cavity: It is triangular in shape with smooth borders. The upper border, the fundus, may be convex or saddle shaped, and the cornua are generally pointed.

Hysterosalpingography is not accurate in differentiating a bicornuate from a septate uterus because external contour of uterus is not visible. Since both have completely different surgical interventions, a correct diagnosis is very important. An additional investigation by means of three-dimensional ultrasound is recommended.[3]

HYSTEROSONOGRAPHY

Hysterosonography or saline infusion sonohysterography (SIS) is a technique in which a catheter is placed into the endometrial cavity and sterile saline is instilled to separate the walls of the endometrium (Fig. 1.8). It is best performed between cessation of menses and day 10 of menstrual cycle when the endometrium is at its thinnest, and focal lesions such as polyps are best seen. During the secretory phase there may be false-positive findings from folds of thickened endometrium. For

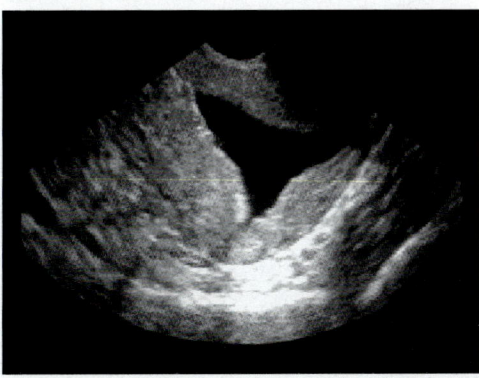

Fig. 1.8: Endometrial cavity seen on hysterosonosalpingography

evaluation of uterine cavity, approximately 5 to 30 ml of warm sterile saline is injected via a catheter (See Chapter 2 for details).

Complete sonographic evaluation of the endometrial cavity is performed in both coronal and sagittal planes. In addition, 3-dimensional (3D) imaging has been advocated to get a better global view of the uterine cavity.[4] The balloon is then deflated, and evaluation of the lower uterine segment and endocervical region is performed. Doppler evaluation is helpful in distinguishing blood clots from polypoidal lesions.[5]

Saline infusion sonohysterography and HSG had similar results in detecting intrauterine adhesions. Both methods had a sensitivity of 75%, while the specificity was 93% and 95%, respectively (Fig. 1.9).

Saline infusion sonohysterography can distinguish focal lesions from diffuse endometrial thickening. Polyps are focal lesions, which project into the lumen of the endometrial cavity (Fig. 1.10). The anechoic saline outlines the polyp which is echogenic (Figs 1.10 and 1.11).

Fibroids appear as hypoechoic masses with respect to the myometrium, in contrast to endometrial polyps, which are usually hyperechoic.

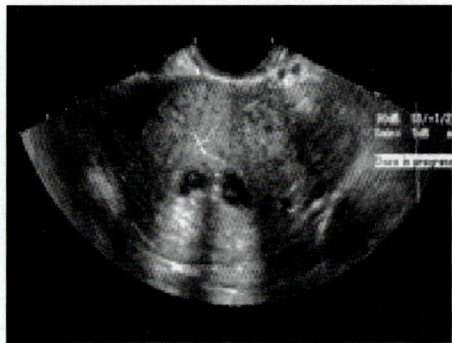

Fig. 1.9: Intrauterine adhesions as visualized by sonohysterosalpingography

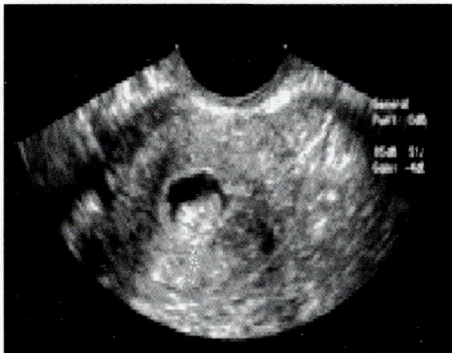

Fig. 1.10: Polyp seen in endometrial cavity on SIS

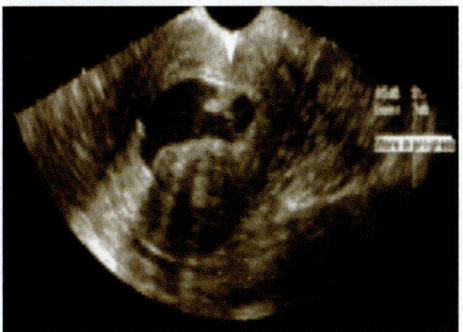

Fig. 1.11: Submucous fibroid in posterior wall projecting into the cavity as seen in saline infusion sonohysterography

Accuracy of the hysterosonography was superior to hysterosalpingography (90.9 and 85.2% respectively). The hysterosonography had a higher diagnostic accuracy in the detection of uterine cavity anomalies and it was better tolerated by the patients when compared to hysterosalpingography and hysteroscopy.[6] The sensitivity and specificity of sonohysterography were the same as that for hysteroscopy.[7]

Advantages of Hysterosonography over the HSG

1. It uses no ionizing radiation
2. The entire uterus including fundus is visualized rather than the outline of the endometrial canal
3. It is well tolerated by the patient and has few complications
4. It has higher accuracy.

Saline infusion sonohysterography (SIS) is a simple examination that yields additional information over TVS of the uterus. As the walls of the endometrium are separated by saline infusion, they can be evaluated individually. Focal abnormalities are accurately detected by this technique. This information can thus be used to direct therapeutic intervention.

MAGNETIC RESONANCE HYSTEROGRAPHY

Magnetic resonance hysterography has been reported in the literature as a new technique for evaluating uterine abnormalities. Magnetic resonance imaging gives excellent soft tissue contrast in the uterus. Saline is instilled into the endometrial canal as in SIS. MRI of the uterus is then done using a fluid-attenuated inversion recovery sequence to null the signal from water. This technique may be useful for evaluation of endoluminal lesions. It remains to be seen whether this technique adds any additional information over SIS or conventional MRI of the female pelvis.[8]

HYSTEROSCOPY

Hysteroscopy is the endoscopic visualization of the endometrial cavity. Two techniques have evolved panoramic and contact hysteroscopy. Panoramic hysteroscopy is performed after the uterine cavity has been distended with medium. Contact hysteroscopy is achieved without uterine distension, instead the objective lens of the telescope is held in contact with the structure under scrutiny. Diagnostic hysteroscopy should be used routinely in the work-up of infertile women, even in the presence of eumenorrhea. Persistent functional endometrial polyps, usually located at uterotubal junction were present in

13% of women who had no cause for infertility. These even if small, are likely to impair fertility in this select group of patients. Removal of such lesions may improve subsequent reproductive performance in 50% of these patients.[9] Routinely when hysteroscopy was performed in women undergoing IVF, 38% had abnormalities, of which 32% were polyps.[10]

Instruments

Panoramic Hysteroscope

The viewing system consists of a telescope with a stainless steel sheath. Telescope ranges from 4 to 6 mm in diameter. For diagnostic hysteroscope a calibrated probe is required to assess size of intrauterine lesions. For surgical hysteroscopy suction irrigation cannulas, soft tubal probes, biopsy forceps, scissors and well insulated cautery is needed.

Light Sources

A standard halogen bulb will provides adequate illumination. The light is transmitted by a fibroptic cable and light system.

Distension Media

1. **Low viscosity solution:**
   - 5% dextrose
   - 3% sorbitol
   - 1.5% glycine

   They are instilled via ½ to 3 liter infusion bag. Infusion pressure is controlled by gravity or a pressure cuff inflated between 80 to 120 mm Hg. Approximately 150 ml is used in 10 minutes. Net amount should not be more than 2000 ml.

Disadvantage

i. There is uterine cramping because of a high volume low rate system of delivery.

ii. This media mixes with blood obscuring vision. Therefore a continuous flow hysteroscope with isolated inflow outflow channels is utilized. With this system, the uterus is irrigated continuously and blood and cellular debris are flushed out.

Advantage

i. They are readily available at a low cost
ii. Due to continuous inflow and outflow a clear view is maintained.

2. **Carbon dioxide:** Carbon dioxide is instilled at a flow rate of 25 to 100 ml/min upto a maximum pressure of 200 mm Hg. This medium is perfectly suited for diagnostic procedures outpatient setting.

Advantage

Appearance of the tissue is more true to life than other media.

Disadvantage

• There is less magnification than with 5% dextrose or dextran because of lower index of refraction of carbon dioxide.
• A patulous cervix may limit ability to maintain uterine distension
• Some procedures may require larger amount of carbon dioxide leading to shoulder pain.

3. **Dextran:** Dextran can be used as distension medium. There are two form of dextran:
   • Dextran 40, a 10% dextran solution (molecular weight 40,000) in 5% dextrose
   • Dextran 70, a 32% dextran solution (molecular weight 70,000) in 10% dextrose. Volume used should not exceed 250 ml.

Advantage

• Since it is immiscible with blood it provides excellent visualization. The view, however, is not sharper than when CO_2 is used.
• Intermittent delivery of 5 to 10 ml causes less uterine cramping.
• It is electrolyte free and nonconductive.

Disadvantage

- The medium is very difficult to remove from instruments as it solidifies when it dries. Instruments need to be soaked in warm water before cleaning
- Rarely may cause anaphylaxis.

Method

Hysteroscopy is best performed 2 to 3 days after cessation of menstrual flow as endometrium is thin and visualization is best. Also pregnancy is ruled out. Premenstrually endometrial growth can obscure tubal ostia. Vaginal misoprostol can be given for cervical priming in nulliparous women before hysteroscopic surgery and is more effective than dinoprostone.[11] Patient is placed in lithotomy position. Bimanual examination is done to determine the position of the uterus. Anterior lip of the cervix is grasped with a tenaculum. It can also be done in office setting without general anesthesia. A paracervical block may be given. The uterine cavity is sounded after dilating the cervix between 4 and 7 mm. The cervical occlusion cap is applied if CO_2 is to be used as distension medium. If the fluid medium to be used is 5% dextrose or dextran, it is attached to one of the inflow channels and the sheath is flushed to exclude air bubbles. With the light cable attached the sheath and telescope are inserted through the external OS and fluid medium is gradually injected. The pressure of the distension medium will overcome any residual tightness. The cervical canal is examined as the instrument advances and the uterine cavity is entered safely under vision. An examination of the uterine cavity is performed and tubal ostia are visualized. A 5 mm sheath is used for diagnostic procedures and a 7 or 8 mm sheath is used for operative procedures. The cavity is distended by media to visualize the anterior and posterior walls of the uterus which were in apposition. After inspection accessory were instruments can be introduced through operating channel of hysteroscope.

Contraindications

1. Acute pelvic infection
2. Active uterine bleeding
3. Pregnancy
4. Recent uterine perforation
5. Uterine cancer.

The contact hysteroscope has been used to examine pregnant patients in the first trimester and patients with uterine perforation. The danger of tumour dissemination does not apply when contact hysteroscopy or carbon dioxide for panaromic hysteroscopy is used.

Complications

1. *Pain:* Pain is usually mild to moderate and may persist for a few hours after the procedure. Cramps increase substantially if the procedure time exceeds 20 to 30 minutes. Cervical block, diazepam and prostaglandin synthatase inhibitors are used to decrease pain.

2. *Bleeding:* Bleeding may be due to cervical laceration, severing of uterine artery or its branches, or following incision of septum, extensive dissection of synechiae, resection of polyps or submucous myoma.

3. *Infection:* It occurs if some subclinical infection was pre-existent.

4. *Uterine perforation:* It usually occurs when there is extensive dissection of intrauterine adhesions. In such cases a laparoscopy should be done simultaneously. Central perforations can be managed by observation. If perforation does occur abdominal contents are visualized immediately.

5. *Endometrial dislocation:* The development of endometrial implants on peritoneal surfaces is a theoretical risk.

6. *Anesthetic accidents:* These can occur because of the anaesthetic agents.

7. *Complications related to the medium*
   - Allergic reactions: These occur but are seen rarely with dextran.
   - Circulatory overload: Circulatory overload occurs if large amount of dextran enters the venous circulation.
   - Acute non-cardiogenic pulmonary edema and disseminated intravascular coagulation: It is seen when more than 500 ml of dextran are used. Absorption of 200 to 300 ml interferes with platelet function and inhibits factors V, VIII and IX.
   - Fluid overload: When large volumes of glucose in water, saline or sorbitol are used fluid overload may be seen
   - Hyperglycemia and hyponatremia: It is seen if large volumes of glucose in water have been absorbed
   - Ammonia retention: It occurs where large amounts of glycine have been used in patients with limited hepatic function.

Caution: If the field of vision is cloudy or obscured, the hysteroscope should not be advanced , since it may be in contact with the uterine wall.

Contact Hysteroscopy

It is used for diagnostic, not therapeutic purposes. Its simplicity lies in that distending medium is not necessary. There are two sizes 6 mm and 8 mm. It can be accompanied by a biopsy or grasping forceps. Its use requires patience as it does not provide a panoramic view of the uterine cavity. It can be used for amnioscopy and has been successful in identifying meconium staining and congenital anomalies. It has been used to stage endometrial cancer and for examination of the bladder.

Hysteroscopic Findings

Normal Uterine Cavity

The normal endometrium is pink or tan and has very few blood vessels in the proliferative phase. The opening of the endometrial glands are defined by punctuate, pale whitish area, and the tubal ostia are easily seen. The secretory endometrium is pink or tan with a velvety appearance. Small submucous blood vessels are easily visualized.

Polyp

When visualized, polyps need to be differentiated from dislodged strips of endometrium and from submucous myomata. Myomata are fixed whereas polyps undulate with the ebb and flow of the distension medium[12] (Fig. 1.12).

Adhesions

They occur in 14 to 24% of infertile women. They can be diagnosed and treated in the same sitting.

Myoma

Myomas are seen in upto 6.5% of infertile women. They tend to bulge in the uterine cavity over a thin endometrium. They are smooth, firm, pale and rounded. They do not move with the distension medium (Fig. 1.13).

Septa

Appearance of the septa is typical. The paired uterine cornua are divided by a fibrous band.

Adenomyosis

There is increased vascularity with dark appearing blobs on the endometrial surface.

Others

These include cervical stenosis, cesarean section scar defects, vascular abnormalities and endometritis.

Other Uses of Hysteroscopy in Infertility

1. Selective hydrotubation
2. Removal of intratubal stents

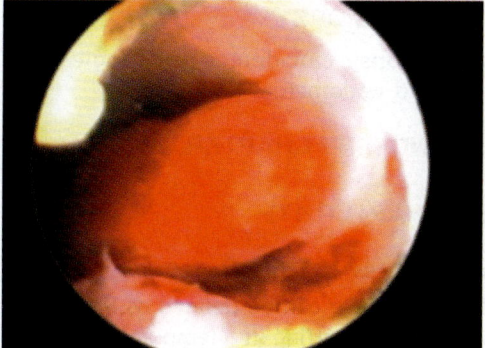

Fig. 1.12: Polyp as seen on hysteroscopy

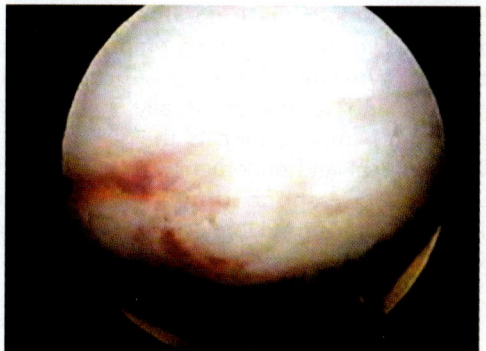

Fig. 1.13: Myoma seen on hysteroscopy

3. Tuboscopy
4. Selective cannulation of fallopian tube.

Hysteroscopy has become an important diagnostic procedure in the infertile patient. When combined with laparoscopy it offers a very thorough survey of the lower female genital tract. It has an important role in diagnosis and treatment of intrauterine adhesions and septa in patients of infertility and recurrent pregnancy loss.

ENDOMETRIAL BIOPSY

Endometrial biopsy can detect pathologies like chronic endometritis and endometrial tuberculosis.

ULTRASOUND (SEE CHAPTER 17)

MRI (SEE CHAPTER 17)

II. Tests to Assess Uterine Receptivity

Endometrial receptivity can be defined as the histological and molecular changes occurring in a temporal and spatial manner in the endometrium so as to facilitate embryonic implantation. Under the influence of estrogen and progesterone, the endometrium undergoes these important changes so as to make it receptive to the implanting embryo. This period is known as the 'Window of Receptivity'[13] and lasts for approximately 4 days in women usually from day 20 to 24. The key factor for implantation is the synchrony between embryo development and endometrial receptivity. The ability of the decidua to respond optimally to the invading trophoblasts is determined by endocrine and endorgan interactions that long precede ovulation.

TESTS THAT ASSESS ENDOMETRIAL CHANGES

Endometrial Histology

A. *Endometrial histopathology:* This is done by endometrial biopsy taken during the late luteal phase. This has been the gold standard to assess endometrial maturity. There are certain limitations to this procedure, namely:
   a. It is preformed in the late luteal phase and hence may give information only of invasion phase.
   b. It is representative of the endometrial changes within the cycle and cycle variations are well known.
   c. Does not reflect the endometrium as a whole, regional variations being frequently encountered.

    d. Cannot be carried out in the cycle in which the patient is undergoing ART.

B. *Study of Pinopodes:* Pinopodes are studied by scanning electron microscopy (SEM). Though a better indicator of endometrial receptivity, it is expensive, not universally available and cannot be carried out during a IVF cycle.

Ultrasound and Doppler

Transvaginal sonography is a simple non-invasive modality that is being increasingly used to assess endometrial receptivity. Both endometrial thickness and echogenic pattern have been studied as potential markers of endometrial receptivity. Using Doppler the impedance to blood flow of the uterine artery is expressed as the pulsatility index (PI) and is the lowest at the time of implantation.

a. *Endometrial thickness*: It is generally accepted that if the thickness is < 7 mm on ultrasound the implantation is poor. Similarly endometrial volume of <2.5 ml is associated with a poor pregnancy rate.

b. *Echogenicity*: Endometrial character is hypoechoic compared to the surrounding myometrium in the proliferative phase. As thickness increases a distinct triple line/multilayered pattern is seen and is considered to be predictive of implantation (Fig. 1.14). Further under the influence of progesterone the endometrium undergoes secretory changes and becomes more isoechoic and then hyperechoic. A non-multilayered endometrium is associated with poor implantation.

    The endometrium and periendometrial area is divided into 4 zones (Table 1.2).These zones give it the typical preovulatory triple line appearance which is an indicator of good uterine receptivity.

c. *Endometrial vascularity*: Sub- and intra-endometrial vascularity is a prognostic factor for implantation once endometrium is more than 7 mm irrespective of the morphological index.

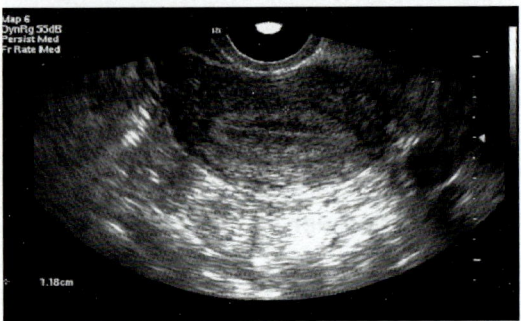

Fig. 1.14: Typical triple layer endometrium

Table 1.2: The endometrial and periendometrial areas have the following four zones	
• **Zone 1**	2 mm thick area surrounding the hyperechoic outer layer of the endometrium
• **Zone 2**	Hyperechoic outer layer of the endometrium
• **Zone 3**	Hypoechoic inner layer of the endometrium
• **Zone 4**	Endometrial cavity

Uterine perfusion is maximum during the midluteal phase. PI < 3 is associated with increased pregnancy rate. Absence of sub-endometrial blood flow on the day of LH surge is related to implantation failure.

Spiral artery perfusion is evaluated by color Doppler and the endometrium has been divided into 4 zones (Fig. 1.15).

Zone 1   -   Only myometrial vessels surrounding endometrium are seen

Zone 2   -   Vessels penetrate through the hyperecho-genic endometrial edge

Zone 3   -   Vessels reach the internal endometrial hyperechogenic zone

Zone 4   -   Vessels reach upto the endometrial cavity

A good vascularity in zone 3 or 4 which relates to the surface of the endometrium suggests good endometrial receptivity.

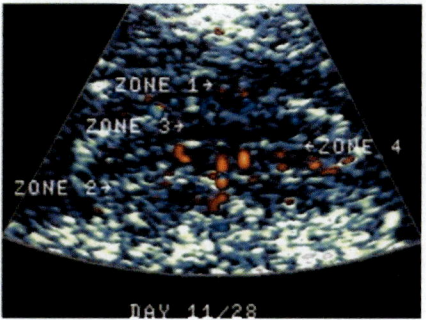

Fig. 1.15: Vascular penetration on power Doppler to zone 4

Hormonal Levels

These are of not much use for assessment of endometrial receptivity.

Markers of the Embryo-endometrial Dialogue

Evaluations of the various biomarkers are mostly research tools. Kits for evaluation of integrins and mucins are now commercially available (Table1.3).

Table 1.3: Molecules at three stages of implantation

1. Apposition—Chemokines
    Interleukin—8(IL - 8)
    Monocyte chemoattractant protein - 1 (MCP - 1)
    Regulated on activation T-cell expressed and secreted
    (RANTES)

2. Adhesion—Cytokines
    LIF
    IL - 1
    HBGF
    Integrins
    HOXA10

3. Invasion—Proteolytic enzymes
    Serineproteases
    Metalloproteases
    Collagenases

Despite progress and research in the field of infertility the rate of live birth rate with IVF has not gone beyond 30%. In 75 % of the failed cases there is no cause for failure other than implantation forming a major obstacle to ART. The complexities of embryo apposition to invasion of the epithelium are only partly understood at the molecular level and still present a challenge to infertility specialist.

REFERENCES

1. Davies AC, Keightlev A, Borthwick-Clark A, Walters HL. The use of low osmolality contrast medium in hysterosalpingography: A comparison with conventional contrast medium. Clin Radiol 1985; 36: 533-6.
2. Baramki TA. Hysterosalpingography. Fertil Steril 2005;83(6):1595-606.
3. Braun P, Grau FV, Pons RM, Enguix D. Is hysterosalpingography able to diagnose all uterine malformations correctly? A retrospective study. Eur J Radiol 2005 ;53(2):274-9.
4. Bonilla-Musoles F, Raga F, Osborne NG, Blanes J, Coelho F. Three-dimensional hysterosonography for the study of endometrial tumors: Comparison with conventional transvaginal sonography, hysterosalpingography, and hysteroscopy. Gynecol Oncol 1997; 65:245-52.
5. Bree RL, Bowerman RA, Bohm-Velez M, et al. US evaluation of the uterus in patients with postmenopausal bleeding: A positive effect on diagnostic decision making. Radiology 2000; 216:260-4.
6. Guimaraes Filho HA, Mattar R, Pires CR, Araujo Junior E, Moron AF, Nardozza LM. Comparison of hysterosalpingography, hysterosonography and hysteroscopy in evaluation of the uterine cavity in patients with recurrent pregnancy losses. Arch Gynecol Obstet 2006;274(5):284-8.
7. Valenzano MM, Mistrangelo E, Lijoi D, Fortunato T, Lantieri PB, Risso D, Costantini S, Ragni N. Transvaginal sonohysterographic evaluation of uterine malformations. Eur J Obstet Gynecol Reprod Biol 2006;124(2):246-9.
8. Rouanet De Lavit JP, Maubon AJ, Thurmond AS. MR hysterography performed with saline injection and fluid attenuated inversion recovery sequences: initial experience. Am J Roentgenol 2000; 175:774-6.

9. Shokeir TA, Shalan HM, El-Shafei MM. Significance of endometrial polyps detected hysteroscopically in eumenorrheic infertile women. J Obstet Gynaecol Res 2004;30(2):84-9.

10. Hinckley MD, Milki AA. 1000 office-based hysteroscopies prior to *in vitro* fertilization: Feasibility and findings. JSLS 200;8(2):103-7.

11. Preutthipan S, Herabutya Y. A randomized comparison of vaginal misoprostol and dinoprostone for cervical priming in nulliparous women before operative hysteroscopy Fertil Steril 2006; 86:990-4.

12. Jansen FW, de Kroon CD, van Dongen H, Grooters C, Louwe L, Trimbos-Kemper T. Diagnostic hysteroscopy and saline infusion sonography: Prediction of intrauterine polyps and myomas J Minim Invasive Gynecol 2006;13(4):320-4.

13. Psychosos A. Endocrine control of egg implantation. In Greep RO, Astwood EG, Geiger SR (Eds): Handbook of Physiology, American Physiological Society, Washington DC, USA 1973;187-225.

CHAPTER 2

Tests for Evaluation of Tubal Structure and Function

Surveen Ghumman

Fallopian tube obstruction is thought to play a role in 12 to 33% of subfertile couples.[1] Assessing the patency of the fallopian tubes is, therefore, an important part of the work-up of a subfertile couple. Prevalence of tubal disease varies in different population subgroups. Bilateral tubal block identified by hysterosalpingography is found in 24% of couples with secondary infertility with normal sperm and ovulatory cycle, but is much less in couples with male factor subfertility or anovulation (5 and 7%, respectively). Therefore, in the latter groups, assessment of fallopian tubes could reasonably be delayed in the diagnostic work-up. If these women do not conceive with simple interventions such as clomiphene citrate, then tubal assessment should be combined with effective therapeutic procedures such as ovarian drilling at the time of laparoscopy and dye test.

There are several tests available for this purpose, including hysterosalpingography, laparoscopy and dye test, selective salpingography and hysterosalpingo-contrast sonography. Hysterosalpingography evaluates patency and internal lining. Laparoscopy gives a direct view of the serosal aspect of the tube and its relation with the ovaries and other pelvic organs. When investigating tubal pathology with these tests, it is usually the morphological aspect of the tube which is evaluated and the functional aspect is rarely looked into. There are tests which would assess the function of the tubes (e.g. measurement of tubal perfusion pressures during selective salpingography). Tubal endoscopy has the theoretical advantage of assessing the tubal mucosa responsible for most of the tubal function. However, it is a technically demanding procedure and the clinical significance of its findings are not totally defined.

The tubal status helps to determine the right therapeutic choice. Tubal reconstructive surgery in selected cases improves cumulative probability of pregnancy. However, if tubal pathology is severe tubal reconstruction surgery is contraindicated and salpingectomy improves the results of IVF ET. Tubal pathology needs to be diagnosed and evaluated in order to enable the physician to decide between tubal reconstruction and tubal ablation as mode of treatment.

HYSTEROSALPINGOGRAPHY

Hysterosalpingography is a simple, safe and inexpensive X-ray based contrast study of the uterine cavity and fallopian tubes where medium is injected through the cervical OS in order to opacify and outline the uterine cavity and tubes to establish tubal patency. It should be the preliminary investigation for tubal factor infertility and timed between cessation of menstruation and ovulation.

Oil-soluble or water-soluble contrast medium is used. Water-soluble contrast medium is preferred as it is better tolerated by patient, coats the surface without sticking to them, producing sharp and finely shaded images with greater visual detail. The water soluble contrast medium is eliminated in 30 minutes. HSG is performed under fluoroscopic control. The contrast medium is injected very slowly so as to avoid discomfort, contraction of the uterus, spasm of uterotubal junction and obscuring of the lesion with large quantities of contrast medium. A delayed film after 10 to 20 minutes is taken as it yields information about the external contour of the internal genitalia, shape of ovarian fossa and presence of periadenexal adhesions.

The peritoneal spill from the normal HSG is identified easily. The dispersion of agents in the pelvis depends on:
1. Type and amount of contrast medium used
2. Degree of tubal patency
3. Presence or extent of significant periadenexal adhesions.

Complications

1. Pelvic inflammatory disease 1-3%
2. Uterine perforation
3. Bleeding from tenaculum site
4. Intolerance to iodine.

Limitations

1. Does not indicate the exact nature of intrauterine or intratubal lesion.

2. *False positive results for cornual occlusion:* If confronted with proximal tubal obstruction continue to apply steady pressure with the syringe and simply wait 3 to 5 minutes. Often the spasm passes. If not a smooth muscle relaxant and a tranquilizer are given as it may be due to stress or irritation caused by the contrast media.

3. *Poor accuracy for prediction of periadenexal adhesions and endometriosis:* Adhesions are discernable as a collection of contrast in the lateral pelvic wall. It may be difficult to differentiate between these localized pelvic collections and hydrosalpinges. Sharply defined borders suggest the contrast medium is confined within the tube, whereas a halo configuration indicates periadenexal adhesions that allow some of the fluid to surround and outline the tubal wall.

A Normal Salpingography should Display

1. A smooth proximal portion and isthmus without irregularities.
2. A progressive enlargement of the tubal lumen at the ampullary level with regular parietal coating and presence of mucosal folds.
3. A peritoneal spillage obtained without accumulation of contrast medium in the tube with good diffusion in abdomen outlining intestinal loops and other pelvic structures.
   Pathological findings on HSG are seen in Table 2.1.

Abnormal features of the fallopian tube:

1. Hydrosalpinx (Fig. 2.1).
2. Clubbing or irregular contour at the distal end of obstructed tube.
3. Destruction of longitudinal mucosal folds.
4. Proximal or distal tubal obstruction (Fig. 2.2).
5. Beaded or lead pipe appearance of the tube (Fig. 2.3).
6. Loculated spill around the tube.
7. Extravasation of dye (Fig. 2.4).
8. Diverticular outpouching seen in salpingitis isthmica nodosa.
9. Calcified lymph nodes.

The distal tubal disease can be classified into various stages (Table 2.2).

Table 2.1: Pathological findings in the fallopian tube seen on HSG

1. In the proximal part of the tube
    i. *Tubal polyp:* Pear shaped enlargement of the tube with a small globular or elongated vacuole surrounded by contrast medium usually not big enough to obstruct the tube.
    ii. *Salpingitis isthmica nodosa:* Diverticulae and irregularities in the lumen or spicules of contrast radiating from the lumen.
    iii. *Proximal obstruction:* Sudden arrest in the progression of contrast medium after normal opacification for a few millimeters or centimeters. This flame shaped tubal image differentiates real obstruction from cornual block.
2. In the distal part of the tube
    i. *Hydrosalpinx:* Total obstruction with hydrosalpinx may be seen.
    ii. *Phimosis of distal tubal ostium:* Partial distal obstruction where peritoneal spillage is obtained only after accumulation of contrast medium in the ampulla.
    iii. *Intraluminal adhesions:* Mucosal pathology appears under the form of parietal irregularities and disorganization of mucosal folds.
3. Intraperitoneal spread
    i. Adhesions are seen as localized pooling and loculation of contrast in the distal end of oviduct.

Table 2.2: Classification of distal tubal disease based on HSG findings	
Stage I	Distal phimosis
Stage II	Occlusion without tubal dilation
Stage III	Occlusion with dilation to 15 to 25 mm
Stage IV	Occlusion with dilation of [is greater than] 25 mm

Diagnostic Accuracy

In a meta-analysis using laparoscopy with chromotubation as a gold standard HSG is found to have a 65% sensitivity and 83% specificity for detecting tubal blockages.[2] Reliability

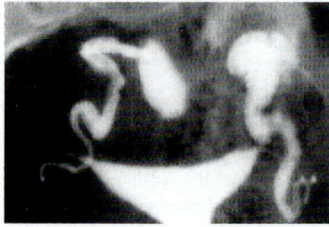

Fig. 2.1: HSG with bilateral hydrosalpinx

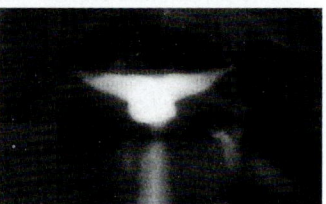

Fig. 2.2: Bilateral cornual block

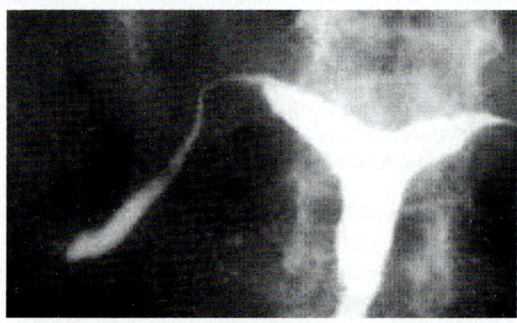

Fig. 2.3: Lead pipe appearance of tube

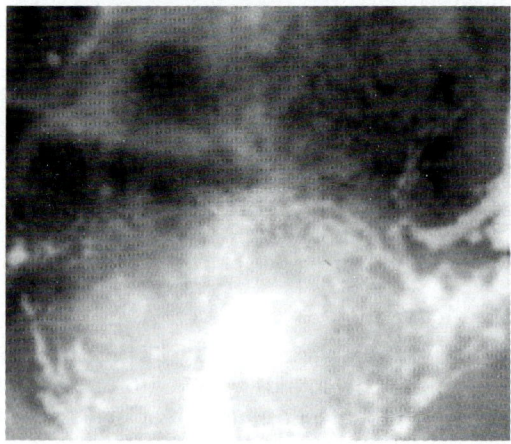

Fig. 2.4: Extravasation of dye

between observers (inter-observer reliability) is almost perfect for proximal occlusion, substantial for distal obstruction and hydrosalpinx and moderate to poor for adhesions.[3] The routine use of HSG at an early stage in the fertility workup prior to laparoscopy and dye does not influence pregnancy rate.[4]

> *Recommendation:* Women who are not known to have comorbidities (such as pelvic inflammatory disease, previous ectopic pregnancy or endometriosis) should be offered screening with hysterosalpingography before laparoscopy to rule out tubal occlusion.[5]

Selective Salpingography and Tubal Cannulation

If HSG demonstrates a cornual or proximal tubal block, selective salpingography with or without tubal cannulation is the next step. Transcervical tubal cannulation is done under hysteroscopic, sonographic or fluoroscopic guidance. In due to salpingography, each tube is cannulated and then flushed with a contrast agent. The high pressure due to direct injection helps to overcome obstruction due to mucus plugs and minor synechiae. If proximal tubal blockage is identified, a guide-wire is passed through the selective salpingography catheter into the fallopian tube to achieve recanalization (tubal catheterization). Thus, a see-and-treat approach is possible in an outpatient setting with selective salpingography and tubal catheterization.

Tubal patency was achieved in 78% out of which 28.6% achieved spontaneous pregnancy within 1 year of treatment. The procedure should be universally accepted, taught and practiced in the diagnosis and treatment of the fallopian tube occlusion, especially in infertility units which are not located in tertiary care hospitals.[6]

Accuracy: Accuracy of selective salpingography is better than laparoscopy and dye test in predicting proximal tubal occlusion; both tests are equivalent in predicting distal tubal occlusion; while laparoscopy and dye test is better than selective salpingography in predicting peritubal disease.[7]

Tubal perfusion pressure: Although tubes may be shown to be patent anatomically, they may still have poor function. Tubal perfusion pressure, which may be an indicator of tubal function, has been shown to have prognostic value in predicting conception. Reductions in tubal perfusion pressure with tubal catheterization are associated with improved conception rates.[8] Tubal perfusions pressures (TPP) measured at selective salpingography can classify women into three prognostic groups (Table 2.3).

Table 2.3: Prognostic classification according to tubal perfusion pressure	
	Tubal perfusion pressure
Good	Both tubes <300, or one tube <300 and the other 300-500 mm Hg
Mediocre	Both tubes 300-500, or one tube<300 and the other >500 mm Hg
Poor	Both tubes >500, or one tube 300-500 and the other >500 mm Hg

Age-adjusted 4 year, cumulative non-IVF/ICSI conception rates in the three groups were 74%, 56% and 30% respectively.[9]

Complications: No major complications have been reported with selective salpingography and tubal catheterization, and most minor complications can be managed conservatively.

Recommendation: Transcervical tubal cannulation should be considered as first line treatment for patients with proximal tubal block as it is a simple outpatient procedure with a success rate of 80-90% in restoring the patency of at least one fallopian tube and a 30% pregnant rate in the first three to six months after the procedure.

HYSTEROSALPINGOSONOGRAPHY

By ultrasonography, tubes are not clearly visible and the examination is not precise enough to give an idea of the internal lining of the tube. Hysterosalpingosonography involves the transcervical injection of isotonic saline, the course of which is followed in real time by transvaginal ultrasound to check the patency of the tube. There is no anesthetic requirement and there is no ovarian irradiation.

Technique

Patient preparation for the examination is minimal. The patient is placed in the lithotomy position. A brief bimanual examination can aid in locating the cervix. A sterile speculum retracts the posterior vaginal wall and the cervix is brought into view. The catheter is placed at the external cervical os, and then advanced into the endometrial canal. Once in the endometrial canal, the balloon is inflated so that the catheter does not become dislodged. The speculum is carefully removed, and the endovaginal probe is inserted beside the catheter.

Under direct sonographic visualization, the balloon is gently retracted to occlude the internal cervical os. Again, under sonographic guidance, warm sterile saline is injected. Complete sonographic evaluation of the endometrial cavity is performed in both the coronal and sagittal planes. Fallopian tube patency is assessed. Finding a normal cavity and bilateral fill and spill of saline is reassuring, but where there is doubt, hysterosalpingography or a laparoscopy and dye hydrotubation test should be done.

Complications

The rate was 1% for serious complications. Pelvic pain was also cited as a complication, with a rate of 1%. Abdominal and shoulder pain from peritoneal irritation were the most common complaints.

Accuracy

The accuracy of hysterosalpingosonography is not as good as hysterosalpingograpy, for assessment of tubal patency. The concordance value is 83.5%. The use of color Doppler improved the sensitivity from 82 to 91% and specificity from 86 to 100% and is recommended as a supplement to gray scale imaging in cases of suspected tubal occlusion.[10]

In a study the sensitivity of 3D-contrast hystero-salpingosonography (3D-HyCoSy) for detecting tubal patency was 100% with a specificity of 67%. The positive and negative predictive values were 89 and 100%, respectively. 3D-HyCoSy with its advantage of having no ovarian radiation may be recommended as an initial investigation for tubal patency.[11]

LAPAROSCOPY

Laparoscopy and dye test (chromopertubation) is widely considered the gold standard test for investigating tubal patency (Fig. 2.5). The passage of the dye is followed and the nature of the spill is examined by viewing the fimbriae to determine fimbrial phimosis or fine fimbrial adhesions which may impede ovum pickup. Dye may be seen to extravasate (Fig. 2.6). There may be adhesions seen on laparoscopy (Fig. 2.7).

Indications

1. Whenever tubal pathology is suspected because of previous history of PID, chronic pelvic pain, pelvic surgery.
2. Abnormal findings on HSG.
3. Unexplained infertility.

Advantage

1. Allows assessment for peritubal disease, adhesions and endometriosis.
2. Laparoscopy has the advantage of providing means of surgical procedures like adhesiolysis, salpingo-neostomy, fimbrioplasty and tubal cannulation alongside.
3. It has a better prognostic value in predicting fertility compared with hysterosalpingography, thus supporting the use of laparoscopy and dye test as the reference test for studies evaluating tests for tubal patency[12] (Table 2.4).

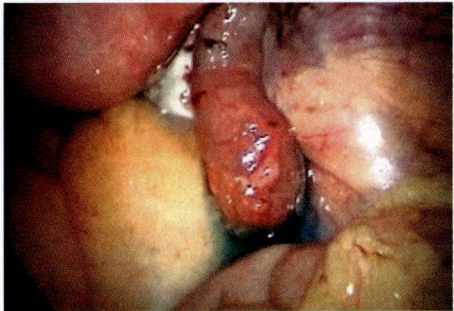

Fig. 2.5: Chromotubation of tube on laparoscopy

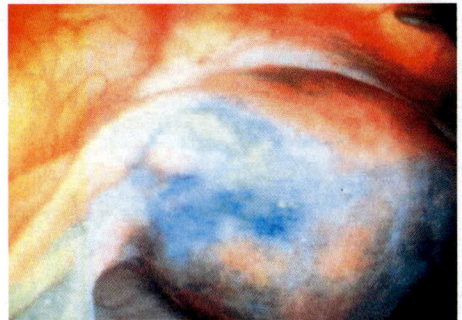

Fig. 2.6: Extravasation of dye on chromotubation

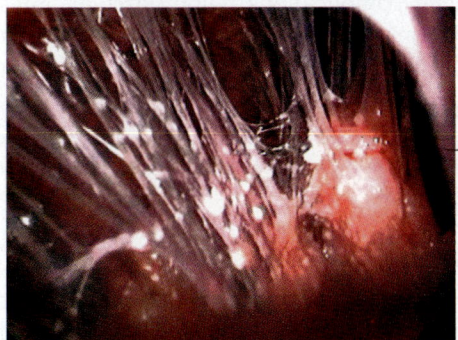

Fig. 2.7: Adhesions in pelvis

Table 2.4: Comparison of hysterosalpingography and laparoscopy with chromotubation

Hysterosalpingography	Laparoscopy andchromotubation
• Outpatient procedure	• Day surgery procedure
• Analgesia adequate	• General anesthesia required
• Simple and inexpensive	• Expensive
• Gives uterine cavity information	• Shows outer contour of the uterus only
• Tubal patency tested	• Shows outer appearance of tubes and their patency; Ovaries and pelvic perito- neum can also be assessed
• Screening test	• Definitive test
• Not particularly sensitive for mild distal tubal disease or endometriosis	• Distal tubal disease or endo- metriosis can be diagnosed and treated

Disadvantage

1. Laparoscopy is an invasive procedure and is associated with morbidity.[13]
2. It requires anesthesia
3. Complication rates for diagnostic laparoscopy have been reported to be between 0.06 and 0.20%, with the most significant complications being vascular, intestinal and urological injuries. Anesthetic complications and methylene blue toxicity have also been reported, but are rare.[14]

Recommendation: Women suspected of having comorbidities (such as endometriosis and pelvic inflammatory disease) should undergo laparoscopy so that both pelvic and tubal pathology can be assessed.[5]

TUBAL ENDOSCOPY

Advances in fiberoptic technology make it possible to evaluate the tubal lumen endoscopically. Salpingoscopy and falloposcopy are the two basic procedures used.

Salpingoscopy: Salpingoscopy is a transfimbrial approach allowing visualization from the ampullary-isthmic junction to the fimbriae.

Falloposcopy: Falloposcopy is a transcervical approach allowing assessment of the tubal lumen from the uterotubal ostium to the fimbriae.

These procedures provide more sensitive information than laparoscopy with chromotubation or hysterosalpingo-graphy alone. Findings provide a strong correlation with conception. Technical shortcomings make falloposcopy more difficult than the more straightforward transfimbrial technique.[15] Falloposcopy predicted salpingoscopic status correctly in 84% of cases.[16]

Falloposcopy

It is the transvaginal microendoscopic access of oviductal lumen from uterotubal ostium exploring the entire length of the tube especially the intramural or isthmic segments. Kerin described in 1990 the first successful endoscopic evaluation of the tube from intramural to distal segment.[17] The falloposcope is a flexible high-resolution microendoscope of 0.5 mm diameter and 1.73 m length that contains a bundle of 2000 optical fibers and 8 to 12 illuminating fibers. The falloposcope is capable of magnifying up to 50 times.

Anesthesia: General anesthesia was used when suspected abnormal tubes were examined by falloposcopy, especially if concurrent laparoscopy was also performed. Office falloposcopy under sedation, however, is gaining greater acceptance.

Time: The optimal time for performing falloposcopy is during the mid-follicular phase of the menstrual cycle, because the ostium can be visualized most easily in the absence of blood and a thick endometrial lining.

Steps of the Procedure

Step I: Gaining access to the uterotubal ostium:
Hysteroscopic guidance competes with the tactile impression for this. Advantage of using hysteroscopic guidance is that it

allows visual control of the catheterization process as well as detection of ostial spasm that may simulate proximal tubal obstruction.

Step II: Tubal catheterization:

Two methods can be used

1. *Coaxial catheter system:*[18] In order to prevent kinking within the uterine cavity hysteroscope is kept close to ostium or a larger guide wire is used for the intrauterine distance. The tip of the hysteroscope is directed to within 3 mm of the uterotubal junction. A flexible, platinum tipped tapered guidewire is then introduced into the junction till either a point of resistance, increase in patient discomfort, or a distance of 15 cm is reached. A catheter is introduced over the wire for a similar distance and the guidewire is withdrawn.

2. *Linear everting balloon catheter*: It uses a pressurized tubular polyethylene 'balloon' which carries the endoscope along the tube, protecting the tube and endoscope from damaging one another and negotiating the curves and strictures without exerting shear force on the tubal wall.[19]

   Use of the linear everting balloon catheter system with sedation is now usually regarded as an office procedure that does not need laparoscopy or hysteroscopy. It consists of inner and outer catheter bodies (of diameters 0.8 mm and 2.8 mm, respectively) that are joined circumferentially at their distal tips by a distensible polyethylene membrane (Fig. 2.8). The falloposcope is advanced within the inner catheter and the membrane and introduced into the uterus. Once the ostium is identified, the outer catheter is held in position and pressure is applied to the membrane by using the fluid filled syringe; the inner catheter is pushed forward, resulting in the linear eversion of the balloon into the fallopian tube. As a result, the falloposcope is carried forward at twice the speed of the balloon. The balloon and falloposcope are advanced into the fallopian tube up to a distance of 10 cm or till resistance is encountered.

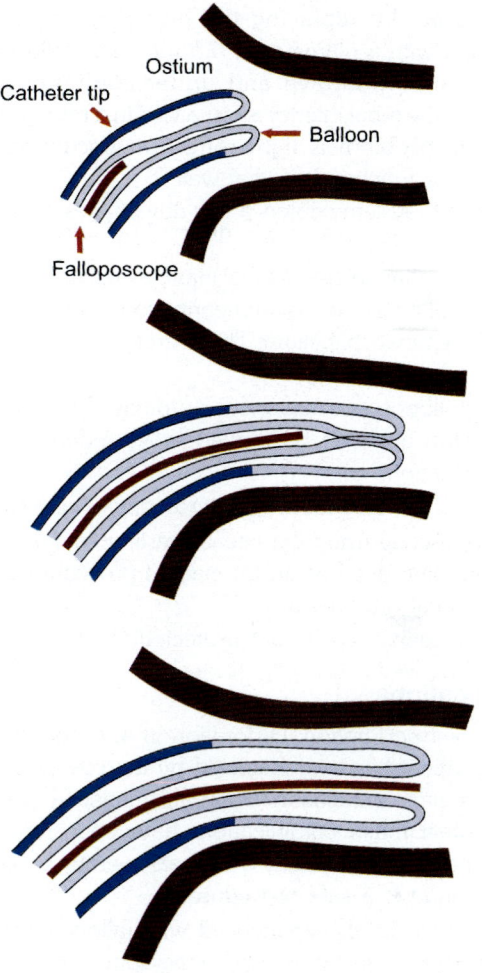

Fig. 2.8: Falloposcopy using linear everting balloon catheter

Step III: Visualization of the endosalpinx:

This is done by replacing the guidewire by a miniature endoscope with a diameter of 0.5 mm. The falloposcope and catheter are withdrawn and under continuous irrigation distension, the tubal interior is visualized in a retrograde manner. The main problem is light reflection occurring when the falloposcope touches the tubal wall.

The LEC system confers a few advantages over the coaxial system:

1. There is minimal risk of tubal injury associated with guidewire cannulation as there is no shearing force between the balloon and the tubal epithelium. The everting balloon will negotiate any tubal tortuosity.

2. The falloposcope advances automatically during balloon eversion and can be moved independently to optimise visualization.

3. There is no need for any hysteroscopy or cervical dilatation.

4. Falloposcopy using the linear everting catheter system can be accomplished as an out-patient procedure that requires only local anesthesia.

5. The falloposcope is well protected inside the balloon.

Complications

1. *Pinpoint perforation*: Perforation in 4.9% per tube and 8% per patient has been detected by the coaxial system using guide-wire cannulation. They are managed conservatively. No other major complications have been reported. Thus, falloposcopy particularly with linear everting balloon catheter technique is a safe procedure.[21]

2. *Pain*: Pain levels experienced with falloposcopy are lower compared with hysterosalpingography.

3. *Failure rate*: In 10% patients cannulation may not be possible.[20]

Salpingoscopy

It is the endoscopic examination of the ampullary portion of the tubal lumen via the fimbrial end. The fimbria is held by an atraumatic forceps. Irrigation allows distension and facilitates visualization. The optics are then advanced more proximally but cannot go beyond the isthmo-ampullary junction. Endosalpinx is examined.

Since normal vascularity is difficult to observe being situated under the mucosal surface description concentrates on the patency parameter, intraluminal findings such as synechiae, polyp or debris and mucosa surface pattern. The normal mucosa is low in reflex, smooth and velvet-like with a white rose to pink color (Table 2.5). Atrophied mucosa gives a mirror like appearance. There are many ways of classifying the severity of the disease based on these findings (Tables 2.5 and 2.6).

Table 2.5: Normal appearance of tubal mucosa
i. *Ampullary mucosa:* It has extensively ramified and vascularized fold structures with secondary folds freely floating in distension medium
ii. *Isthmic segment:* 4 or 5 longitudinal folds which are flatter
iii. *Intramural part:* Fold structure is absent

Table 2.6: Classification depending on severity
Grade I : Normal mucosal fold pattern
Grade II : Separation and flattening of both major and minor mucosal folds which are largely preserved
Grade III: Focal lesions like small adhesions between folds
Grade IV: Adhesive or destructive lesions over entire ampulla
Grade V : Fibrosis and complete loss of folds

One to three points are assigned according to degree of pathologic change (Table 2.7). Other tubal findings such as mucus plug, debris, polyps, endometriosis, salpingitis isthimica nodosa, inflammatory, neoplastic conditions or absent tubal segment are categorized as moderate or severe tubal segments.

Table 2.7: Normal appearance of tubal mucosa

Site of disease	Right Tube				Left Tube			
	Intramural	Isthmic	Ampullary	Fimbrial	Intramural	Isthmic	Ampullary	Fimbrial
Patency Patency .... 1 Stenosis .... 2 Fibrotic obstruction 3								
Epithelium Normal .... 1 Pale, atrophic .... 2 Flat, featureless 3								
Vascularity Normal .... 1 Intermediate .... 2 Poor pallor 3								
Adhesions None .... 1 Thin, weblike .... 2 Thick 3								
Dilation None .... 1 Minimal .... 2 Hydrosalpinx............. 3 Other 2-3								
Cumulative Score								
Total Score	Right Tube:		(Normal = 20)		Left Tube:		(Normal = 20)	

Then a cumulative score is calculated for the entire tube and the disease is graded. The prognosis depends on the grade of the disease (Table 2.8).

The overall result and pregnancy rate after reconstructive surgery for tubal blockage is disappointing. It has been suggested that the selection criteria for tubal surgery rather than the surgical technique determines the success of the outcome.[18]

Winston and Margara have classified the hydrosalpinx into four stages[23] (Table 2.9).

Tubal surgery is warranted only in patients with mild to moderate tubal disease; for those with severe disease, *in vitro* fertilization is better. With falloposcopy a more accurate

Table 2.8: Pregnancy rate according to scoring[22]

Score	Grade of disease	Spontaneous pregnancy rate
20	Normal tubal lumen	28%
20 to 30	Moderate tubal lumen disease	12%
> 30	Severe endotubal disease	0%

Table 2.9: Classification of hydrosalpinx

Stage	Hydrosalpinx	Pregnancy rate after tubal surgery
Stage I	A thin-walled hydrosalpinx with little or no fibrosis	39%
Stage II	A thick-walled hydrosalpinx with good mucosa	20%
Stage III	A thick-walled hydrosalpinx with marked mucosal damage, or a thick fibrous adhesion	9%
Stage IV	A tubo-ovarian mass or fibrosis, or an adherent hydrosalpinx with incarcerated ovary and/or isthmic damage	6%

assessment of the tubal status can be made before subjecting the patient to tubal surgery, and helps to decide the optimal mode of treatment. Falloposcopic findings can lead to a change in patient management in more than 60% of cases.[18] The increased accuracy of the tubal assessment helps in the allocation of patients to the most appropriate treatment.

Transvaginal Hydrolaparoscopy

Access to the peritoneal cavity is gained by needle puncture through the posterior fornix to the pouch of Douglas and space is filled with 200 cc of saline solution. 3 mm optics allows inspection of pelvic structures under water. In such cases salpingoscopy has been possible without manipulating the structures.

Tests Designed to Assess Tubal Function

1. *Biodegradable microspheres*: Biodegradable micro-spheres have been introduced into the pouch of Douglas by either cul-de-sac puncture or laparoscopy. These microspheres were recognizable by fluorescence and were collected in a cervical cup 24 hours later.

2. *Radionucleotide HSG*: A solution containing 99 m Tc labeled albumin microspheres is squirted towards the external OS of cervix and upper vagina. The transport through uterus and tubes is monitored by gamma camera. The transport depends on the anatomic patency and functional integrity of the uterus and tubes.

   In patients who show a negative hysterosalpingoscintio-graphy (HSSG) the pregnancy rate achieved spontaneously or by intrauterine insemination is significantly reduced compared to the patients who showed an intact transport mechanism confirmed by positive HSSG.[24]

3. *Tubal perfusion pressure*: It has been shown to be of prognostic value (Table 2.3).

Infection Screening

Chlamydia antibody testing is a simple and cheap screening test for the likelihood of tubal subfertility. The predictive value of testing will depend on the cut-off level of the immunoglobulin G titer chosen and the criteria applied for tubal factor subfertility. Recent studies concluded that the optimum cut-off titer should be 16 because it gives the best combination of sensitivity and specificity. However, high titers of chlamydial antibodies in infertile women indicate the need for early laparoscopy to assess tubal status. A systematic review summarizing the a vailable evidence showed chlamydial antibody titers to have a diagnostic accuracy that was similar to that of hysterosalpingography.[25]

Complications of tests used to assess tubal status are shown in Table 2.10.

Table 2.10: Complications of tests used to assess tubal status

Test	Complications
HSG	Pelvic infection (1-3%)
	Extravasation (6.9%)
	Lipo-granuloma
	Anaphylaxis
	Death
Laparoscopy and dye test	Vascular injury: 0.2/1000
	Bowel injury: 0.4–0.7/1000
	Urological injury: 0.1/1000
	Methylene blue toxicity.
	Anesthetic complications.
Selective salpingography and tubal catheterization	Tubal perforation
	Minor bleeding
	Vasovagal reactions
	Ectopic pregnancy
	Risks of cancer for women due to the radiation exposure is estimated at 4 to 13 per million procedures
Hysterosalpingo-contrast sonography	Abdominal and shoulder pain
	Vasovagal reaction
Falloposcopy	Pinpoint perforation of the tube

Guidelines for investigating tubal disease

- Where there is no suspicion of tubal disease with anovulation investigation can be delayed till clomiphene induction has been tried.
- Hysterosalpingography, being a reliable, reasonably accurate and safe test with the potential of improving pregnancy outcome in its own right, should be the screening test in women with no other suspected comorbidities such as endometriosis and pelvic infection.
- If such comorbidities are suspected, then laparoscopy and dye test may be a more suitable test, as it would also allow a complete assessment of the pelvis, and treatment if indicated.
- In women with proximal tubal blockage, selective salpingography with tubal catheterization should be offered.
- Chlamydia serology is the most cost-effective and least invasive diagnostic test for tubal disease.

A systematic step by step approach is needed to diagnose and treat tubal pathology (Fig. 2.9).

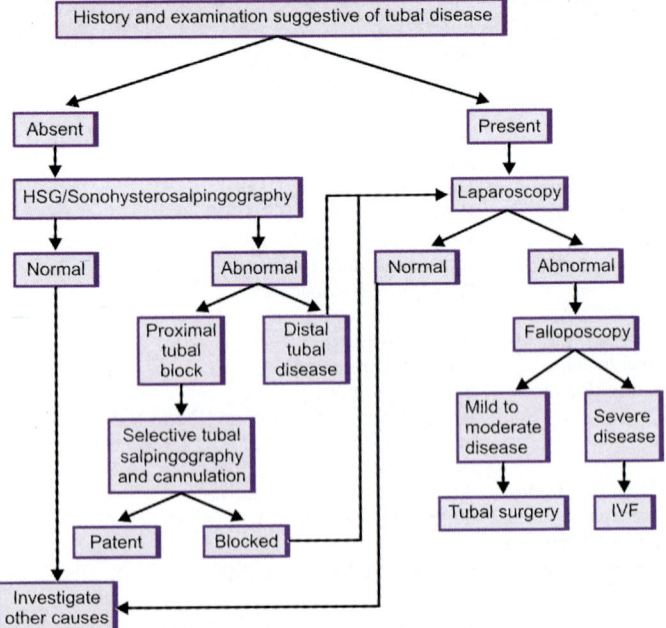

Fig. 2.9: Step by step approach to diagnosis of tubal pathology

REFERENCES

1. Snick HK, Snick TS, Evers JL, Collins JA. The spontaneous pregnancy prognosis in untreated subfertile couples: The Walcheren primary care study. Hum Reprod 1997;12:1582-8.

2. Swart P, Mol BW,Van der Veen F, Van Beurden M, Redekop WK, Bossuyt PMM. The accuracy of hysterosalpingography in the diagnosis of tubal pathology: A meta-analysis. Fertil Steril 1995; 64:486-91.

3. Glatstein IZ, Sleeper LA, Lavy Y, et al. Observer variability in the diagnosis and management of the hysterosalpingogram. Fertil Steril 1997;67:233-7.

4. Perquin DA, Dorr PJ, de Craen AJ, Helmerhorst FM Routine use of hysterosalpingography prior to laparoscopy in the fertility workup: A multicentre randomized controlled trial. Hum Reprod 2006;21(5):1227-31.

5. National Institute for Clinical Excellence, NHS. Fertility: Assessment and Treatment for People with Fertility Problems—Full Guideline. London: RCOG Press, 2004.

6. Rawal N, Haddad N, Abbott GT. Selective salpingography and fallopian tube recanalisation: Experience from a district general hospital. J Obstet Gynaecol 2005;25(6):586-8.

7. Woolcott R, Fisher S, Thomas J, Kable W. A randomized, prospective, controlled study of laparoscopic dye studies and selective salpingography as diagnostic tests of fallopian tube patency. Fertil Steril 1999;72: 879-84.

8. Johnson N. Tubal flushing for subfertility. Cochrane Database Syst Rev 2004;1.

9. Papaioannou S, Afnan M, Girling AJ, Coomarasamy A, McHugo JM, Sharif K. The potential value of tubal perfusion pressures measured during selective salpingography in predicting fertility. Hum Reprod 2003;18: 358-63.

10. Kalogirou D, Antoniou G, Botsis D, Kassanos D, Vitoratos N, Zioris C. Is color Doppler necessary in the evaluation of tubal patency by hysterosalpingo-contrast sonography. Clin Exp Obstet Gynecol 1997; 24(2):101-3.

11. Chan CC, Ng EH, Tang OS, Chan KK, Ho PC. Comparison of three-dimensional hysterosalpingo-contrast-sonography and diagnostic laparoscopy with chromopertubation in the assessment of tubal patency for the investigation of subfertility Acta Obstet Gynecol Scand 2005;84(9):909-13.

12. Mol BW, Collins JA, Burrows EA, van der Veen F, Bossuyt PM. Comparison of hysterosalpingography and laparoscopy in predicting fertility outcome. Hum Reprod 1999;14:1237-42.

13. Wang PH, Lee WL, Yuan CC. Major complications of operative and diagnostic laparoscopy for gynecologic disease. J Am Assoc Gynecol Laparosc 2001;8:68-73.

14. Bilgin H, Ozcan B, Bilgin T. Methemoglobinemia induced by methylene blue pertubation during laparoscopy. Acta Anaesthesiol Scand 1998;42:594-5.

15. Surrey ES. Microendoscopy of the human fallopian tube. J Am Assoc Gynecol Laparosc 1999;6(4):383-9.

16. Scudamore IW, Dunphy BC, Bowman M, Cooke ID. Comparison of ampullary assessment by falloposcopy and salpingoscopy. Hum Reprod 1994;9(8):1516-8.

17. Kerin JF, Daykhovsky L, Segalowitz J. Falloposcopy a microendoscopic technique for visual exploration of the human fallopian tube from the uterotubal ostium to fimbria using a transvaginal approach. Fertil Steril 1990;54:390-400.

18. Surrey ES, Adamson GD, Nagel TC, et al. Multicentre feasibility study of a new coaxial falloposcopy system. J Am Assoc Gynecol Laparosc 1997;4:473-8.

19. Bauer O, Diedrich K, Bacich S, et al. Transcervical access and intraluminal imaging of the fallopian tube in the non-anaesthetized patient; preliminary results using a new technique for fallopian tube access. Hum Reprod 1992;7:7-11.

20. Dunphy BC, Office falloposcopic assessment in proximal tubal occlusive disease. Fertil Steril 1994;61:168-70.

21. Kerin JF, Williams DB, San Roman GA, Pearlstone AC, Grundfest WS, Surrey ES. Falloposcopic classification and treatment of fallopian tube lumen disease. Fertil Steril 1992;57:731-41.

22. Kerin JF. Falloposcopy: Antegrade Imaging in the Management of Oviductal Disease. J Am Assoc Gynecol Laparosc 1996;3(4, Supplement):S21.

23. Winston RM, Margara RA. Microsurgical salpingostomy is not an obsolete procedure. Br J Obstet Gynaecol 1991;98:637-42.

24. Kissler S, Wildt L, Schmiedehausen K, Kohl J, Mueller A, Rody A. Predictive value of impaired uterine transport function assessed by negative hysterosalpingoscintiography (HSSG). Eur J Obstet Gynecol Reprod Biol 2004;113(2):204-8.

25. Mol BW, Dijkman B, Wertheim P, Lijmer J, van der Veen F, Bossuyt PM. The accuracy of serum chlamydial antibodies in the diagnosis of tubal pathology: A meta-analysis. Fertil Steril 1997;67:1031-7.

CHAPTER 3

Fibroid

Surveen Ghumman

Uterine myomas are benign tumors composed mainly of smooth muscle cells but also containing variable amount of fibroconnective tissue. They are the most common tumors of the reproductive tract. Since uterine myomata increase in frequency in advancing reproductive years and with current tendency of women to delay pregnancy into these years, the occurrence of fibroids in patients desiring pregnancy have increased. Today this commonly encountered condition poses a great challenge to the infertility specialist.

PREVALENCE

They occur in 20 to 25% of women of reproductive age. 40% of women with myomas in the reproductive age have infertility.[1] Conversely 5% of infertility patients have fibroids although in only 2 to 3% cases would myomas be responsible for it. The application of gross serial sectioning at 2 mm intervals in hysterectomy specimens revealed an incidence of 77%.[2]

Hysteroscopic series have reported finding submucous fibroids in 6-34% of women investigated for abnormal uterine bleeding, in 2-7% of women investigated for infertility, and in only 1.5% of asymptomatic women undergoing hysteroscopic sterilization, suggesting that the site of the fibroid may be important in determining symptoms.[3-5]

CLASSIFICATION

Uterine fibroids are classified according to their location:
1. Submucous (spanning the uterine cavity and wall);
2. Intramural (in the uterine wall);
3. Subserous (outer part of the uterine wall);
4. Pedunculated (connected to the uterus by a stalk).

SYMPTOMS

Abnormal bleeding: Menorrhagia, metorrhagia or menometorrhagia occurs in one-third of the patients. It is due to increased endometrial surface, local hyperestrogenism, hyperplasia, anovulation and interference with myometrial contractility as well as contractility of spiral arteries.

Pressure symptoms: Pressure on the urinary bladder may cause frequency, incontinence and retention. There may be silent ureteral obstruction from pressure against the pelvic brim. Rarely pressure on the bowel will lead to constipation or intermittent intestinal obstruction.

Pain: Abdominal discomfort, heaviness and dyspareunia occur in one-third of patients. The cause may be a twist in subserous fibroid, infection or acute carneous or red degeneration.

Abdominal mass: Abdominal mass may be palpable in large fibroids. A growth in size of more than 6 weeks is an indication for surgery as there may be a malignancy.[6]

Infertility: Causes of infertility in a fibroid uterus (Fig. 3.1).
1. Ovarian compression.
2. Anovulation.
3. Prostaglandin induced uterine contractions.
4. Bilateral cornual obstruction due to manual compression.

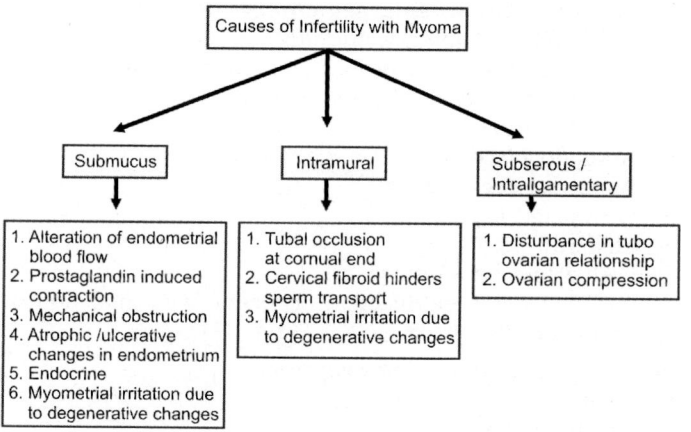

Fig. 3.1: Causes of infertility with fibroid uterus

5. Fibroids distort the endometrium and interfere with endometrial blood flow in a manner which inhibits appropriate nidation and implantation.[7] There was a significant negative impact on implantation rate in the intramural myomata groups versus the control groups, 16.4 vs. 27.7% in a study.

6. Interference with sperm transport by distortion and increase in surface area within the uterine cavity and impingement of leiomyomata on endocervical canal or interstitial portion of fallopian tube. Also there is interference with prostaglandin induced uterine contraction.

7. Myometrial irritation may occur from degeneration of intramural or submucous fibroid.

8. Cervical fibroids alter position of the cervix and affect fertility.

Pregnancy complications: There is an increased risk of:

1. *Spontaneous abortion:* This is because of:
   a. Alterations in blood supply of the endometrium
   b. Uterine irritability
   c. Rapid growth and degeneration of leiomyomata during pregnancy
   d. Difficulty in enlargement of uterine cavity to accommodate growing fetus
   e. Interference with proper implantation and placental growth because of poorly developed endometrium.

2. Premature delivery

3. Abruptio placentae

4. Abnormal presentation

5. Obstructed labour

6. Stillbirth

7. Postpartum hemorrhage

8. Red degeneration, infection or torsion with infarction of subserous fibroid.

Miscellaneous signs and symptoms

- Ascitis
- Uterine inversion
- *Polycythemia*: Marked erythropoietin activity is found within the leiomyomata.

INVESTIGATIONS

The accurate assessment of the number, size and location of fibroids, is important to assess whether the fibroid is causing the infertility. It is especially important when myomectomy is planned, because it often influences the type of surgical approach. There is no single correct approach to evaluating uterine fibroids. A number of options are available which vary considerably both in cost and convenience.

The role of imaging studies in women with fibroids is:

a. To confirm the clinically suspected diagnosis of fibroids.
b. Exclude other associated causes of uterine enlargement or pelvic masses such as adenomyosis, uterine malignancy, and benign or malignant ovarian masses.
c. To identify normal ovaries in the presence of an enlarged uterus.
d. Examine the kidneys and urinary tract for obstruction due to the pelvic mass.
e. Precise determination of the number, size and location of the fibroids.

Various imaging modalities are used.

1. **Ultrasonography:** It is considered the most important initial investigation for evaluation of size shape, echotexture, evidence of degenerative changes and exact distance from endometrial cavity or serosa of the fibroid. The fibroids appear as hypoechoic areas but may vary in their degree of echogenicity; being heterogeneous or hyperechoic, depending on the amount of fibrous tissue and/or calcification. Fibroids may have an anechoic components resulting from necrosis.

> Abdominal ultrasonography should always be performed before transvaginal sonography which may miss fundal and subserosal fibroids.

If fibroids are small and isoechoic relative to the uterus, the only ultrasonic sign may be a bulge in the uterine contour. The echogenic endometrial stripe may be displaced by a fibroid. Diffuse leiomyomatosis appears as an enlarged uterus with abnormal echogenicity. Ultrasound has a sensitivity of 60%, a specificity of 99%, and an accuracy of 87%. In fewer than 5% of patients, fibroids if necrotic, may mimic normal pelvic structures (especially the ovaries) and pathologic pelvic conditions, including uterine variants and pregnancy-related conditions. TVS was better at mapping and sizing submucous and intramural fibroids than hysteroscopy.

Color Doppler may be able to detect a malignant change or uterine malignancy.

3-D ultrasonography is very accurate in detecting location and number of fibroids.

2. **Saline infusion sonography:** This would detect a polyp or submucous fibroid. Transvaginal sonohysterography avoided the need for diagnostic hysteroscopy in 47% of women who could then proceed to planned operative hysteroscopy.[8]

3. **Hysterosalpingography:** Observing early uterine filling under fluoroscopic visualization while slowly injecting the contrast medium will provide greater detail of the uterine cavity. The size of the lesion cannot be accurately assessed because position of the lesion from the X-ray plate may vary thus altering the size of the image on the plate. An abnormal HSG needs to be followed by a hysteroscopy.

4. **CT scan:** It has a limited role in the diagnosis of uterine fibroids. On CT scans, fibroids are usually indistinguishable from healthy myometrium unless they are calcified or necrotic. Calcifications may be more visible on CT scans than on conventional radiographs because of the superior contrast differentiation with CT. It is not as specific as ultrasound in differentiating uterine masses from ovarian masses or the surrounding bowel. CT scan provides complete visualization of the female pelvis including non-gynecological structures, but offers limited resolution of the internal architecture of the female pelvic organs and requires the use of ionising radiation.

There is insufficient evidence to recommend CT scanning in the assessment of fibroids.

5. **MRI:** It is the most accurate imaging technique for detection and localization of leiomyomata. Various degrees of cellularity, degeneration, necrosis and calcification can be identified. Fibroids are sharply marginated areas of low-to-intermediate signal intensity on both T1- and T2-weighted MRIs. An inhomo-geneous area of high signal intensity may be depicted on T2-weighted images; this results from hemorrhage, hyaline degeneration, edema, or highly cellular fibroids.

    The intravenous administration of gadolinium-based contrast material usually is not required, however, if it is administered, fibroids usually enhance later than the healthy myometrium. Fibroid enhancement can be hypointense (65%), isointense (23%), or hyperintense (12%) in relation to that of the myometrium. MRI has a sensitivity of 86-92%, specificity of 100%, and accuracy of 97% in the evaluation of probable fibroids.

    Advantages of MRI are that it is accurate in:
    a. Detection of small myoma of upto 3 mm in size.
    b. Localization of myoma within the uterus
    c. Assessment of impingement on endometrial cavity
    d. Differentiation between adenomyosis, leiomyomata and diffuse leiomyomatosis.
    e. Identification of ovaries with a large uterus
    f. Provides imaging planes permitting better visuali-zation of more lateral and posterior areas of the pelvis.

    MRI is the most accurate imaging technique for fibroids when the location or nature of the fibroids remains uncertain after transvaginal ultrasound and transvaginal sonohystero-graphy (TVSH) or for those who wish to avoid the possible discomforts of a TVSH

6. **Diagnostic hysteroscopy:** On diagnostic hysteroscopy myomata are fixed whereas polyps undulate with the ebb and flow of the distention medium. Submucous myoma tends to bulge in the uterine cavity over a thin endometrium.

They are smooth, firm, pale and rounded. To categorize the degree of intramural extension, the classification system for submucous myomas by the European Society of Gynaecological Endoscopy is used (Table 3.1).

Table 3.1: Classification system for submucous myomas by the European Society of Gynaecological Endoscopy	
Type	*Degree of intramural extension*
Type 0	Pedunculated submucous myomas without intramural extension
Type I	Sessile submcous myoma with the intramural part less than 50%
Type II	Sessile submucous myoma with an intramural extension of 50% or more

If the myoma is completely in the uterine cavity it is very easy to resect but the deeper it goes into the myometrium the more difficult it is to remove and the risks become higher for the hysteroscopic route. Hence preoperative assessment and classification is very important in order to decide feasibility of the operation.

7. ***Diagnostic laparoscopy:*** Fibroids may be coincidentally discovered at laparoscopy. However since at that time it is not confirmed that the fibroid is responsible for infertility they should not be treated in the same sitting without determining their position with respect to the endometrial cavity.

8. ***Intravenous pyelogram and barium enema:*** This is to diagnose pressure effects. It is indicated if the uterine mass is extending laterally or there is compromise of ureteral function. It is useful preoperatively to trace the course of the ureter if fibroid is large.

Indications for Therapy of Uterine Myoma in Infertile Patients

In an infertile patient a fibroid is treated if it is an established cause of infertility. If indications exist for therapy of fibroids irrelevant to the presence of infertility these conditions would apply to the infertile patients too. Thus, infertile patient with pain and menorrhagia not responding to treatment must be treated. Therapy in these cases should be designed so as to optimize future fertility (Table 3.2).

> Uterine myoma which do not interfere with tubal structure nor with endometrium and its underlying myometrial architecture are unlikely to result in infertility and are best left alone. Submucous fibroids and large fibroids that are symptomatic in patients who want to become pregnant should be removed.

The presence of myomata uteri in the setting of infertility does not always suggest an etiological association. Since removal of fibroid may lead to fertility compromising pelvic adhesions, before undertaking treatment for fibroids to improve fertility two conditions must be met.

1. All other causes of infertility must be ruled out.
2. It should be proven that uterine myomata present are affecting the reproductive function either because of size or position.

Table 3.2: Indications for myomectomy in infertile patients

Conditions irrelevant to infertility not responding to treatment
- Fibroid related pain
- Fibroid related menorrhagia / anemia
- Complication of large pelvic masses like hydronephrosis

Conditions relevant to infertility
- Submucus fibroid with significant distortion of endometrial cavity
- Occlusion of tubal orifices
- Large Intramural fibroid resulting in significant uterine cavity distortion.

Effect of location of fibroid on pregnancy rates after myomectomy was studied by Casini in 181 women showing the importance of position of the fibroid in determining success of surgery[9] (Table 3.3).

Table 3.3: Effect of location of fibroid on pregnancy rates after myomectomy

Position of fibroid	Pregnancy rate after myomectomy	Pregnancy rate where surgery was not done
Submucosal	43.3%	27.2%
Intramural	56.5%	41%
Submucosal-intramural	40%	15%
Intramural-subserosal	35.5%	21.43%

The location and size of the myomas are the two parameters that influence the success of a future pregnancy. Subserosal myomas seem to have little, if any, effect on reproductive outcome, especially if they are up to 5 to 7 cm in diameter. Intramural myomas that do not encroach upon the endometrium and are smaller than 4 to 5 cm also can be considered to be relatively harmless to reproduction. Myomas that compress the uterine cavity significantly reduce pregnancy rates, and should be removed before assisted reproductive techniques are used.[10] Rakbow felt that fibroid location, followed by size, is the most important factor determining the impact of fibroids on IVF outcomes.[11] Any distortion of the endometrial cavity seriously affects IVF outcomes as there is a lower implantation rate, and myomectomy is indicated in this situation. Patients with intramural fibroids have a lower implantation rate per cycle.[8] Myomectomy should also be considered for patients with large fibroids, and for patients with unexplained unsuccessful IVF cycles.

MANAGEMENT

In the recent years management of fibroids has undergone many advancements. Management may be expectant, medical or surgical.

Expectant Management

Asymptomatic patients with subserosal or small intramural fibroid can be managed expectantly. Conservative management may also be used for a submucous fibroid which is not causing infertility. Uterine size must be evaluated 3 months after initial examination to detect rapidly growing tumors. If the uterine size is stable follow-up examination must be scheduled every 6 months or as indicated by change or increase in symptoms. Patient must be counseled on the increased risk of complications associated with myoma during pregnancy if she conceives.

Medical Therapy

Since fibroid growth and maintenance are stimulated by estrogen and are affected by hormonal cyclic changes, many of these treatments are based on the suppression of estrogen. Treatment options for women with large or symptomatic uterine fibroids have traditionally been hysterectomy or myomectomy. As many women are delaying child-bearing into their thirties or forties and there is a desire for less invasive treatment, alternative options to surgery have been developed. Medical therapy is an option if the woman is not considered fit for surgery or does not wish to undergo surgery; however, fibroids will return to pre-therapy size within 6 months of stopping therapy.

> The medical management of myomas cannot replace surgery for symptomatic infertile women or one with recurrent abortion because the effect of drugs is temporary and with return of ovarian function the fibroids also reach their original size.

Progestins: Fibroids contain progesterone receptors and, as such, progestins should in theory be effective; however, there is little evidence to support the use of progestins in the treatment of uterine fibroids.[12]

Combined oral contraceptives: No effect was seen in fibroid size but duration of menstrual period was decreased when oral contraceptives were given.

GnRH Agonist: The GnRH agonist therapy has allowed effective medical management of the fibroid. It is given in doses adequate to suppress endogenous estrogen levels to < 45 pg/ml. The average shrinkage of myoma is 50%, the maximum occurring by 8 to 12 weeks. Reduction in the tumor mass is primarily due to alterations in the cellular matrix rather than reduction in number or volume of cells in myoma. The reduction in total fibroid/uterine volume seems to be dependent on the level of estrogen suppression with heavier women (having elevated levels of circulating estrone) requiring larger doses of GnRH analogues.[13] Regrowth of the tumor occurs rapidly once the therapy is stopped.

Advantages of GnRH therapy
1. Allows definitive therapy to be delayed until iron reserves are replenished and there is preoperative normalization of hematocrit.
2. Reduction in intraoperative blood loss.
3. Simplification of surgical approach due to shrinkage in size.
4. Increased probability of hysteroscopic approach.

Disadvantages
1. Since tumor response is variable not all patients are benefited.
2. It requires 2 to 3 months of expensive therapy before maximum response occurs.
3. It regrows on stoppage of therapy.
4. It makes development of tissue planes more difficult during surgery making the overlying myometrium adherent to the myoma.
5. Severe hemorrhage has been encountered in women where GnRH therapy has caused necrosis of submucous myoma.[14]
6. Small myomas may become too small to be noticed at surgery thus leaving behind myomas which grow later.
7. Mean reduction in trabecular bone density of 1% per month occurs in women treated for 6 months. This bone loss is usually reversible but some of it may be permanent.

Addback therapy of estrogen progestogen may be used if treatment extends beyond 3 months. With combined addback therapy (estrogen plus progestin), the reduction in uterine and fibroid size is maintained while the annoying side effects of GnRH analogue treatment are controlled. Addback therapy is usually administered at about 12 weeks after the beginning of GnRH analogue treatment by which time the maximum reduction in uterine size has occurred.

Use of GnRH agonists in treatment of myoma in the infertile patient: There are a few data regarding the use of GnRH agonist in treatment of infertility associated myoma. Therapy obviously induces a state of anovulation preventing pregnancy for the duration of therapy. If concomitant ovulation induction is required when patient is on GnRH agonist therapy human menopausal gonadotropins can be used as replacement therapy.[15] Usually ovulatory menses resume 3 to 24 weeks after last depot GnRH injection. During which time the uterus may increase to pretreatment size. Short-term treatment to reduce size before surgery specially to make hysteroscopic removal feasible can also be done.

Mifepristone (RU 486): Mifepristone in a dose of 25 mg per day can cause a decrease of 49% in the myoma size.[16] Side effects were mild and bone density was not affected.

Gestrinone: It is a synthetic derivative of ethynyl nortestosterone with antiestrogenic and antiprogesterone properties. It was most effective when given intravaginally for a period of 6 to 12 months. Uterine volume decreased in 73% of women and regression of large leiomyomata lasted upto one year. Most women experienced androgenic side effects such as acne, hirsutism and weight gain although these reversed on cessation of treatment. The long-lasting effects of reduced fibroid volume after stopping treatment may be a major advantage for gestrinone.[17]

Danazol:

Danazol causes a regression in fibroids but its usefulness as a treatment option is limited because of its androgenic side effect profile which restricts duration of use to 6 months.

Non-steroidal anti-inflammatory drugs: NSAIDs can be useful in reducing heavy menstrual bleeding not associated with uterine fibroids but they are not effective as a treatment for women with fibroids.[18]

> Calcified myomas and myomas that are fibrous and avascular do not respond to medical treatment.

Surgical Therapy

Basic surgical options are:

- Hysterectomy
- Myomectomy.

Choice of therapy in the infertile patient is myo-mectomy although in the era of surrogacy and egg donation hysterectomy is now being considered as an alternative. Fibroids have a primitive type of blood supply with little resistance to ischaemia (disruption of blood supply). They may be supplied by one uterine artery, or may have a bilateral supply.

Prerequisites

1. Counseling patient on the possibility that conversion of surgery to hysterectomy may occur.
2. Other factors for infertility have been ruled out.
3. Blood should be arranged.
4. An endometrial sample is a must if abnormal bleeding occurred.

Surgical Methods for Myomectomy Include

- Hysteroscopy
- Laparoscopy
- Laparotomy
- Robotic myomectomy.

Choice of Method

The method used depends on many factors like (Table 3.4).

Table 3.4: Factors determining route of myomectomy
1. Fertility
2. Uterine size
3. Previous surgery or suspected adhesions
4. Location of the fibroids
• Deep intramural
• Lateral
5. Number of the fibroids
6. Size of the fibroids - > 8 cm consider laparotomy
7. Any additional surgery

- *Size, location, and number of fibroids.*
  - Hysteroscopy can be used to remove submucosal fibroids in the uterus that have not grown deep into the uterine wall.
  - Laparoscopy is usually reserved for removing a few fibroids, up to about 5 to 8 cm across, that are subserosal or intramural but not deep in the myometrium.
  - Laparotomy is used to remove large fibroids, multiple fibroids, or fibroids that have grown deep into the uterine wall. With multiple fibroids there is a chance of leaving smaller myomas behind.

Laparotomy is preferred for multiple small fibroids which need to be palpated to be located.

- *Concomitant surgery:* Concomitant surgery like need to correct urinary or bowel problems, may require a laparotomy.
- *Size of uterus:* If size is greater than 20 weeks it may be difficult to do a myomectomy through a laparoscope.
- *Fertility:* A critical part of successful myomectomy is optimal reconstruction of the uterus after the fibroids have been removed. Laparoscopy is not recommended for very large fibroids in an infertile patients because:

1. Meticulous placement of multiple sutures are needed to repair the irregular defects in uterine wall caused by removal of fibroids which is difficult and time consuming by laparoscopy. Consequently too a few sutures may be applied. Suboptimal reconstruction can lead dead spaces which are potential sites of bleeding and infection. This results in:
   i. Weakned uterine wall which can rupture in subsequent pregnancy.
   ii. Postoperative bleeding requiring an emergency hysterectomy.
   iii. Poor hemostasis leading to adhesion formation, tubal occlusion and infertility.
2. Also endoscopic myomectomy requires considerable manual dexterity and hand eye coordination. There is less flexibility in choosing the site for the uterine incision and it is difficult to perform delicate movements or use very fine sutures.
3. The operating time is frequently longer than if the procedure were performed by laparotomy.
   In a woman who intends to have children, or who is undergoing an evaluation for infertility, a laparotomy may be the more prudent choice with large fibroids. There are also reports of uterine rupture during pregnancy following laparoscopic myomectomy but vaginal delivery can be accomplished safely, provided that delivery is managed as in vaginal birth after cesarean.[19]

There was no evidence of a difference in outcome in terms of clinical pregnancy rate and live birth rate when fibroids were removed via laparotomy or laparoscopy for infertility. There were some non-fertility benefits of removal via laparoscopy including shorter hospital stay, less febrile illness and a smaller drop in preoperative hemoglobin concentration when compared to laparotomy.[20]

While deciding the route of surgery, the surgery which gives the best results should be done, as it is the quality of surgery not quicker recovery which determines the success in an infertile patient. Decision for approach of myomectomy should be taken after looking through the laparoscope.

Role of Preoperative GnRH

Hormone treatment with GnRH agonists, may be used preoperatively to decrease the size of the fibroid and the bleeding, promoting improvement in hemoglobin if the patient is anemic.[21]

Disadvantages
1. The fibroids become much more difficult to separate from the surrounding uterine tissue making the myomectomy technically more difficult.
2. GnRH treatment may shrink small fibroids which could, therefore, be missed at surgery only to enlarge again and cause problems later.

Administration of GnRH analogues for 2 to 4 months prior to surgery for uterine fibroids is recommended for women with a large uterus (> 18 weeks size) or preoperative anemia

Vaginal Myomectomy

Myomectomy can be done vaginally depending on location and size of fibroid.

Avulsion of polyp

Pedunculated fibroid polyp can be removed by twisting it free with an Allis clamp. If bleeding occurs a 26 French Foley's catheter is inserted through cervix and inflated for tamponade.

Hysteroscopic removal

Higher submucus pedunculated myomata can be accessed by hysteroscopy. Morcellation may be required to remove very large tumors. One should avoid too much downward traction on the tumor because the uterine fundus may invert (See Chapter 4).

Vaginal myomectomy

Vaginal myomectomy may also be done in intramural and subserosal leiomyomas. An open myomectomy can be performed through anterior or posterior colpotomy.

Technique: Posterior vaginal wall is retracted with a Sims speculum (Fig. 3.2). Anterior lip of cervix is held by a volsellum (Fig. 3.3). A transverse incision is given on the vagina mucosa anteriorly on the cervix (Fig. 3.4). The cervix is pulled downwards with a volsellum while the bladder is pushed up with a gauze to expose the UV fold (Fig. 3.5). The UV fold is defined by lifting it with an artery forceps (Fig. 3.6). An incision is given on the UV fold to open the anterior peritoneum (Fig. 3.7). The anterior wall of uterus becomes accessible. An incision is given on the fibroid which is accessible anteriorly and fibroid is enucleated (Fig. 3.8). The base is stitched as in abdominal myomectomy and serosal sutures are applied. The fibroid can be approached from the posterior pouch if it is located on the posterior wall. The posterior lip of the cervix is held with a volsellum and a transverse incision is given on the vagina (Figs 3.9 and 3.10). The posterior fold of peritoneum is lifted (Fig. 3.11). Pouch of Douglas is opened after giving an incision on the peritoneal fold (Fig. 3.12). The posterior surface of the uterus is visualized. Myomectomy of fibroids accessible posteriorly is done in a similar manner to that shown anteriorly. Preoperative criterion included:

1. Uterine size less than or equal to 16 weeks
2. Good uterine mobility
3. Adequate vaginal access
4. Absence of adnexal pathology.

Three patients out of 10 in a study who had a transvaginal myomectomy through a colpotomy conceived.[22]

Vaginal myomectomy is recommended as the most appropriate initial treatment for pedunculated submucous myomata.

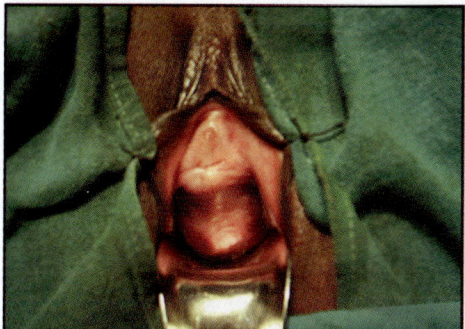

Fig. 3.2: Posterior vaginal wall is retracted by Sims speculum

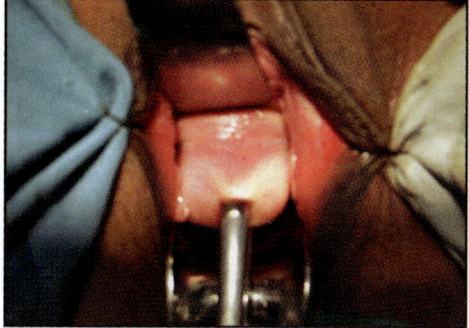

Fig. 3.3: Anterior lip of cervix held with a volsellum

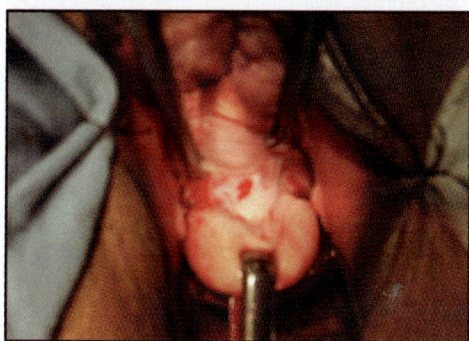

Fig. 3.4: Transverse incision given anteriorly on cervix

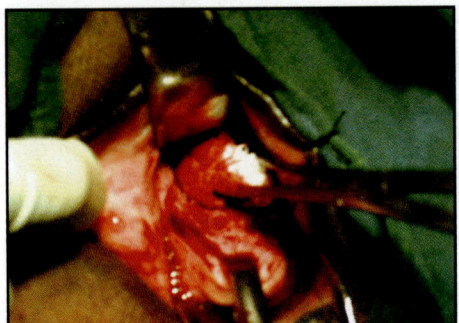

Fig. 3.5: Traction given on cervix with volsellum while bladder is pushed up

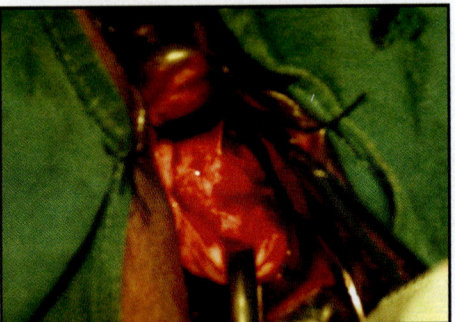

Fig. 3.6: Uterovesical fold lifted with an artery forceps

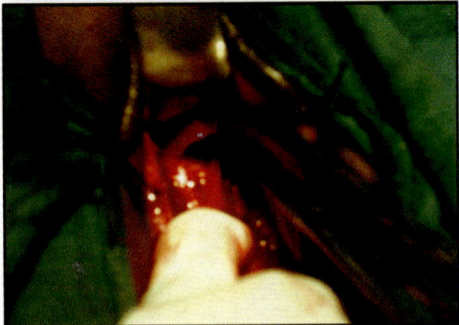

Fig. 3.7: Transverse incision given to open UV fold

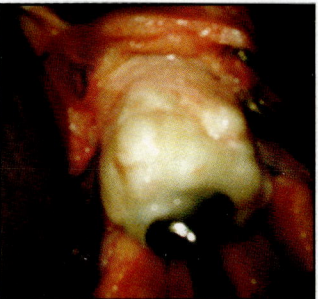

Fig. 3.8: Enucleation after giving incision on the fibroid through anterior pouch

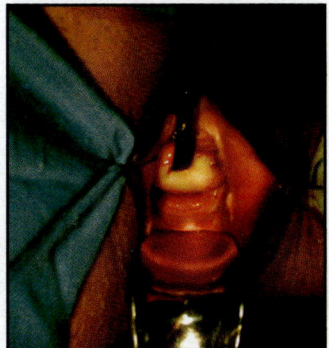

Fig. 3.9: Posterior lip of cervix held with a volsellum

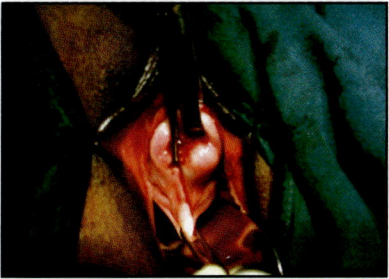

Fig. 3.10: Picking posterior vaginal wall with Allis forceps to give a transverse incision

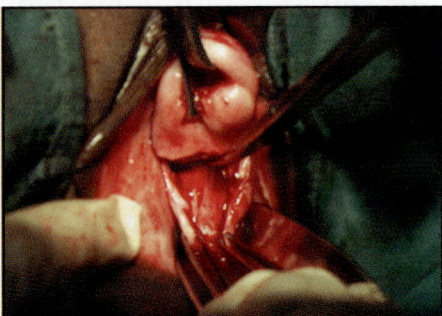

Fig. 3.11: Posterior fold of peritoneum defined

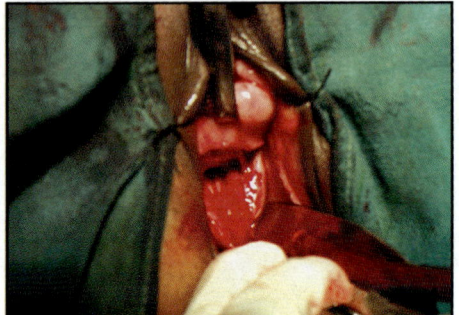

Fig. 3.12: Pouch of Douglas opened

Abdominal Myomectomy

Myomectomy can be done abdominally either by lapartromy or laparoscopically.

Time: The surgery is usually done in the proliferative phase of the cycle.

Indications for open surgery

1. Uterus size more than 22 weeks.
2. Fibroids more than 14 weeks in size with a broad base (Pedunculated fibroids of this size or even greater can be removed laparoscopically).

3. Myoma which occupies all of one uterine surface.
4. Deep seated multiple myomas.
5. Unfavorable location of the fibroid(s) such as intra-ligamental, deep in the pouch of Douglas, or posterior. Myomectomy in these locations tend to be more difficult
6. Multiple fibroids throughout the uterus.
7. Previous history of extensive abdominal surgery like endometriosis, adnexal pathology, or adhesions of the gastrointestinal tract due to abdominal tuberculosis.
8. High risk medical conditions not permitting pneumo-peritoneum.

During this surgery there are two major technical concerns

1. Minimization of blood loss
2. Prevention of postoperative adhesions: The overall incidence of postoperative adhesions has been reported to be between 14 to 53%.

Hemostasis: Hemostasis during surgery can be achieved by good surgical technique.

1. Penrose drain or elastic rubber tourniquet passed through the avascular plane of the broad ligament (Fig. 3.13). It is important that arterial blood supply is occluded otherwise blood loss will be increased with only venous occlusion. The mean blood pressure should be reduced to 60 mm Hg. The higher the blood pressure the tighter the tourniquet has to be tied to occlude the circulation.
2. Bringing the uterus up to the abdominal incision provides a stretch on uterine arteries and decreases bleeding.
3. Atraumatic clamps applied on infundibulopelvic ligaments or uterine artery which are released every 20 minutes (Fig. 3.14).
4. Local infiltration with vasopressin 20 units in 20 ml of saline. The effect lasts for 30 minutes. It is as effective as

mechanical vascular occlusion. Care should be taken in avoiding injecting directly into the vascular channel and no more than 30 ml should be used because of potential side effects. It is contraindicated in vascular disease and patients on tricyclic anti-depressants.

5. Good surgical technique, careful dissection in the right plane between the myoma and the pseudocapsule and prompt suturing

6. Preference for a vertical midline incision which is the least vascular plane.

7. Electrocautry or laser may cause decreased blood loss from superficial vessels in comparison to the knife.

8. Preoperative GnRH agonists in cases with uterine volume greater than 600 cm^3 or 16 weeks size.

After reconstruction of the uterus is complete the determination of adequate hemostasis in the uterus cannot be made until all tourniquets are released and blood pressure has returned to normal.

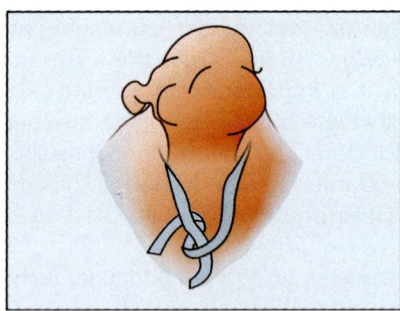

Fig. 3.13: Elastic rubber tourniquet through broad ligament

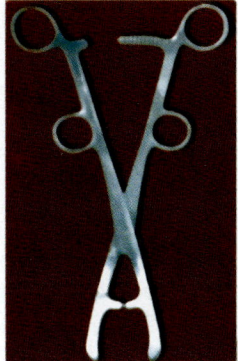

Fig. 3.14: Bonneys uterine artery clamp–1920's

Prevention of Postoperative Adhesions

Patients at a higher risk of adhesion formation must be identified (Table 3.5). Postoperative adhesions may be prevented in a number of ways.

1. Keeping incisions to a minimum number
2. Vertical midline incision
3. Avoidance of posterior incision. Posterior myoma is removed by fundal incision or if cavity has been entered already a transcavity approach can be done.
4. Proper closure and suturing which ensures hemostasis.
5. Minimal surface damage should be there.
6. Avoid digital blunt dissection of fibroids.
7. Sutures on serosal surface should be fine absorbable non-reactive material
8. Running suture lines are preferred to avoid knot volume.
9. Operative field is kept moist and free of clots
10. Omental or peritoneal grafts are used.
11. Uterine suspension if there is a posterior incision.
12. Physiological solution is used to irrigate the pelvis.
13. Absorbable (Interceed – oxidized regenerated cellu-lose) or non-absorbable (Gore-Tex – polytetra-fluoroethylene surgical membrane) barriers.

Table 3.5: Risk factors for adhesion formation
1. Existence of adhesions before operation
2. Additional surgical procedures carried out at the same time
3. Posterior location of myoma.
4. Uterine suturing: It may cause inflammatory change inducing adhesion formation

The choice of cutting instruments includes electrocautry, laser or sharp knife. There is decreased blood loss from tiny superficial vessels using electrocautery or laser but these methods of cutting may cause greater local tissue damage, specially when operating near tubal insertions. The advantage of the greater precision is offered by a sharp scalpel.

CO_2 laser has been used as a tool that decreases bleeding, tissue injury and adhesion formation. Myomata of 1 cm diameter can be vaporized directly by laser.

Principles of Successful Myomectomy for Infertility

1. Prior to start of the surgery it is important to determine the relative position of the fibroids to tubal ostia and endometrial cavity.
2. Use of as a few incisions as possible with care to avoid intramural portion of the fallopian tube.
3. The direction of dissection for significant fibroids is from lateral to a medial direction and from inferior to superior direction. This decreases blood loss and avoids damage to the lateral blood vessels.
4. The natural contour of the uterine cavity should not be altered by the procedure
5. The tubes should not be damaged by the operation. The fibroids located at the cornua will be difficult to resect without damage to the fallopian tubes.
6. Rough or deperitonealized surfaces should be avoided on the uterine surface, especially on the posterior wall where these changes may promote adhesion formation with the adnexae.
7. Meticulous hemostasis in order to avoid adhesions.

Method

Choice of abdominal incision: It is the surgeon's option but it is important that there is adequate exposure to deal with deep or posterior fibroids. One would need greater exposure for extensive myomectomy than hysterectomy.

Planning the uterine incision: The uterus is lifted through the incision. Before starting see if myomectomy is feasible, in what sequence the leiomyomata will be removed and how the uterus will be reconstructed. Careful planning of uterine incision is important to restrict the incision to a minimum number and preferably anteriorly and in the midline to avoid vascular areas of the uterus and the broad ligament.

Myometrial incision: Incision is made on the myoma and it is dissected at the plane of the capsule. Usually a vertical midline incision is given. It is placed in such a manner that maximum number of tumors are obtained (Fig. 3.15).

Developing a cleavage plane: The myoma is grasped by a tenaculum or myoma screw and digitally dissected to exposure the base. Bleeding points are coagulated (Fig. 3.16). A Kelly's clamp is placed at the base and the fibroid removed followed by ligation of the pedicle. This avoids tissue retraction leading to blind placement of deep sutures. If the myoma is slightly protruding into the endometrial cavity the myoma can usually be dissected free from endometrial cavity without incising the endometrial cavity. When it is deep in the myometrium , it is appropriate to palpate endometrial cavity to detect pedunculated fibroids. The endometrial cavity can be stained with methylene blue to aid in identifying it.

Repairing the Myometrial Defect: After myomectomy the redundant hypertrophic uterine tissue should be partly removed because it involutes. The myoma bed is usually closed with interrupted figure of eight or mattress 2-0 delayed absorbable sutures (Figs 3.17A and B). Large defects may be closed by purse string sutures to obliterate dead space. Excess myometrial tissue may be removed to allow adequate closure. Multilayer closure is done and several layers of sutures may be required. It is important to close all deep dead space. However, locking sutures devitalize tissue.

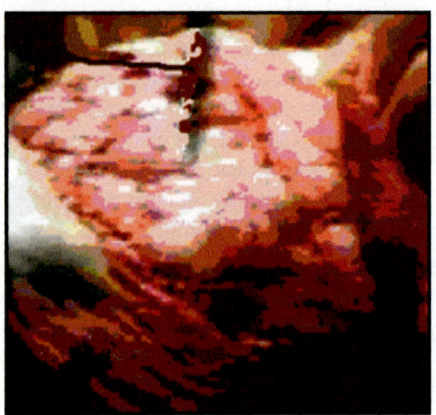

Fig. 3.15: Incision given on the myoma

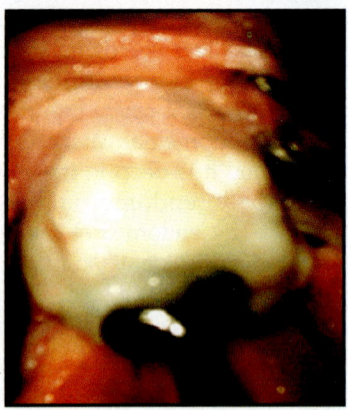

Fig. 3.16: Traction given to fibroid by tenaculum or myoma screw while separating it from its capsule

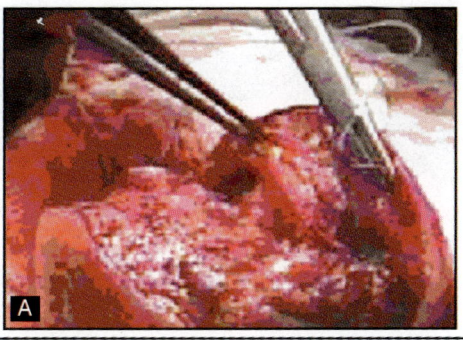

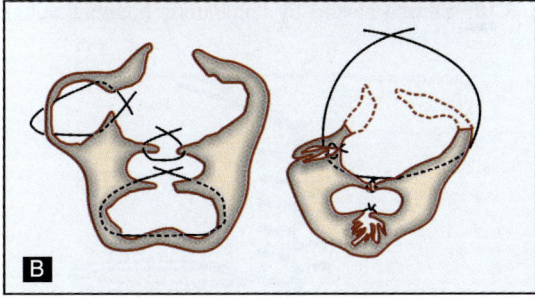

Figs 3.17A and B: Repairing myometrial defect by interrupted figure of 8 sutures

Serosal Sutures

Suture on serosal surface should be of fine absorbable non-reactive material. Running suture lines are preferable to avoid extra knot volume. Serosa is closed by continuous baseball suture of 5-0 or 6-0 non reactive absorbable material (Figs 3.18 and 3.19).

Tips:
1. In reconstructing the uterus, the surgeon should refer to fixed points such as attachment of the round ligament and fallopian tube on each side of the corpus.
2. If blood vessels are cut or left on the surface of the myoma, it usually means that the dissection has been carried out in an improper plane.

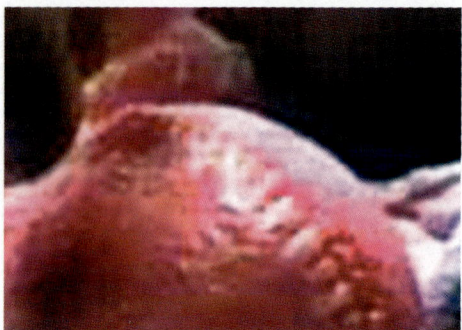

Fig. 3.18: Serosa closed by continuous baseball sutures

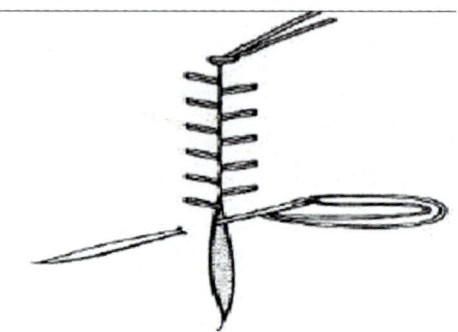

Fig. 3.19: Closing serosa with baseball stitch

Occasionally adenomyomatosis is encountered where tumor consists of nodules of adenomyosis with associated uterine scarring and induration. These do not have clear tissue planes and are difficult to dissect specifically from the uterus. Cytoreductive surgery to eliminate the more severe areas may be necessary. Since clear tissue planes are not available it is only possible to eliminate the central endometriotic core of these lesions.

Results

1. *Menorrhagia:* Menorrhagia is relieved in 80% of cases.
2. *Dysmenorrhea:* Pelvic discomfort and dysmenorrhea are relieved to a lesser extent as often other gynecological disease is present.
3. *Infertility:* Usually 60% of patients with no other cause for infertility conceive and mostly during the first 2 years.[23]
4. *Miscarriage:* The abortion rate decreased from 41 to 19%.[24]
5. *Uterine size:* Decrease in uterine size occurred in first 3 months.
6. *Recurrence:* Fibroids return after surgery in 10 to 50% of women, depending on the how many fibroids were originally present. Fibroids that were larger and more numerous are most likely to recur.[25] Treatment options for recurrence is expectant, GnRH agonists, repeat myomectomy or hysterectomy.

Subsequent Pregnancy

Because fibroids can grow back, it is best to try to conceive as soon after a myomectomy as is safely possible.[25]

- Wait 4 to 6 months after surgery to allow the uterus to heal before pregnancy.
- A hysterosalpingogram may be done after 4 months to check the uterus and fallopian tubes before any infertility treatment is started.

Pregnancy After Myomectomy

Usually a pregnancy rate of 40% is seen after myo-mectomy. When incisions have been made into the uterine wall to remove fibroids, future pregnancy may be affected. Sometimes, placental problems develop, such as placenta abruptio or placental accreta.

1. *LSCS*: Indication for LSCS after myomectomy
   - Multiple incisions on the uterine cavity.[26]
   - Entry into endometrial cavity.
   - Postoperative infection

A small incision into the endometrial cavity may not require a cesarean section. Risk of rupture is 0.5%. This decision should be made by the operating surgeon and communicated to the patient.

2. *Cervical cerclage*: If cervical myomectomy has been performed there may be need for elective cervical cerclage in second trimester.

Complications

Early Complications

- Persistent bleeding
- Intraoperative damage to bowel or ureter.
- Ileus (bowel obstruction)
- Conversion to hysterectomy
- Pelvic infection.

Late Complications

- Uterine rupture at delivery. This depends on the site, number and size of the uterine incision as well as the quality of the uterine closure
- Adhesion formation
- Late intestinal obstruction
- Infertility
- Repeat surgery due to recurrence of the fibroids.
- Rare chance of malignancy (1:200 to 1: 500).

Robotic Myomectomy

The surgical robot is a major advance in the ability to precisely operate through small incisions. The surgeon sits at a console and looks through a 3-dimensional video camera. The hand movements in the surgeon are duplicated in the patient by the robot. Most importantly, the instruments duplicate the wrist movements of the surgeon, allowing the instruments to change angles to allow precise suturing. This is an important advantage over laparoscopic or hysteroscopic myomectomy. The robotic surgery does not always eliminate the need for abdominal myomectomy, when there are multiple or very large myomas and/or many myomas.

Myolysis

Myolysis is the destruction of fibroids by the application of a laser probe or electric current to heat-coagulate symptomatic uterine fibroids. Cryomyolysis is a similar treatment, but instead of using a laser or electrical current, a probe is used to deliver a freezing agent such as liquid nitrogen directly to the fibroid to cause it to shrink and necrose. The probe is inserted into fibroids through the laparoscope and the electrical, laser or freezing apparatus is activated, resulting in necrosis of the affected portions inside the fibroid. This is repeated several times, at different locations inside the individual fibroid, until the extent of the necrosis inflicted in a certain fibroid is considered sufficient.

These methods are time consuming and usually limited to the treatment of moderate size fibroids. The patient may be first treated with Lupron injections over several months prior to the procedure in order to reduce fibroid size and vascularity.

Complications

a. *Pelvic infection and adhesions:* Following the procedure the site of perforation created by the probe on the uterine surface tend to ooze sero-sanguinous fluid leading to pelvic infection and adhesions.
b. *Fibrosis and weakening of myometrium:* The procedure may destroy large portions of the uterine muscle leading to uterine rupture in subsequent pregnancy.
c. *Persistence of symptoms:* Failure of the myolysis procedure to solve abnormal bleeding, pain or other clinical problems happens frequently and additional surgery like hysterectomy may then be required.

Myolysis is no longer considered the treatment of choice for fibroids.

Laparoscopic Clipping of the Uterine Arteries

Another treatment for uterine fibroids is laparoscopic clipping of the uterine arteries. It is a minimally invasive technique and has results similar to uterine artery embolization. It is not recommended in infertility.

Uterine Artery Embolization (UAE)

The embolization, consisting of introducing tiny particles of polyvinyl alcohol (500 to 700 micron size), into the uterine artery on both sides through a properly placed catheter (Fig. 3.20). This causes blockade of feeding vessels to fibroid leading to ischemic necrosis and degeneration, reducing the size over a period of weeks and months.

There are several concerns like reduced fertility as a consequence of injury to the uterus and ovaries, placental insufficiency resulting from inadequate blood flow to the uterus and uterine rupture during pregnancy because of UAE induced myoma necrosis. However no infertility has been reported after this procedure in practice.[27] The ideal candidate for UAE is a post-fertility, premenopausal patient with symptomatic uterine fibroids who strongly desires to avoid hysterectomy or have a contraindication to general anesthesia.

Although there is no fixed size limitation, patients with pedunculated subserosal fibroids are not considered ideal candidates.

Procedure

The procedure is done with intravenous sedation under local anesthesia. A small nick of 1/4th inch is given below the inguinal ligament. The access to the femoral artery is made and an angiographic catheter is introduced (Fig. 3.20). This is advanced till uterine artery or major feeding vessel is reached. An arteriogram at this stage provides precise arterial mapping of blood supply to uterus and fibroid. Subsequently polyvinyl alcohol (PVA) particles 500 μm in diameter are introduced slowly. The vessel is completely blocked after a few minutes (Fig. 3.21). PVA flows into the hypervascular uterine fibroids, blocking small arteries and causing ischemic necrosis. Normal myometrium is unharmed because it is supplied by multiple collateral arteries. The procedure is continued till complete blockade is ensured and is repeated on the other side. It takes approximately 1-2 hours and the post procedure stay is usually 6 to 8 hours. Most women can return to work 7 days after the procedure.[28]

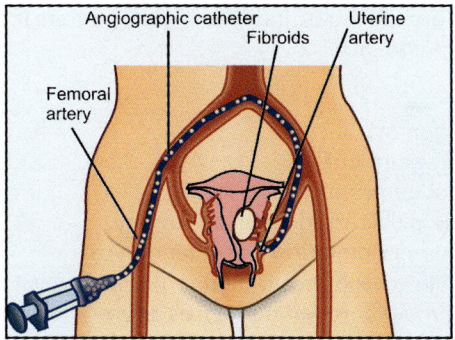

Fig. 3.20: Catheterization of femoral artery and injection polyvinyl alcohol particles

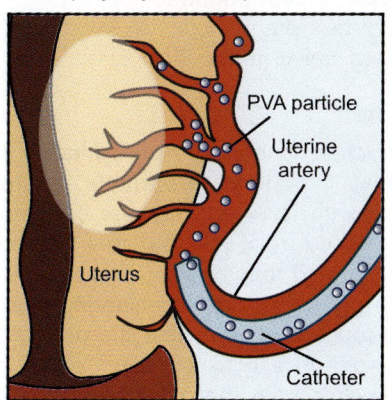

Fig. 3.21: PVA particles of 500 µm in diameter enter the abnormal arteries in the uterus

Contraindications

UAE is contraindicated in women with any of the following conditions:

Absolute

- Women with a current/ past history of pelvic malignancy
- Pelvic infections
- Rapid growth of fibroid or postmenopausal women with fibroid growth (may indicate development of sarcoma)
- Viable pregnancy.

Relative

- Coagulopathy.
- Renal impairment.
- Immunocompromise.
- Previous pelvic irradiation or surgery.
- Extensive endometriosis or adenomyosis.
- Pedunculated subserosal uterine fibroid (attachment point less than 50% of diameter) as there is risk of uterine detachment.
- Contrast medium allergy.
- Arteriovenous malformation.
- Desire for future pregnancy.
- Undiagnosed pelvic mass.

Complications

1. *Postembolization syndrome*: Approximately 15 to 30% of patients may experience a variable "postembo-lization syndrome," with fever and malaise occurring during the first post-procedure week, but this syndrome resolves spontaneously and may be related to the release of tissue-breakdown products from degenerating uterine fibroids.[29]

2. *Severe postoperative pain:* After the procedure, almost all patients experience 6 to 12 hours of variably intense, cramping pelvic pain that may be treated with oral or intravenous analgesia. Epidural analgesia may be used in

patients who experience severe pain. The pain diminishes during the first week following UAE, and patients can be maintained on oral analgesics.

3. *Groin infection:* bleeding or hematoma.
4. *Contrast induced:* renal and vascular damage.
5. *Target organ defects:* Uterine infection, perforation, sexual dysfunction and myoma sloughing.
6. *Infection:* Occasionally, submucosal fibroids become necrotic and may be expelled from the uterus following UAE. 0.7% of patients had infection or severe ischemia requiring hysterectomy.[30,31] One death from sepsis has been reported in the literature out of approximately 6,500 procedures performed worldwide.[32] Less severe infections may occur more commonly and is managed without hysterectomy.
7. *Non-target organ embolization*: Ovarian sequelae, sciatic nerve effects and gluteal muscle pain.
8. *Radiation exposure*: An average of 14 rads exposure occurs but may be as high as 20 cGy with the use of continuous fluoroscopy.[23] This amount is equivalent to approxi-mately five computed tomographic (CT) scans of the pelvis. A few cases of temporary amenorrhea and post-procedure menopause have occurred and, although the incidence of these conditions is low, they must be considered a possible risk.[28] Using modern intermittent fluoroscopy, however, much lower doses would be expected, and much larger absorbed radiation doses have not caused an increase of genetic defects in offspring.
9. *Premature menopause*: Although only uterine artery blood supply is interrupted some cases of premature menopause have been reported.
10. Uterine cavity and myoma communication.[33]

Results
1. *Technical success:* Technical success rate is 96 to 98%.[30,34]
2. *Menorrhagia:* Improvement in menorrhagia, bulk related symptoms occurred in 80 to 90% patients.[30,34]

3. *Reduction in volume*: Average fibroid volume reduction is approximately 50% in three months and 65% at one year. Uterine volume decreases by approximately 40% in three months. The reduction in the fibroid's size leads to a decrease or resolution in the symptoms they cause.[30,34]

4. *Patient satisfaction*: It was reported that 86% patients indicated satisfaction with the results of the procedure. [31]

5. *Long-term results*: The long-term effectiveness of UAE is unknown at present. Recent study over a six year period showed no recurrences. However, longer follow-up is needed to draw definitive conclusions.

6. *Repeat surgery*: It has been shown that if the procedure is not successful and surgery is needed, this surgery is rendered easier, with a likelihood of less bleeding.

UAE vs Myomectomy

There is no evidence of benefit of UAE compared to surgery (hysterectomy/myomectomy) for satisfaction. There are more minor complications, unscheduled visits and readmission rates after discharge in the UAE group compared to hysterectomy. However, there are no differences between major complication rates and UAE is associated with shorter hospital stay. More randomised controlled trials are needed before any definite conclusion can be drawn. It is not preferred in infertile patient.[35]

UAE has several potential advantages over hyster-ectomy, myomectomy:

1. Unlike myomectomy or hysterectomy, UAE involves virtually no blood loss or risk of blood transfusion

2. General anesthesia and surgical incisions are avoided.

3. Recovery is weeks shorter than recovery from hysterectomy or open myomectomy (7 to 10 days versus six weeks),

4. All fibroids are treated at once, which is not the case with myomectomy.

5. UAE recurrence rates appear to be lower than those of myomectomy.

6. There are no differences between major complication[35]
7. Satisfaction rate is similar

Disadvantage over surgical treatment

1. More minor complications, unscheduled visits and readmission rates after discharge in the UAE group compared to myomectomy/hysterectomy.
2. Effect on fertility and subsequent pregnancy still uncertain.

Embolization of uterine fibroids may be an effective alternative to myomectomy or hysterectomy but randomized control trials are awaited.

Fertility and UAE

In a review on percutaneous UAE for the treatment of symptomatic fibroids, Lupattelli et al stated that although randomized trials are still underway, UAE appears a good option for those patients who wish to conserve their fertility or when surgery is contraindicated.[36,37] There is insufficient data at this time to ensure that UAE is safe for women who may wish to become pregnant in the future, the report notes. Moreover, few studies have assessed the effect of embolization on pregnancy-related outcomes. For these reasons, ACOG (American College of Obstetricians and Gynaecologist) considers the procedure investigational or relatively contraindicated in such women.[38,39]

There have been numerous reports of pregnancies following uterine fibroid embolization; however, prospective studies are needed to determine the effects of uterine fibroid embolization on the ability of a woman to have children. In a study of 26 completed pregnancies after UAE, 27% ended in miscarriage; there were two terminations and one ectopic pregnancy. Of 16 deliveries after 24 weeks, first and second trimester bleeding occurred in 40% and 33% respectively, 25% had preterm deliveries and the cesarean section rate was 88%. The rate of primary postpartum hemorrhage was 20%. There was 6.7% cases with fetal growth restriction.[40] Compared with the general obstetric population; there is a significant increase in delivery by cesarean section, preterm delivery, postpartum hemorrhage and miscarriage.

MRI-guided Ultrasound Ablation

This is the first non-invasive outpatient, procedure that uses high intensity focused ultrasound waves to ablate the fibroid tissue. The patient lies on her front and ultrasound waves are focused with the guidance of Magnetic Resonance Imaging into the center of a particular fibroid (Fig. 3.22). The treatment is limited only to those fibroids where the focused ultrasound energy does not traverse bowel or bladder on its way to reach the fibroid (Fig. 3.23). Otherwise, the bladder or bowel may sustain damage. The focused ultrasound energy is continued long enough to produce thermablation of the center of the sonicated fibroid. MRIs provide a three-dimensional view of the targeted tissue, allowing for precise focusing and delivery of the ultrasound energy. MRI also enables the physician to monitor tissue temperature in real-time to ensure adequate but safe heating of the target. Immediate imaging of the treated area following MRI guided ultrasound ablation helps the physician determine if the treatment was successful. This volume will become necrotic and eventually shrink.

Presently, the procedure is allowed to continue for two or three hours and is limited to fibroids smaller than 7 cm.

Frequently, it has to be discontinued because of the patient's inability to lie still on her back for such a long time. It may cause skin burns at the treatment site and possibly some damage to adjacent tissues such as nerves. Long-term results and complications are unknown.

Results

Currently, there is very little information regarding the effectiveness of MRI-guided ultrasound ablation for the treatment of uterine leiomyomata. Recent studies by Tempany and Stewart suggested that MRI-guided focused ultrasound surgery appeared to be safe and effective for the treatment of uterine leiomyomas.[41,42] The treatment leads to a modest reduction in the fibroid volume of about 13%. However, improvement in the quality of life, such as bleeding, pain, and

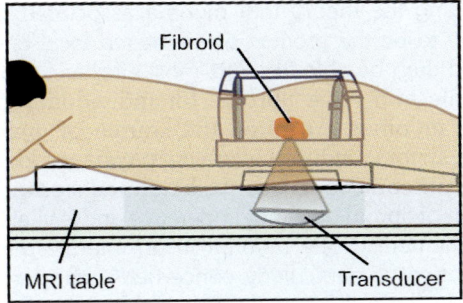

Fig. 3.22: Patient lying while ultrasound rays are focused with guidance of MRI

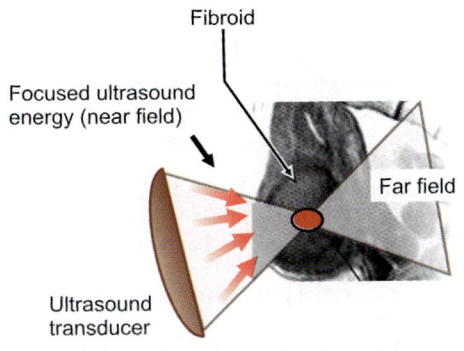

Fig. 3.23: Focused ultrasound energy on the tumor avoiding bowel and bladder

pressure is apparently more significant. In a multi-center 71% of women undergoing MRI guided ultrasound ablation. reached the targeted symptom reduction at 6 months and it was concluded that MRI guided ultrasound ablation treatment, results in short-term symptom reduction for women with symptomatic uterine leiomyomas, with an excellent safety profile.[43] Uneventful pregnancy was reported after focused ultrasound surgery for adenomyoma of 84 cm.[44]

Accepting the theory that myoma associated infertility is most likely to be the product of an altered local environment, one would then be able to select most effectively patients who are infertile and have fibroids for individualized therapy. Although myomas are often the source of gynecological complaint, myoma induced infertility, pregnancy loss and poor obstetric outcome are less well defined conditions. The localization of fibroid becomes imperative and is vital in deciding the management of the myoma in an infertile patients. The infertile patient is particularly concerned with uterine sparing options and their effect on fertility (Table 3.6). The infertility specialist must have complete knowledge of these options in order to counsel the patient in the most appropriate manner (Fig. 3.24).

REFERENCES

1. Vollenhoven B. Introduction: the epidemiology of uterine leiomyomas. Clin Obstet Gynaecol 1998;12:169-76.
2. Cramer SF, Patel A. The frequency of uterine leiomyomas. Am J Clin Pathol 1990;94:435-8.
3. Vercellini P, Cortesi I, Oldani S, et al. The role of transvaginal ultrasonography and outpatient diagnostic hysteroscopy in the evaluation of women with menorrhagia. Hum Reprod 1997;12: 1768-71.
4. Cramer DW. Epidemiology of myomas. Sem Reprod Endocrinol 1992;10:320-4.
5. Cooper JM, Houck RM, Rigberg HJ. The incidence of intrauterine abnormalities found at hysteroscopy in women undergoing elective hysteroscopic sterilization. J Reprod Med 1983;28:659-61.
6. Buttram VC, Reiter RC: Uterine leiomyomata: etiology symptomatology and management . Fertil Steril 1981; 36:433.
7. C Benecke, TF Kruger, TI Siebert, JP Van der Merwe, DW. Steyn Effect of Fibroids on Fertility in Patients Undergoing Assisted Reproduction A Structured Literature Review Gynecologic and Obstetric Investigation 2005;59:225-30.
8. Bronz L, Suter T, Rusca T. The value of transvaginal sonography with and without saline instillation in the diagnosis of uterine pathology in pre-and post-menopausal women with abnormal bleeding or suspect sonographic findings. Ultrasound Obstet Gynecol 1997;9:53-8.

Table 3.6: Uterine-sparing treatment of fibroids

Treatment	Advantages	Effect on fertility	Disadvantages
GnRH therapy	Shrinkage of uterine fibroids may allow removal with less blood loss, or removal by laparoscope or hysteroscope	Infertility therapy needs to be postponed till completion of course	Induces premature menopause-like symptoms; Loss of bone mineral density. Rapid regrowth of fibroids when therapy is discontinued
Abdominal myomectomy	Allows uterine conservation, usually in women who desire fertility	60% pregnancy rate	Postoperative recovery – 6 weeks; General anesthesia required; Transfusion rate of 3 to 20% Adhesions recurrence rate - 10 to 27%
Laparoscopic myomectomy	Much shorter recovery period than with abdominal myomectomy; best suited for pedunculated and subs-erosal fibroids or smaller intramural fibroids[7,8]	Weaker scar leads to higher incidence of scar rupture in subsequent pregnancy	Large, multiple or deep uterine fibroids are problematic adhesion formation General anesthesia required. Higher incidence of scar rupture in subsequent pregnancy
Laparoscopic myolysis	Treated uterine fibroids may shrink up to 40% by 6 months follow-up	Rupture reported due to weakening of wall	Dense and fibrous adhesions

Contd...

Contd...

Treatment	Advantages	Effect on fertility	Disadvantages
Hysteroscopic resection and/or endometrial ablation	Outpatient procedure for bleeding patients; short recovery period		Failure rate at 2 years post-ablation 32% Adenomyosis in 52%, Synechiae formation 13%
Uterine fibroid embolization	Symptoms improved in 80 to 90% Surgical incision and general anesthesia not required No blood loss All fibroids treated at once;[13] No recurrences noted Return to normal activities in 7 to 10 days	Effect on fertility uncertain Subsequent pregnancy shows higher rate of PPH and LSCS	Effect on fertility uncertain Delayed infection may occur Availability limited, Long-term follow-up data unavailable
MRI Guided Ultrasound ablation	Non-invasive technique	Effect on fertility uncertain	No RCT Injury to bowel and bladder Skin burns
Laparoscopic uterine artery ligation	Minimally invasive	Effects on fertility uncertain	Long-term trials required

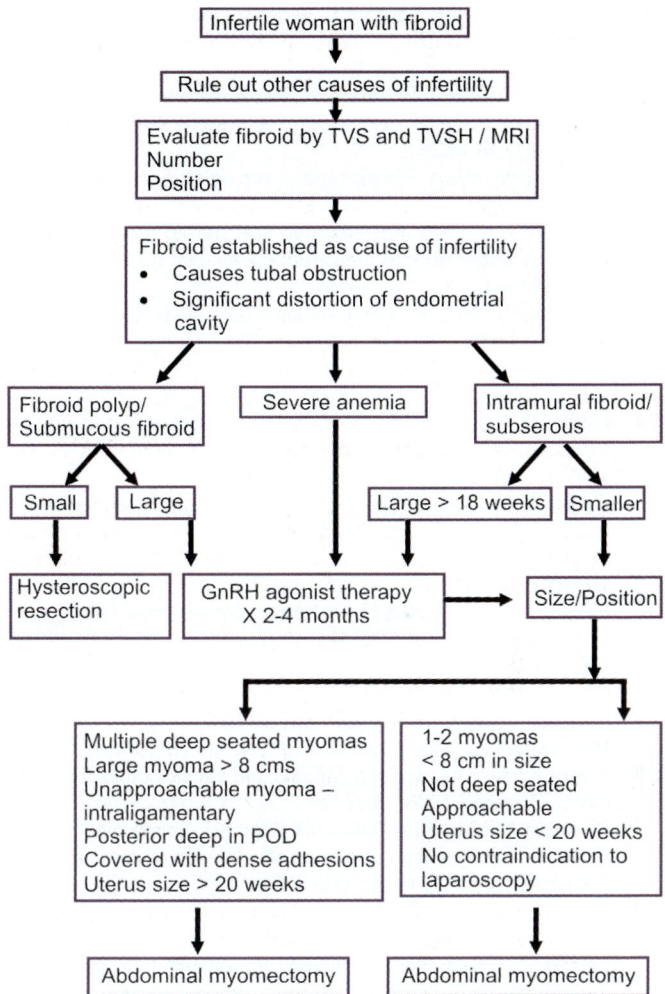

Fig. 3.24: Management of fibroid in the infertile patient

9. Casini ML, Rossi F, Agostini R, Unfer V. Effects of the position of fibroids on fertility. Gynecol Endocrinol. 2006;22(2): 106-9.

10. Kolankaya A, Arici A. Myomas and assisted reproductive technologies: when and how to act? Obstet Gynecol Clin North Am. 2006;33(1):145-52.

11. Rackow BW, Arici A. Fibroids and in-vitro fertilization: which comes first? Curr Opin Obstet Gynecol 2005;17(3):225-31.

12. Soules MR, McCarty KS. Leiomyomas: steroid receptor content. Variation within normal menstrual cycles. Am J Obstet Gynecol 1982;143:6-11.

13. Friedman AJ, Daly M, Juneau-Norcross MJ, Rein MS. Predictors of uterine volume reduction in women with myomas treated with a gonadotropin-releasing hormone agonist. Fertil Steril 1992;58:413-5.

14. Freidman AJ. Vaginal hemorrhage associated with degenerating submucus leiomyomata during leuprolide treatment. Fertil Steril 1989;52:152-4.

15. Gagliardi CL, Emmi AM, Weiss G, Schmidt CL. Gonadotropin releasing hormone agonist improves the efficiency of controlled ovarian stimulation / intrauterine insemination . Fertil Steril 1991;55:939- 44.

16. Murphy A Morale A, Kettel L et al Regression of uterine leiomyomata to the antiprogesterone RU 486: dose response effect. Fertil Steril 1995;64:187.

17. Coutinho EM, Goncalves MT. Long-term treatment of leiomyomas with gestrinone. Fertil Steril 1989;51:939-46.

18. Makarainen L, Ylikorkala O. Primary and myoma-associated menorrhagia: role of prostaglandins and effects of Ibuprofen. Br J Obstet Gynaecol 1986;93:974-8.

19. Kumakiri J, Takeuchi H, Kitade M, Kikuchi I, Shimanuki H, Itoh S, Kinoshita K. Pregnancy and delivery after laparoscopic myomectomy. J Minim Invasive Gynecol. 2005;12(3):241-6

20. Griffiths A, D'Angelo A, Amso N. Surgical treatment of fibroids for subfertility. Cochrane Database Syst Rev. 2006 Jul 19;3:CD003857.

21. Lethaby A, Vollenhoven B, Sowter M. Pre-operative GnRH analogue therapy before hysterectomy or myomectomy for uterine fibroids (Cochrane Review). The Cochrane Database of Systematic Reviews 2001, Issue 2. Art. No.: CD000547. DOI:10.1002/14651858.CD000547.

22. Rovio PH, Heinonen PK. Transvaginal myomectomy with screw traction by colpotomy. Arch Gynecol Obstet. 2006;273(4):211-5.

23. Hart R (2003). Unexplained infertility, endometriosis, and fibroids. BMJ, 327(7417): 721–4.

24. Practice Committee of the American Society for Reproductive Medicine. Myomas and reproductive function. Fertil Steril 2004; 82(Suppl 1): S111–S6.

25. Wallach E, Vlahos NF Uterine myomas: An overview of development, clinical features, and management. Obstet Gynecol 2004;104(2): 393-406.

26. Stewart EA. Uterine fibroids. Lancet 2001, 357(9252): 293–8.

27. McLucas B, Goodwin S, Adler L, Rappaport A, Reed R, Parrella R: Pregnancy following uterine fibroid embolization: Int J Gynecol Obstet 2001;74:1-7.

28. Worthington-Kirsch RL, Popky GL, Hutchins FL. Uterine arterial embolization for the management of leiomyomas: quality-of-life assessment and clinical response. Radiology 1998;208:625-9.

29. Goodwin SC, Vedantham S, McLucas B, Forno AE, Perrella R. Preliminary experience with uterine artery embolization for uterine fibroids. J Vasc Interv Radiol 1997;8:517-26.

30. Spies JB, Scialli AR, Jha RC, Imaoka I, Ascher SM, Fraga VM, et al. Initial results from uterine fibroid embolization for symptomatic leiomyomata. J Vasc Interv Radiol 1999;10:1149-57.

31. Hutchins FL, Worthington-Kirsch R, Berkowitz RP. Selective uterine artery embolization as primary treatment for symptomatic leiomyomata uteri. J Am Assoc Gynecol Laparosc 1999;6:279-84.

32. Vashisht A, Studd J, Carey A, Burn P. Fatal septicaemia after fibroid embolisation. Lancet 1999;354:307-8.

33. Ogliari KS, Mohallem SV, Barrozo P, Viscomi F A uterine cavity-myoma communication after uterine artery embolization: two case reports.Fertil Steril 2005; 83(1):220-2.

34. Hallez JP. Myomectomies by endo-uterine resection. Curr Opin Obstet Gynecol 1996;8:250-6.

35. Gupta JK, Sinha AS, Lumsden MA, Hickey M. Uterine artery embolization for symptomatic uterine fibroids (Cochrane Review). The Cochrane Database of Systematic Reviews 2006, Issue 1. Art. No.: CD005073. DOI:10.1002/14651858.CD005073.

36. Lupattelli T, Basile A, Garaci FG, Simonetti G. Percutaneous uterine artery embolization for the treatment of symptomatic fibroids: Current status. Eur J Radiol. 2005;54:136-47.

37. Goodwin SC, Bradley LD, Lipman JC, et al. Uterine artery embolization versus myomectomy: A multicenter comparative study. Fertil Steril. 2006;85:14-21.

38. American College of Obstetricians and Gynecologists (ACOG) ACOG issues opinion on uterine artery embolization for treatment of fibroids. Press Release. Washington, DC: ACOG; January 30, 2004.

39. National Institute for Clinical Excellence (NICE). Uterine artery embolisation for fibroids (second consultation). Interventional Procedure Consultation Document. London, UK: NICE; June 2004.

40. Carpenter TT, Walker WJ Pregnancy following uterine artery embolisation for symptomatic fibroids: a series of 26 completed pregnancies BJOG 2005;112: 321

41. Tempany CM, Stewart EA, McDannold N, et al. MR imaging-guided focused ultrasound surgery of uterine leiomyomas: A feasibility study. Radiology. 2003;226:897-905.

42. Stewart EA, Gedroyc WM, Tempany CM, et al. Focused ultrasound treatment of uterine fibroid tumors: Safety and feasibility of a noninvasive thermoablative technique. Am J Obstet Gynecol. 2003;189(1):48-54.

43. Stewart EA, Rabinovici J, Tempany CM, et al. Clinical outcomes of focused ultrasound surgery for the treatment of uterine fibroids. Fertil Steril. 2006;85(1):22-9.

44. Rabinovici J, Inbar Y, Eylon SC, Schiff E, Hanane A, Freundlich D. Pregnancy and live birth after focused ultrasound surgery for symptomatic focal adenomyosis: a case report. Hum Reprod. 2006;21(5):1255-9.

CHAPTER 4

Endoscopic Management of Fibroid

Neena Singh Kumar
Surveen Ghumman

Fibroids are common benign tumors seen in the reproductive age group. When a myoma is observed during laparoscopic surgery they should only be touched if there is a clear indication for therapy, like significant symptoms or if they are responsible for infertility, as there is always a risk of postoperative adhesion formation. Hence, the risks and benefits have to be evaluated before taking a decision (See Chapter 3). Fibroids can occur at various locations fundal, cervical, broad ligament or in the rudimentary horn (Figs 4.1A to D). They may be subserous, intramural or submucus.

A fibroid should only be treated surgically at the time of diagnostic laparoscopy if there is a favorable risk to benefit ratio in the therapy for the infertile patient.

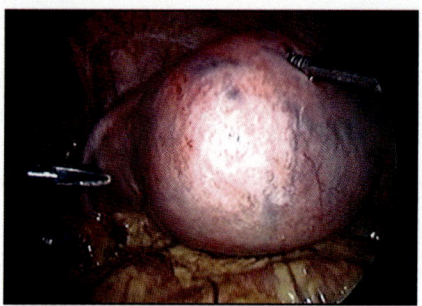

Fig. 4.1A: Posterior wall fibroid

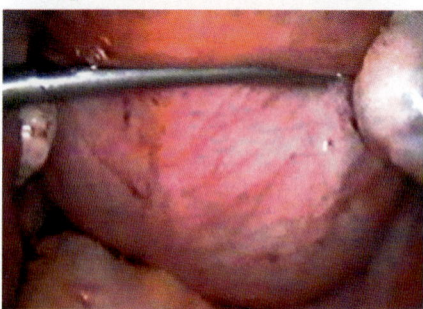

Fig. 4.1B: Cervical fibroid

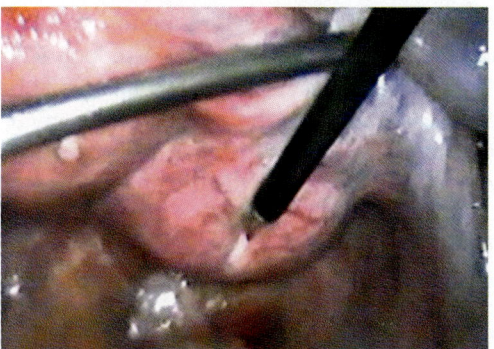

Fig. 4.1C: Broad ligament fibroid

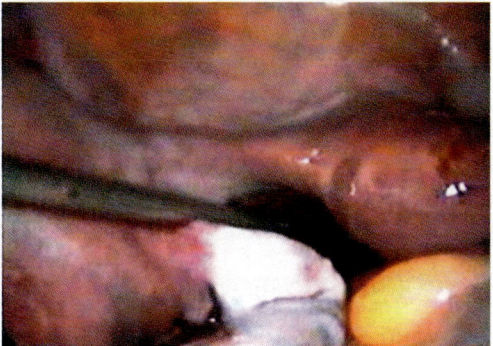

Fig. 4.1D: Fibroid in rudimentary horn of uterus

Principles of Endoscopic Removal of Fibroid

1. Determine the anatomical relation of the myoma with the round ligament and fallopian tubes.
2. Visualize the ureters especially in broad ligament fibroids.
3. Adhere to the principles of atraumatic infertility surgery.
4. Magnification, meticulous hemostasis, and closure of the myometrium is a must to prevent bleeding, adhesions, and postoperative complications.

5. Pedunculated myomas usually require coagulation and electrosection of the pedicle. Rarely are loop sutures used.
6. Sessile myomas require an incision which may be vertical/ horizontal depending on the position of myoma and choice of the surgeon.
7. Submucous myomas are dealt with hysteroscopically.

Preoperative Evaluation

   i. *Hemogram:* Preoperative hemoglobin of more than 10 gm is recommended.
  ii. *Ultrasonography*
      a. To know the size, number and site of myomas.
      b. To differentiate between myoma and adenomyosis
 iii. *Infertility work-up:* The patient should undergo all basic infertility investigations like semen analysis, ovulation studies and a hysterosalpingography to document tubal patency.
  iv. *Pap smear, endometrial biopsy and hysteroscopy:* If she has abnormal uterine bleeding other causes of bleeding need to be ruled out before doing a laparoscopic surgery.

LAPAROSCOPIC MYOMECTOMY

Anesthesia and Positioning of Patient

Laparoscopic myomectomy is performed under general anesthesia. The patient is placed in Trendlenburg's position taking care of pressure points. Diathermy pads are placed below the buttocks. The patient is catheterized as a routine before starting surgery.

Instruments

Instruments to be arranged on the trolley are as follows:
   1. Veress needle (Fig. 4.2)
   2. Trocar cannula 5 mm (Three) (Fig. 4.2)

3. Trocar cannula 10 mm (One) (Fig. 4.2)
4. Scissors (Fig. 4.3)
5. Atraumatic grasper (5 mm) (Fig. 4.3)
6. Traumatic grasper (5 mm) (Fig. 4.3)
7. Bipolar coagulating forceps (Fig. 4.4)
8. Monopolar hook (Fig. 4.4)
9. Needle holder (Two) (Fig. 4.5)
10. Suction irrigation cannula (Fig. 4.6)
11. Port closure needle (Fig. 4.7)
12. Electronic morcellator (Fig. 4.8)
13. CCL ball (Fig. 4.9)
14. Claw forceps (Fig. 4.9)
15. 5 mm myoma spiral (Two) (Fig. 4.9)
16. Injection needle
17. 30° 10 mm for oblique telescope.

Port Placement

One port is placed infraumbilically with a 10 mm 0° or 30° telescope with camera. Two 5 mm ports are placed at the junction of $1/3$ and $2/3$ distance of the spino-umbilical line (an imaginary line joining the umbilicus with the anterior superior iliac spine on either side). The umbilical port and the third ipsilateral port can be placed higher in case of a large fibroid so as to ensure enough space to allow proper traction, tissue dissection and suturing. With two ports on the side of the surgeon the left lower hand uses bipolar and the right hand uses monopolar scissors or spatula. The assistant holds the camera from the other side.

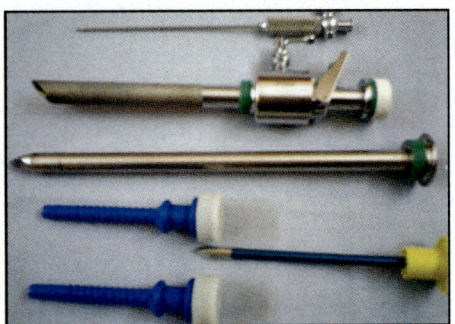

Fig. 4.2: Veress needle, trocar cannula
10 mm, trocar cannula 5 mm

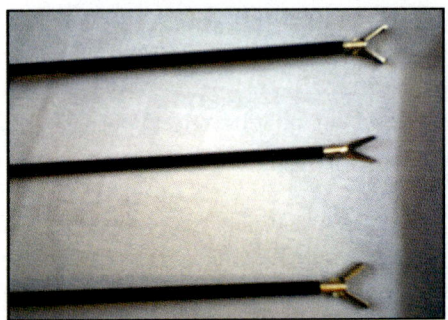

Fig. 4.3: Toothed forceps, scissor, non-toothed grasper

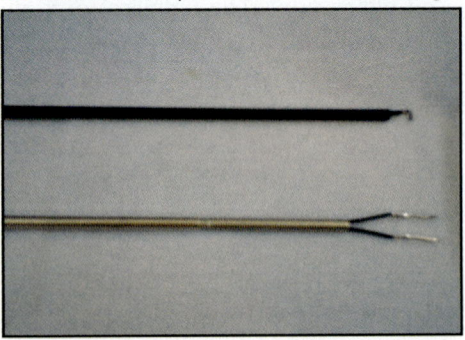

Fig. 4.4: Monopolar hook, bipolar forceps

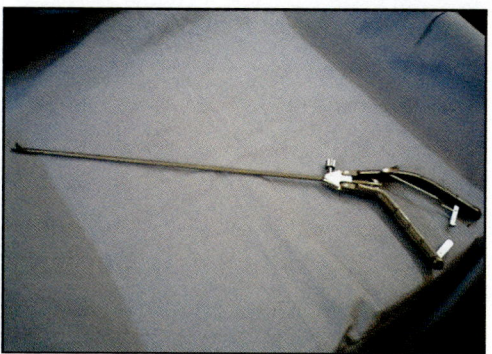

Fig. 4.5: Needle holder

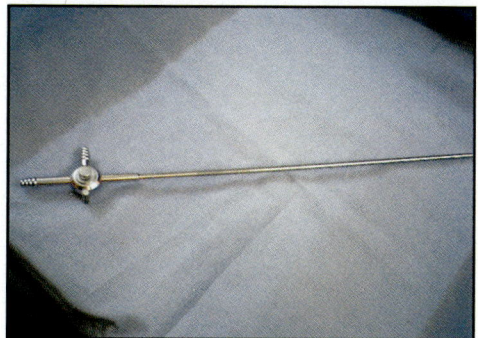

Fig. 4.6: Suction irrigation cannula

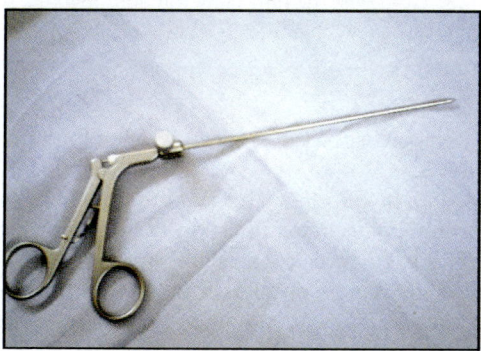

Fig. 4.7: Port closure needle

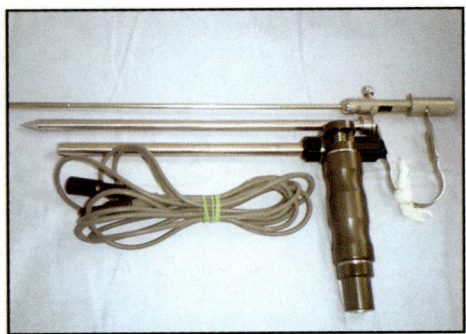

Fig. 4.8: Bipolar forceps, morcellator handle

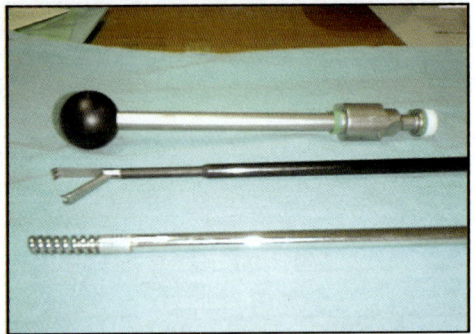

Fig. 4.9: CCL ball, 10 mm claw forceps, myoma screw

Surgical Procedure *(See accompanying DVD ROM)*

Intramural fibroid

The steps of laparoscopic myomectomy of an intramural fibroid are as follows:

- *Positioning of patient:* The patient is placed in supine position until after initial insertion of the Veress needle and the primary 10 mm trocar. The patient is then put in a steep Trendlenburg's position of 20°. A uterine manipulator is inserted to manipulate the uterus to give maximum access to the uterus. A 30° telescope is preferred as it permits better visualization of the site of the operation.

- *Evaluation of the myoma:* After inserting the laparoscope the myomas is evaluated and the course of the ureters is traced especially in broad ligament myomas.
- *Prophylaxis against bleeding:* Injection of a vasoconstrictor agent preferably vasopressin (5 units in 100 cc) at the base of the myoma controls bleeding richly during enucleation (Fig. 4.10A). Bipolar desiccation at the site of incision on the capsule also helps in controlling bleeding.
- *Incision on myoma:* The incision on the myoma is decided depending on the ease of the subsequent suturing and the possibility of postoperative adhesions. The incision should be large enough to deliver the myoma through it. Once the fibroid is seen an incision is made adequate to remove the fibroid with a monopolar spatula, using 100 watts of pure cutting current and 60 watts of coagulating current on monopolar hook (Fig. 4.10B). Incision is widened to view myoma (Fig. 4.11).
- *Enucleation of myoma:* A myoma screw is put in left upper port to fix the fibroid and gently pull it as scissors dissects the surrounding tissue of fibroid (Figs 4.12 and 4.13). Alternatively it can be stabilized with a claw forceps (Fig. 4.14). A firm traction is given on the myoma with the myoma screw or claw forceps and blunt dissection is done with the help of the suction cannula to enucleate the myoma (Fig. 4.15).
- *Control of bleeding:* The bleeding is effectively controlled with bipolar desiccation (Fig. 4.16).
- *Parking the fibroid:* After removal the myoma is parked in the appendicular area as there are least instruments in that area or in pouch of Douglas. In multiple myomas it is important to keep a count of the myomas lest they get lost in the abdominal cavity.
- *Removal of redundant part of capsule:* The excessive capsular tissue needs to be refashioned.

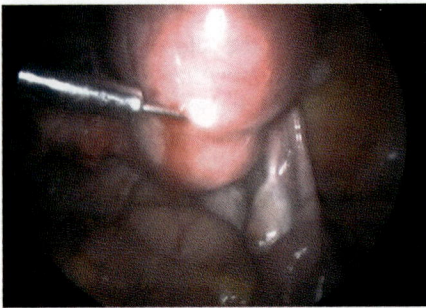

Fig. 4.10A: Injection needle injecting 10 percent vasopressin

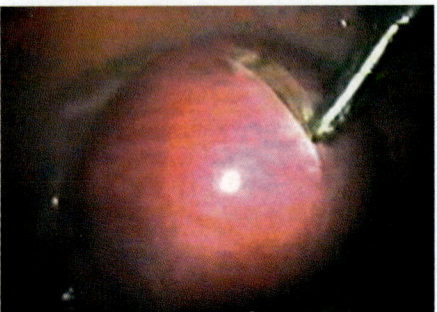

Fig. 4.10B: Vertical incision on capsule of fundal fibroid using monopolar hook

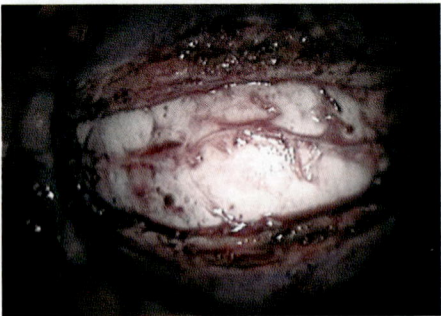

Fig. 4.11: Myoma showing through incision

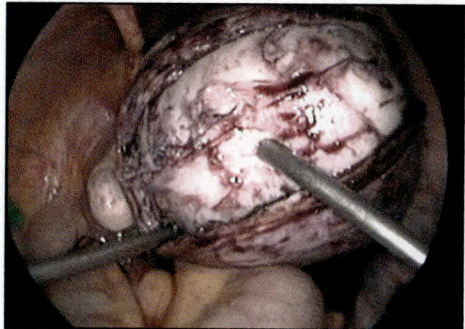

Fig. 4.12: Traction with myoma screw

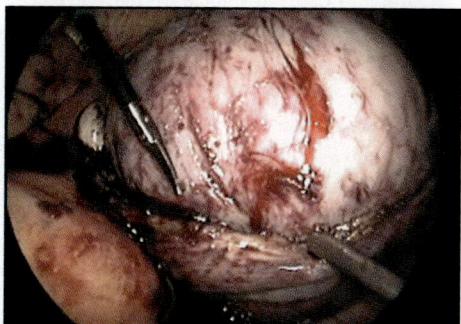

Fig. 4.13: Gradual enucleation of myoma

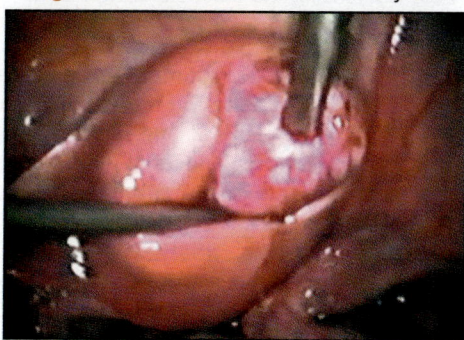

Fig. 4.14: Stabilizing the myoma using claw forceps

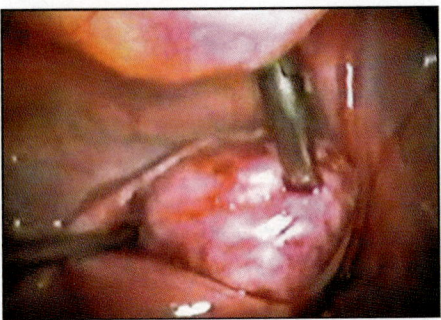

Fig. 4.15: Traction with claw forceps and counter traction used to enucleate the fibroid

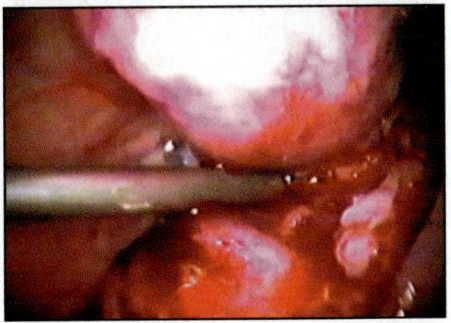

Fig. 4.16: Cauterizing the bleeders using bipolar forceps

- *Suturing of uterine wall:* The uterine wall is sutured so as it reduces the likelihood of rupture of the myometrium and also reduces chances of adhesion formation. Figure of eight sutures with no. 1-0 vicryl in 1-2 layers are taken to obliterate the dead space and reduce chances of intramural hematoma (Fig. 4.17). At the end of the surgery before removing laparoscope the suture line is visualized to ensure hemostasis (Fig. 4.18).[2]

In pedunculated myomas we essentially desiccate and divide the pedicle with bipolar forceps and scissors. After enucleating the myoma the bed is left alone if small or closed with sutures.

• *Removal of myoma:* Earlier, it was achieved by mini-laparotomy or a posterior colpotomy and later by using mechanical morcellator, which made retrieval a cumbersome and lengthy procedure. The advent of electronic morcellator has simplified the removal of myomas and cut short the time taken to complete myomectomy without any additional incisions. One of the accessory ports is simply converted into a 10-15 mm port for morcellation.

  i. *Minilaparotomy:* This method is no longer used. Before the morcellator came into use the myoma used to be removed from a small laparotomy incision

  ii. *Posterior colpotomy using a CCL ball:* Fibroid may be removed through pouch of Douglas using a CCL ball. The ball is inserted in the posterior fornix to delineate the pouch of Douglas (Fig. 4.19). Pouch of Douglas is opened by monopolar needle (Fig. 4.20). The ball becomes visible once pouch is opened (Fig. 4.21). Claw forceps is introduced through the opening (Fig. 4.22). The fibroid is grasped with the claw forceps and the claw forceps is pulled back (Fig. 4.23). The fibroid is removed through the pouch of Douglas (Figs 4.24 and 4.25).

  iii. *Mechanical morcellator (old method):* Using a mechanical morcellator for myoma retrieval is a cumbersome and lengthy procedure (Figs 4.26 and 4.27).

  iv. *Electronic morcellator:* The advent of electronic morcellator has simplified the removal of myomas, making it possible to tackle big myomas and cut short the time taken to complete myomectomy without any additional incisions. Cylindrical serrated morcellator are used to convert big myomas to small strips of tissue which can then be removed (Fig. 4.28). Usually a 10 or 15 mm morcellator and a claw forceps 10 or 15 mm size is used to take out the myoma in long strips. The incision of the left lower port is widened to 15 mm and morcellator is introduced. After ensuring a good grip on the fibroid by the claw forceps the morcellator is started by a foot switch (Fig. 4.29). Morcellation is done in a horizontal manner with the left hand holding the claw to pull the fibroid and the right hand stabilizing the morcellator (Fig. 4.30). Before switching on the morcellator the entry of the sharp rotating blade is ensured. Large myomas are removed in this manner by morcellating into smaller strips of tissue (Fig. 4.31). Uterine myomas can be removed successfully through both culdotomy or electronic morcellator however, because of reduced removal time, the power morcellator is preferred.[3]

Microwave coagulator and electromechanical tissue borer minimizes invasion of the myometrium and abdominal wall. Here we morcellate before removal from the uterus sustaining less myometrial trauma. Horizontal and perpendicular blades hollow out the myoma allowing larger myoma to be removed through smaller incisions.

Irrigation of peritoneal cavity: After the procedure the anatomy of the fallopian tube and uterus is checked and their normalcy ensured. The pelvis is irrigated with fluid. About 300-400 cc of saline is left in the abdomen at the end of the procedure so that scar site remains immersed in the saline at least for a few hours following surgery. This is because the chances of adhesion formation are maximum in first few hours following surgery.

- *Closure of 15 mm accessory port:* The 15 mm accessory port is closed using a port closure needle.

Subserous fibroid

Small subserous fibroids can be ablated. Larger ones are removed laparoscopically. The base of the subserous fibroid is cauterized (Fig. 4.32). The fibroid is removed (Fig. 4.33). Hemostasis is ensured by bipolar cautery (Fig. 4.34).

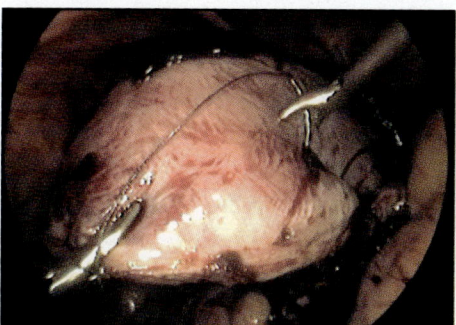

Fig. 4.17: Suturing in progress

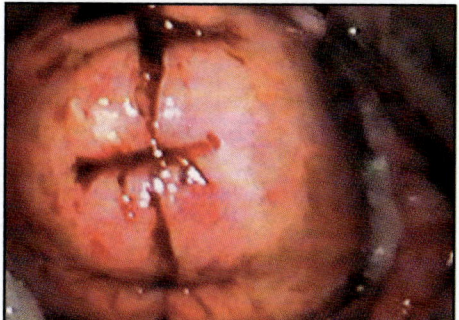

Fig. 4.18: Uterus sutured and complete hemostasis secured

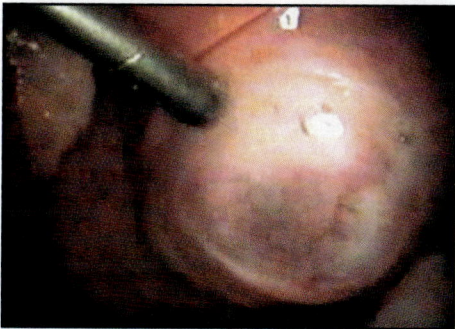

Fig. 4.19: CCL ball inserted in posterior fornix to delineate pouch of Douglas

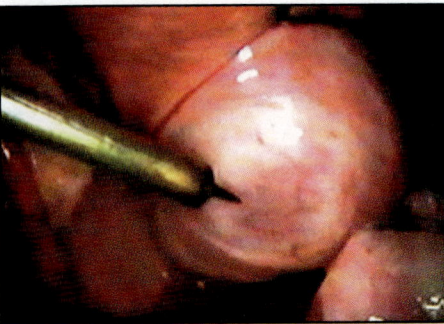

Fig. 4.20: Monopolar needle being used to open pouch of Douglas

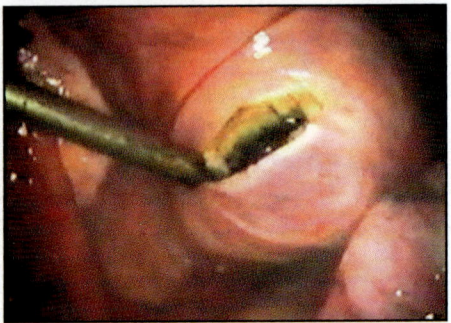

Fig. 4.21: CCL ball becoming visible (black) after giving incision

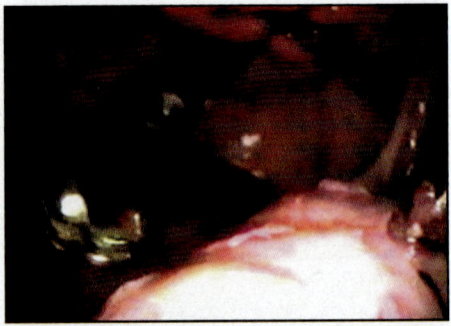

Fig. 4.22: Claw forceps inserted through CCL ball

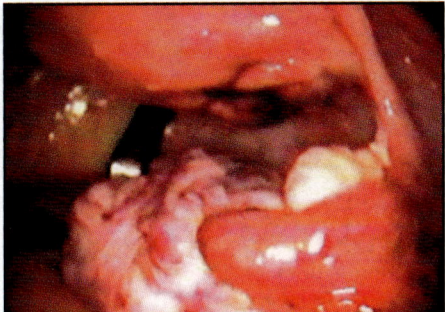

Fig. 4.23: Fibroid held with claw forceps and pulled back towards posterior fornix

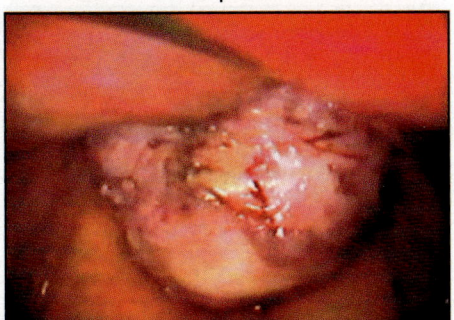

Fig. 4.24: Removing fibroid through pouch of Douglas

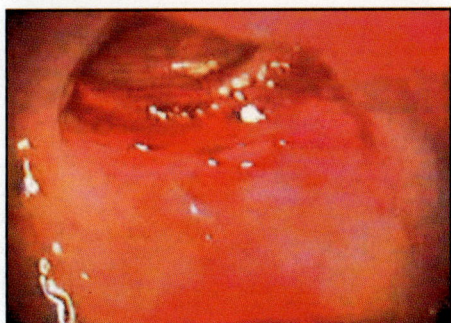

Fig. 4.25: View of pouch of Douglas after removing CCL ball

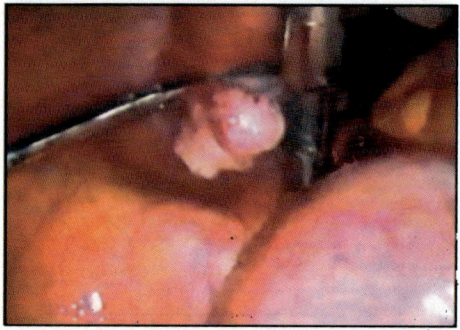

Fig. 4.26: Mechanical morcellation in progress

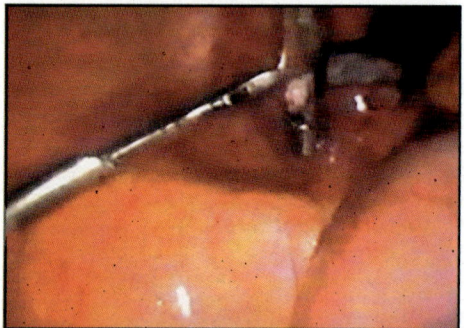

Fig. 4.27: Removal of fibroid with mechanical morcellator

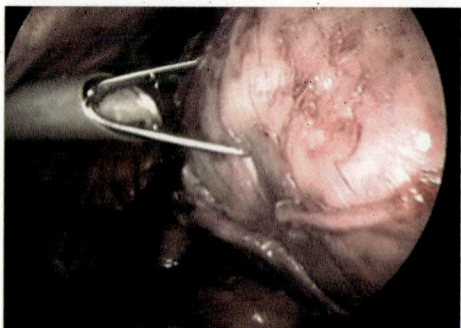

Fig. 4.28: Removal of fibroid with electronic morcellator

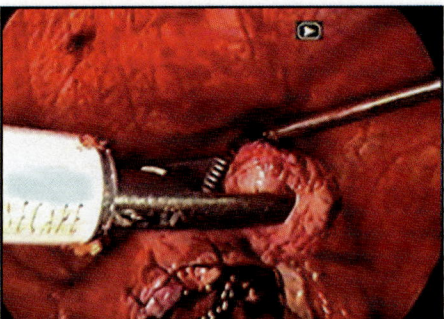

Fig. 4.29: Claw forceps holding the fibroid before morcellation with electronic morcellator

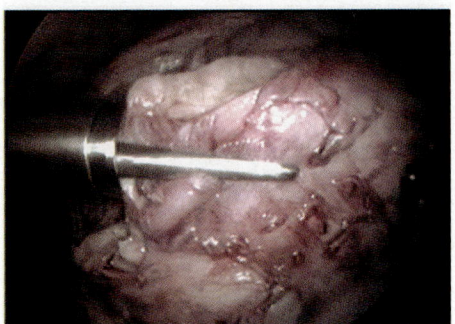

Fig. 4.30: Electronic morcellation in progress removing fibroid piecemeal

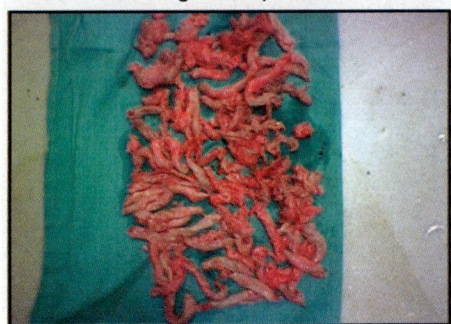

Fig. 4.31: Morcellated myoma pieces

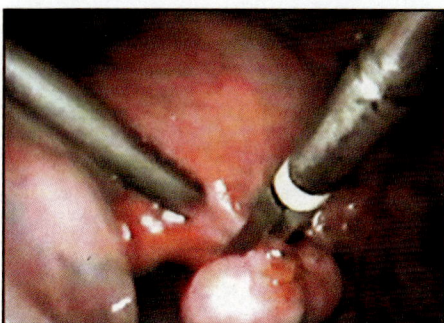

Fig. 4.32: Subserous fibroid cauterized at its base with bipolar cautery

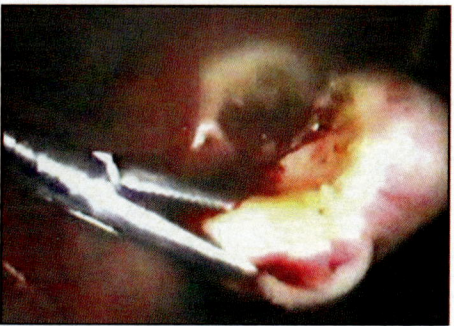

Fig. 4.33: Subserous fibroid removed

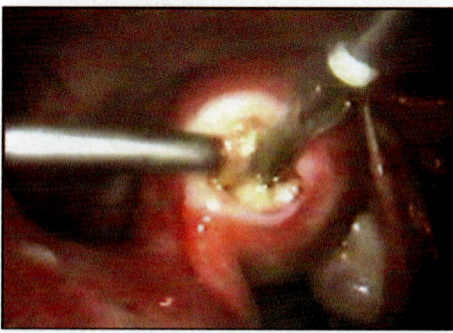

Fig. 4.34: Bipolar forceps used to secure hemostasis

Broad ligament fibroid

In broad ligament fibroid a posterior incision is preferred (Fig. 4.35). Proper visualization of ureters may be necessary as they are lateral and their course may be altered. The fibroid is stabilized with myoma spiral (Fig. 4.36). It is enucleated (Figs 4.37 and 4.38). Many broad ligament fibroids may not require suturing of the bed as they do not involve bulk of the myometrium. Drainage is always posterior.

Multiple fibroids

When there are multiple fibroids it is important to remove fibroids from the most prominent area (Fig. 4.39). The fibroids sitting on each other may then be removed from the same incision.

Postoperative Care

Postoperative analgesia is given along with parenteral antibiotics. Patients are usually discharged within 48 hours.

Risk of Laparoscopic Myomectomy

Besides the risk common to endoscopic surgery there are risks specific to laparoscopic myomectomy:

1. *Operating time:* Time taken for surgery is longer than an abdominal procedure. Hence, there is risk of prolonged anesthesia.
2. *Integrity of the scar in subsequent pregnancy:* The incidence of scar rupture depends on how optimally suturing has been done. Suturing the bed in large fibroids may be difficult (because of a two dimensional movement) leading to weakening of the uterine wall for subsequent pregnancy. Large fibroids or those located posteriorly or on the fundus, are important as this area is stretched maximally during pregnancy.

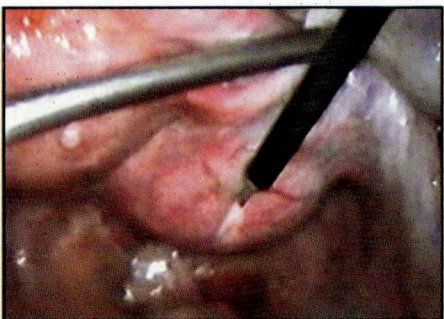

Fig. 4.35: Incision over the broad ligament fibroid

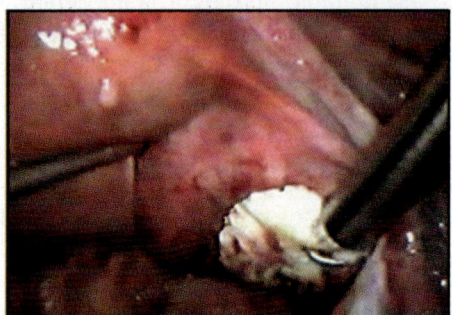

Fig. 4.36: Stabilizing the fibroid with myoma spiral

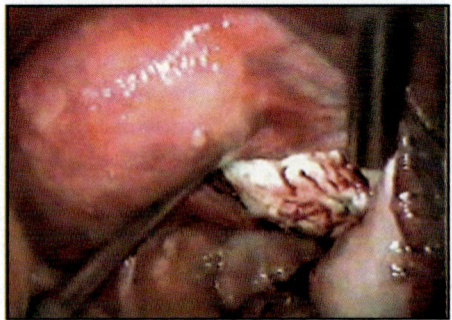

Fig. 4.37: Enucleating the fibroid

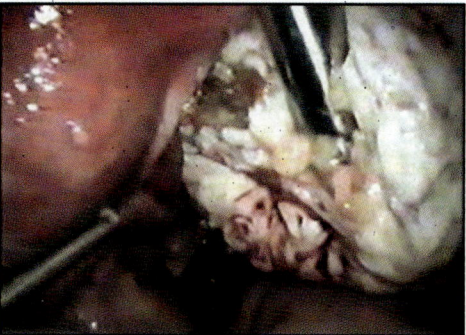

Fig. 4.38: Complete enucleation of broad ligament fibroid

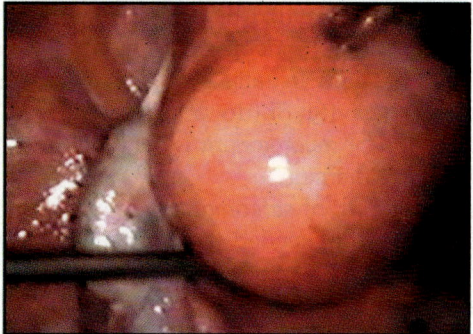

Fig. 4.39: Multiple fibroids

3. *Hemorrhage:* It is seen more with prior treatment with GnRH agonists. The advantage of reduced vascularity is lost by merging of tissue planes making the actual dissection more difficult.

4. *Postoperative residual fibroid:* may go unnoticed during laparoscopic myomectomy which could otherwise be detected by palpation during abdominal hysterectomy. However, the size of these fibroids is too small to have an impact on fertility although they may later grow to cause problems.

5. *Conversion to laparotomy:* Higher conversion rates are seen in bigger fibroids (> 8 cm).[6] Location of fibroids may be such that they are difficult to remove.

6. *Postoperative adhesions:* Postoperative scarring and adhesions which may decrease chances of patients' conception and increase chance of ectopic pregnancy, pain and intestinal obstruction. The incidence of adhesion formation was less with laparoscopic surgery as compared to laparotomy (41% vs. 90%). Prior existence of pelvic adhesions increases chances of postoperative adhesions. They can be prevented by barriers (See Chapter 15).

7. *Accidental adenomyoma/adenomyosis:* It is difficult to deal with and can be avoided by proper imaging technique.

8. *Accidental opening of endometrial cavity during laparoscopic myomectomy:* It is usually unnecessary to suture the endometrial cavity or do a multilayer suturing as approximation of myometrium is sufficient and healing is by secondary intention.

9. *Accidental finding of sarcomatous or malignant change:* A frozen section is needed if malignancy is suspected.

Laparoscopic myomectomy if judiciously employed in properly selected cases definitely offers significant advantages over abdominal myomectomy provided laparoscopic surgeon is skilled.

Laparoscopic Assisted Myomectomy (LAM)

This technique is applied for larger myomas.[4] Myoma enucleation is done laparoscopically (Fig. 4.40). Incision is slightly extended as in mini-laparotomy to remove myoma piecemeal (Figs 4.41 and 4.42). Suturing of the myoma bed is done as in laparotomy thus ensuring hemostasis and subsequent integrity of scar (Fig. 4.43). Laparoscopic portion of procedure allows the diagnosis and treatment of the associated endometriosis or adhesions.

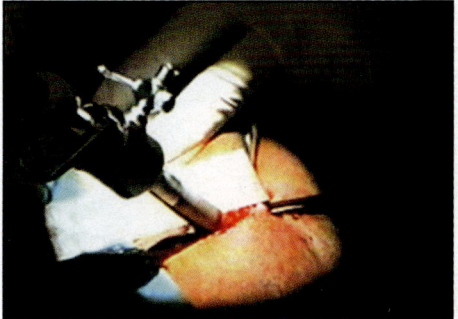

Fig. 4.40: Laparoscopic enucleation of myoma

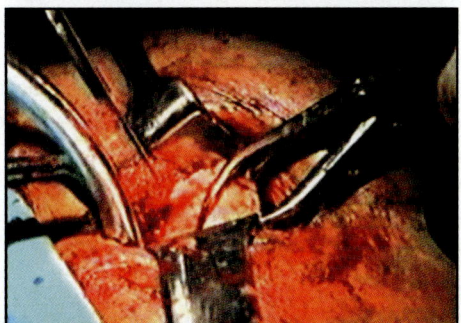

Fig. 4.41: Myoma being removed piecemeal through mini-laparotomy

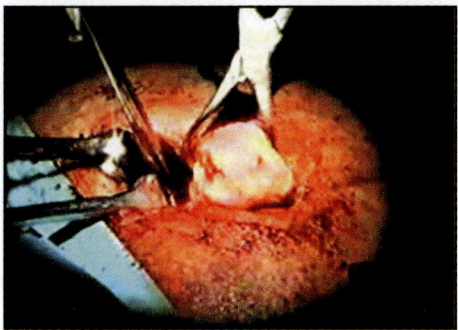

Fig. 4.42: Myoma removal in progress (LAM)

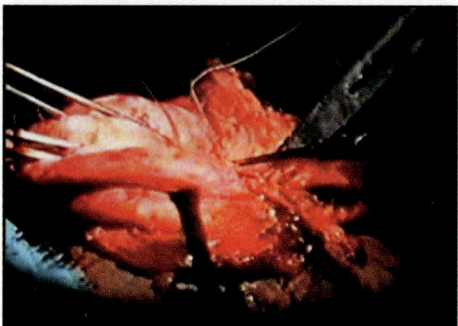

Fig. 4.43: Suturing of myoma bed

Myolysis

Laparoscopic myoma coagulation is termed as myolysis. Various modes are used by different researchers to destroy the stroma and vascular supply of the leiomyoma.

1. Nd YAG laser
2. Monopolar needle
3. Bipolar coagulation needle
4. Cryomyoprobe.

Either Nd YAG laser or bipolar needles are used laparoscopically to penetrate the myomata at multiple sites at 90° angle to the uterus. The myomata ultimately atrophy. The ideal candidates for myolysis are perimenopausal women with myoma of 3 to 10 cm or uterine size of less than 14 weeks. There is a 30 to 50% decrease in myoma size beyond the reduction achieved with GnRH agonists. No regrowth was seen even after several years. There was significant adhesion formation at follow-up laparoscopy due to serosal injury from multiple puncture technique.[7]

Myolysis should not be performed in those cases where patients remain symptomatic or there is less than 25% shrinkage of total uterine volume following GnRH therapy.

Bipolar coagulation myolysis may be less likely to cause damage to the serosa and subsequent adhesion formation. A circumferential technique to destroy vasculature instead of myomatous tissue has been tried with success.

Cryomyolysis has also been described where after verifying placement freezing was performed at an internal probe temperature of -180°C until an iceball encompasses the entire fibroid or reaches the maximum size. A thaw cycle is performed followed by a freeze thaw cycle. In second look laparoscopy adhesion formation was present at freezing site. The role of the therapy in conservative management of uterine myoma in infertile women needs to be defined.[8]

Hysteroscopic Approach

Hysteroscopic treatment of submucous myomas is an attractive option because of avoidance of laparotomy, uterine incision and lengthy hospitalization. Patient can be allowed vaginal delivery.

Prerequisites

1. Uterine cavity should be less than 10 cm in length.
2. Tumor mass should not be more than 3 cm in diameter.
3. At least half of the tumor mass should be protruding into the endometrial cavity.

However experienced hysteroscopic surgeons may approach even larger tumors. Accurate preoperative evaluation of the size and location of submucosal myomas before hysteroscopic myomectomy is important for a safe surgical procedure[9] (See Hysteroscopic Classification in Chapter 3).

Sessile myomas with walls that parallel or convergent respond to removal by hysteroscopy as they are more than 50% intracavitary.

Advantage of GnRH therapy:

1. Shrinking the size of the uterine myoma so that it may be removed hysteroscopically.
2. Thinning the endometrium to make surgery easier.

Procedure (See accompanying DVD ROM)

Submucous myoma

The myoma appears yellowish white tissue in contrast to the pink tan coarse fascicular configuration of the uterine wall (Fig. 4.44). Tubal ostia must be identified at the start of the surgery. Resection may be performed using hysteroscopic scissors, electrocautery or laser (Nd: YAG, KTP or argon). A variety of resectoscopes may be used with cutting current (Fig. 4.45). The myoma is sliced with the loop until the base is reached (Figs 4.46 to 4.49). The resection is begun using 50 W of cutting current. Base is inspected for bleeders. Once the myoma is removed the myometrium contracts to prevent bleeding. For the pedunculated myomas scissor is adequate for surgical management but a resectoscope is needed for myoma which is partially embedded in the uterine wall or larger than 4 cm in diameter. When submucous myomata extent deep into the myometrium only partial resection may be possible removing irregularities and restoring contour of uterine cavity to normal. Hysteroscopic resection of submucous myomata with more than 50% intramural extension should be performed only in selected cases by an experienced surgeon.[10]

Pedunculated Fibroid Polyp

Pedunculated tumors may be grasped and may be avulsed or twisted off (Fig. 4.50). Resectoscope can also be used (Fig. 4.51). Pieces of fibroid are cleared from the endometrial cavity (Fig. 4.52).

> Myomas presenting on opposing uterine wall in an infertile patient may be removed at one month interval of each other to reduce risk of adhesion formation.

Following myomectomy pieces of resected myoma may transiently block the cornual end giving an erroneous impression of tubal blockage.

Postoperative Management

1. If there is postoperative bleeding balloon tamponade may be used. The Foley's is removed after 6 to 12 hours.
2. Exogenous estrogens are given postoperatively to stimulate endometrium and prevent adhesions especially if preoperative GnRH therapy is used. A high dose is needed to obtain rapid endometrial thickening. Therapy may be started at the time of surgery using premarin 1.25 mg twice daily for 6 weeks. Provera 10 mg should be added during the last two weeks. The estrogen re-epithelializes the resected surfaces.
3. Prior to planning pregnancy the cavity is inspected again to rule out adhesion formation and assess its contour which is usually performed two months after initial procedure.

Complications

1. Hemorrhage
2. Uterine perforation
3. Damage to other intra-abdominal structures.
4. Fluid overload from distention medium.

Result: The success of hysteroscopic myomectomy and transabdominal myomectomy is equivalent. Hysteroscopic surgery has better outcome if the uterus is only slightly enlarged

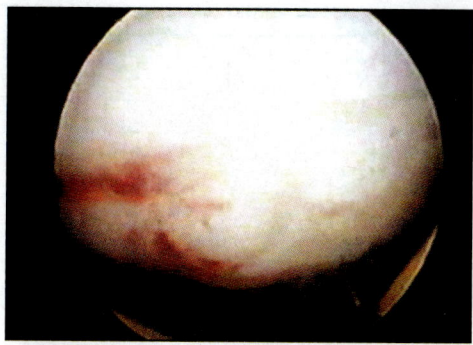

Fig. 4.44: Sessile submucous fibroid visualized by hysteroscope

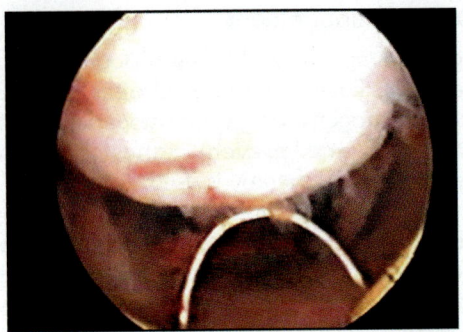

Fig. 4.45: Resectoscope using forward angle loop ready to start resection

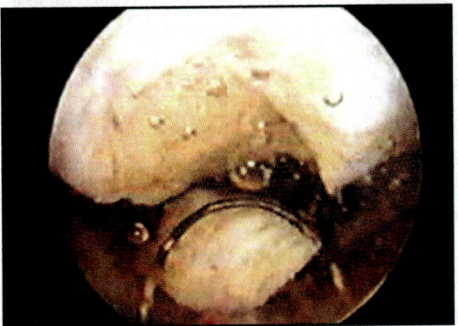

Fig. 4.46: Submucous fibroid being removed piecemeal

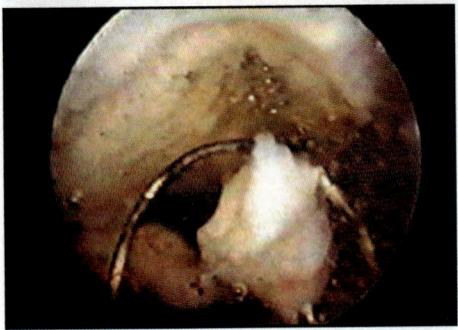

Fig. 4.47: Pieces of fibroid being removed

CHAPTER 5

Uterine Anomalies

Surveen Ghumman

Congenital anomalies of the uterus, although relatively uncommon can have a profound effect on obstetric performance. Pregnancy loss may be the most common presenting symptom. The role of Mullerian anomalies in infertility is still unclear. These anomalies represent a heterogeneous group of congenital malformations that result from arrested development, abnormal formation or incomplete fusion of the Mullerian duct.

DEVELOPMENT

Development occurs in three stages

Stage 1: The uterus starts to form at ten weeks from the Mullerian ducts, the upper end of which becomes the fallopian tubes and the lower ends lie side by side. They will form the uterus by fusing together.

Stage 2: Between 10 to 13 weeks there is widening of the top of this uterine tube to form the fundus. The lower aspect of the central wall dissolves leading to a common uterine cavity at the lower end of the uterus.

Stage 3: Between 13 and 20 weeks dissolution of the whole median septum occurs giving rise to a single, uterine cavity.

Renal anomalies: Renal anomalies associated with uterovaginal anomalies include renal agenesis, ectopic kidney, cystic dysplasia, and a duplicated collecting system. The associated renal anomaly is ipsilateral to the abnormally developed müllerian duct.

INCIDENCE

Exact incidence is difficult to estimate as patients may often remain asymptomatic. In a review of series of HSG the incidence has been calculated as 1 to 3.5%, the most common being variations in double uterus (septate, bicornuate and didelphic).[1]

In the general population, the prevalence of uterine anomalies is 0.5% and of vaginal anomalies is 0.025%. According to Nahum et al, the distribution of uterine anomalies is 4% hypoplastic uterus; 34% septate; 39% bicornuate; 7% arcuate; 11% didelphic; and 5% unicornuate.[2]

SYMPTOMS

Gynecologic
1. Amenorrhea
2. Chronic pelvic pain
4. Dyspareunia.
5. Mass abdomen
6. Infertility – if obstructive transverse vaginal septum

Obstetric
1. Midtrimester abortion
2. Premature delivery
3. Abnormal fetal presentation
4. Retained placenta
5. Postpartum hemorrhage
6. Subinvolution
7. Ectopic pregnancy in rudimentary horn.

ETIOLOGY

A multifactorial or polygenic etiology like ionizing radiations, intrauterine infections, drugs like DES and thalidomide may be responsible. Familial transition of uterine anomalies is known. Fusion defect have been associated with trisomy 13 and 15.

CLASSIFICATION

Uterovaginal anomalies are categorized as disorders of vertical or lateral fusion defects. They are further subcategorized into obstructive or nonobstructive forms, with obstructive uterovaginal anomalies requiring immediate attention because of collection of menstrual blood.

American Fertility Society Classification of Müllerian Anomalies

Class I: Segmental, Mullerian agenesis – hypoplasia (Fig. 5.1)

A. Vaginal
B. Cervical
C. Fundal
D. Tubal
E. Combined

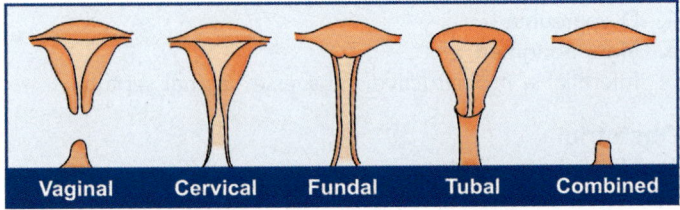

Fig. 5.1: Class I Anomalies of the müllerian duct

Class II: Unicornuate (Fig. 5.2)

A. Communicating
B. Non-communicating
C. No cavity
D. No horn

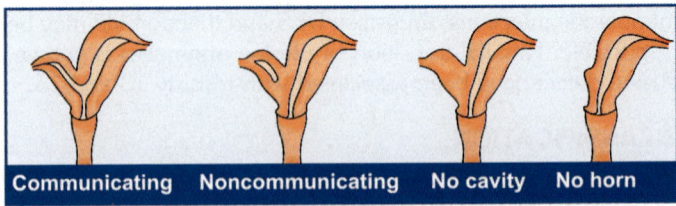

Fig. 5.2: Class II Anomalies of the müllerian duct

Class III Didelphus (Fig. 5.3).

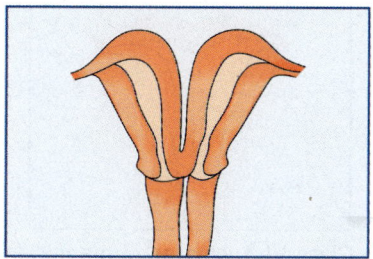

Fig. 5.3: Class III Anomalies of the müllerian duct

Class IV Bicornuate (Fig. 5.4).
    A. Complete (division down to internal OS)
    B. Partial

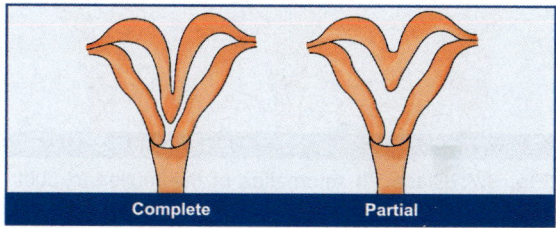

Fig. 5.4: Class IV Anomalies of the müllerian duct

Class V Septate (Fig. 5.5).
    A. Complete (septum to internal OS)
    B. Partial

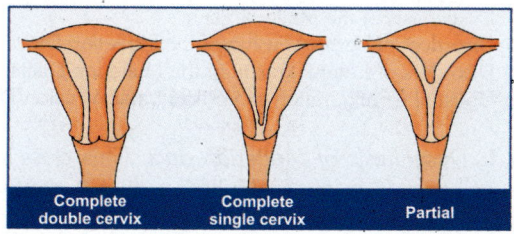

Fig. 5.5: Class V Anomalies of the müllerian duct

Class VI Arcuate (Fig. 5.6).

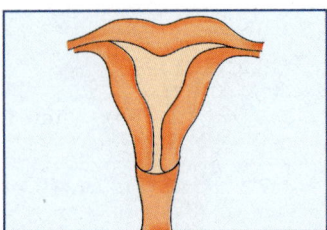

Fig. 5.6: Class VI Anomalies of the müllerian duct

Class VII: Diethylstilbesterol related (Fig. 5.7).

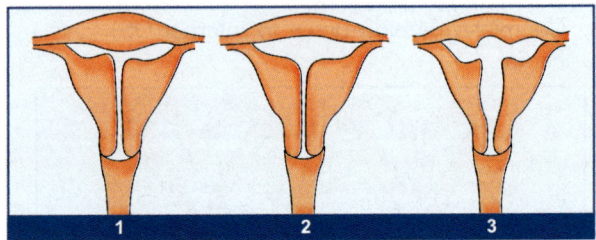

Fig. 5.7: Class VII Anomalies of the müllerian duct

However, this classification was modified to include vaginal anomalies also. (Table 5.1).

Table 5.1: TeLinde's Modification of the American Fertility Society Classification of Uterovaginal Anomalies[3]
Class I   Dysgenesis of the Mullerian Ducts
Class II   Disorders of Vertical Fusion of the Mullerian Ducts
Class III Disorders of Lateral Fusion of the Mullerian Ducts
Class IV   Unusual Configuration of Vertical-Lateral Fusion Defects

CLASS I: *Dysgenesis of Mullerian duct:* This class includes agenesis or hypoplasia of the Mullerian duct derivatives: the uterus and upper two-thirds of the vagina. The most common form is agenesis of the uterus, cervix, and upper portion of the vagina known as Mayer-Rokitansky-Küster-Hauser syndrome.

CLASS II: *Disorders of vertical fusion of the Mullerian duct:* These anomalies are due to failure of fusion of the Mullerian system with the sinovaginal bulb. They include cervical dysgenesis and obstructive and nonobstructive transverse vaginal septa.
A. Transverse vaginal septum
   1. Obstructed
   2. Unobstructed
B. Cervical agenesis or dysgenesis.

CLASS III: *Disorders of lateral fusion of the müllerian ducts:* They result in a duplicated or partially duplicated reproductive tract. Disorders are either due to failure of fusion of the paired müllerian ducts (as in didelphic and bicornuate uteri) and/or failure of midline septum resorption after fusion (as in septate uterus). Disorders due to lateral fusion defects are further sub-classified into:
a. The asymmetric obstructive form
b. The symmetric nonobstructive form
a. Asymmetric obstructed disorder of the uterus or vagina usually associated with ipsilateral renal agenesis
   1. Unicornuate uterus with a non communicating rudimentary horn.
   2. Unilateral obstruction of cavity of a double uterus
   3. Unilateral vaginal obstruction associated with double uterus.
b. Symmetric unobstructed
   1. Didelphus uterus
      a. Complete longitudinal vaginal septum
      b. Partial longitudinal vaginal septum
      c. No longitudinal vaginal septum
   2. Septate uterus
      a. Complete
         1. Complete longitudinal vaginal septum

   2. Partial longitudinal vaginal septum
   3. No longitudinal vaginal septum
  b. Partial
   1. Complete longitudinal vaginal septum
   2. Partial longitudinal vaginal septum
   3. No longitudinal vaginal septum
3. Bicornuate uterus
  a. Complete
   1. Complete longitudinal vaginal septum
   2. Partial longitudinal vaginal septum
   3. No longitudinal vaginal septum
  b. Partial
   1. Complete longitudinal vaginal septum
   2. Partial longitudinal vaginal septum
   3. No longitudinal vaginal septum
4. T - shaped uterine cavity (diethylstilbesterol related)
5. Unicornuate uterus
  i) With a rudimentary horn
   1. With endometrial cavity
    a) Communicating
    b) Noncommunicating
   2. Without endometrial cavity
  ii) Without a rudimentary horn

CLASS IV: Unusual configuration of vertical lateral fusion defects.

Since genital tract aberrations do not necessarily follow any defined and consistent pattern, Class IV is a useful addition embracing any possible unusual configurations or combination of defects. Patients were reported to have cervical duplication with a longitudinal vaginal septum, uterine septum, and a normal fundus. These rare anomalies are not explained by classic embryologic teaching and would fit into Class IV. [4,5]

IMPACT ON FERTILITY

Whether uterine anomalies other than those in class I directly cause primary infertility cannot be conclusively determined.

Primary infertility associated with uterine malformations may be attributed to related disorders such as endometriosis or anovulation. Nickerson found a high incidence of uterine anomalies (74%) in 190 infertile patients with no other cause of infertility. [6] He concluded that there is a correlation between abnormal HSG contour and primary infertility. A congenital defect of steroid receptors in mildly malformed uterus has been postulated as being responsible for the oligomenorrhea seen in these patients.[7]

In a study 6.3% of infertile patients had müllerian anomalies in comparison to 3.8% fertile women. Septate (33.6%) and arcuate (32.8%) uteri were the most common malformations observed. In all these abnormalities, early miscarriages (25-38%) and preterm deliveries (25-47%) were quite common (Table 5.2). The chance of having a live birth was higher in uterus didelphus than unicornuate because of a better blood supply. The septate uterus shows the poorest reproductive potential if untreated. The arcuate uterus presented a live birth rate of 82.7%. Uterine anomalies although relatively frequent in fertile women, are more frequent in infertile patients.[8] However since congenital anomalies like septum, bicornuate or unicornuate uterus usually do not cause infertility, all other causes of infertility should be ruled out before these factors are identified as the cause.

Table 5.2: Rate of pregnancy loss in patients with uterine anomalies		
Study	Spontaneous abortion	Preterm delivery
Raga et al[8]	28%	30%
Michalas et al[9]	36%	22%
Stein et al[10]	14%	25%
Heinonen et al [11]	29%	23%

DIAGNOSIS

1. **Hysterosalpingography (HSG):** HSG is a sensitive and specific test for uterine anomalies and also gives information regarding tubal patency.

Fallacy:
a. Cannot diagnose noncommunicating cavities
b. Cannot differentiate between bicornuate and septate uterus. In a study 94% of patients diagnosed as bicornuate uterus on HSG were subsequently identified as having septate uterus after combined laparoscopy, and hysteroscopy were performed.[12]

2. **Laparoscopy:** Laparoscopy can diagnose non-communicating horn but ultrasonography is more reliable for determining whether the horn is communicating.[13]

3. **Hysteroscopy:** Although hysteroscopy is a useful adjunct to laparoscopy but it cannot differentiate between bicornuate and septate uterus.

4. **Transvaginal ultrasound (TVS):** The sensitivity of transvaginal sonography in diagnosing these anomalies ranges from 42 to 87%. It can diagnose hemato-colpus, hematometra or hematosalpinx.

The more recent three-dimensional (3D) ultra-sonography is less expensive and non invasive compared to hysterosalpingography. The ability to visualize both the uterine cavity and the myometrium on a 3-dimensional scan facilitates the diagnosis of uterine anomalies and enables the differentiation of septate from bicornuate uteri for preoperative surgical planning.[14] Accuracy of 3-dimensional sonograms was 92% for the diagnosis of septate uterus.[13]

Ultrasonography should be done during the luteal phase of the menstrual cycle, when the endometrial echo complex is better identified.[15]

A subseptate uterus is characterized by the normal outer uterine contour. The septum is differentiated from an arcuate uterus because the fundal indentation is an acute angle at the central point whereas in a arcuate uterus it is an obtuse angle (Figs 5.8 and 5.9) (See Chapter 1).

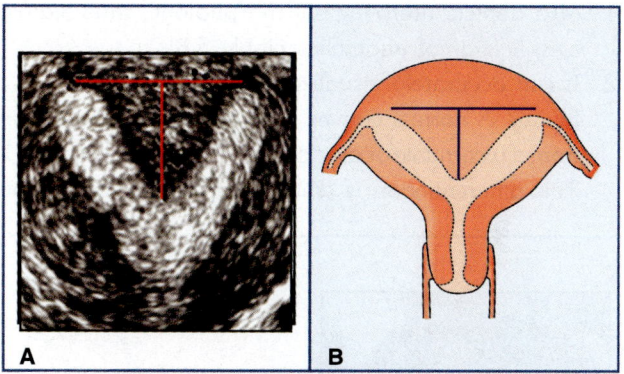

Figs 5.8A and B: Subseptate uterus – Fundal indentation an acute angle at the center

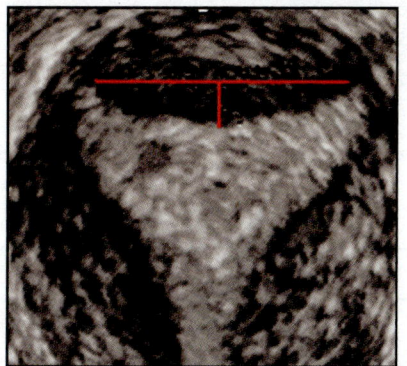

Fig. 5.9: Arcuate uterus with fundal indentation at obtuse angle at the center

5. **Intravenous pylography (IVP):** A thorough evaluation of the urinary system is a must as anomalies of this system often coexist with uterine anomalies.

6. **Magnetic resonance imaging (MRI):** MRI may be the optimal imaging technique available for diagnosis of congenital Mullerian anomalies as:

1. MRI depicts uterovaginal morphology, thus aiding in classification of anomalies (Table 5.3).
2. It can accurately visualize the external contour of the fundus. A normal convex fundus differentiates a septate from a bicornuate or didelphic uterus (Figs 5.10 and 5.11). This differentiation is crucial in treatment, as a septate

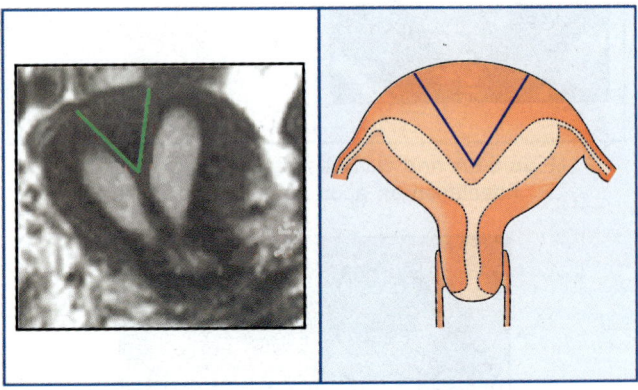

Fig. 5.10: Septate uterus with intercornual distance < 60 degrees

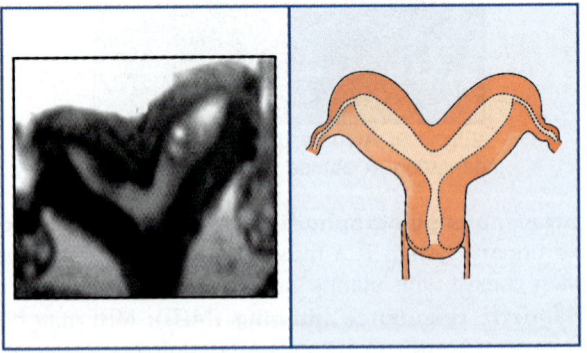

Fig. 5.11: Bicornuate uterus with fundal cleft > 1 cm

uterus requires septectomy, while a bicornuate or didelphic uterus does not usually require any surgical treatment.[16]

3. Avoids purely diagnostic surgery by accurately diagnosing Mullerian abnormalities that are not amenable to surgery.

4. A functioning communicating rudimentary horn can be diagnosed when the endometrial cavity is visualized on MRI.

5. Prediction of the composition of a uterine septum through recognition of its signal pattern and thickness, allows better treatment planning as a fibrous uterine septum is amenable to hysteroscopic resection but a uterine septum containing myometrium because of its vascularity necessitates a transabdominal metroplasty to ensure adequate hemostasis.

6. It also allows concurrent visualization of the urinary system.

MRI findings of the septate uterus, reveal a persistent longitudinal septum partially dividing the uterine cavity with intercornual angle less than 75° (Fig. 5.10). With bicornuate uterus the fundal cleft is more than 1 cm (Fig. 5.11). MRI is typically the most accurate in diagnosis and classification of the anomaly, followed by 3 D and transvaginal ultrasound and hysterosalpingogram (HSG).

The following parameters are recorded in MR images: (Table 5.3).

1. Uterine size

2. External fundal contour

3. Intercornual distance

4. Zonal anatomy

5. Presence of uterine or vaginal septa.

Table 5.3: Findings in uterine anomalies

Anomaly	Uterine size	External fundal contour	Intercornua distance	Zonall Anatomy	Uterine septum
Hypo-plastic	Small	Normal	< 2cm	Poorly differentiated	Absent
Septate	Normal	Convex, flat or < 1 cm Indentation	< 60 degrees	Muscular septum – Isointense and Thick Fibrous septum–Low intensity and Thin	Complete-Reaches internal os Partial– Above internal os
Didelphus	Two uterine bodies with two cervix	Two separate hemiuterus	> 4 cm	Preserved in both the uteri	Absent
Bicornuate	Two uterine bodies and single cervix	Fundal cleft > 1cm	> 4 cm	Tissue separating two horns isointense with myo-metrium	Lower end may have a septum
Unicornuate	Banana shape	Hemiuterus	-	Preserved	

Diagnosis of uterine anomalies by MRI can be done in a stepwise manner (Fig. 5.12).

MANAGEMENT

Management of these conditions typically relates to 3 issues: menstrual problems, fertility problems, and sexual function problems. (Fig. 5.13) The presence and severity of these areas along with the type of anomaly present will help decide the appropriate management.

It is important to discuss with the patient her needs before embarking on any treatment. Often patients with this condition who present with infertility have other causes of infertility like endometriosis, anovulation or male factors. Hence, all other factors of infertility must be ruled out.

The mere presence of an abnormality does not necessitate treatment unless the patient is symptomatic as a result of it.

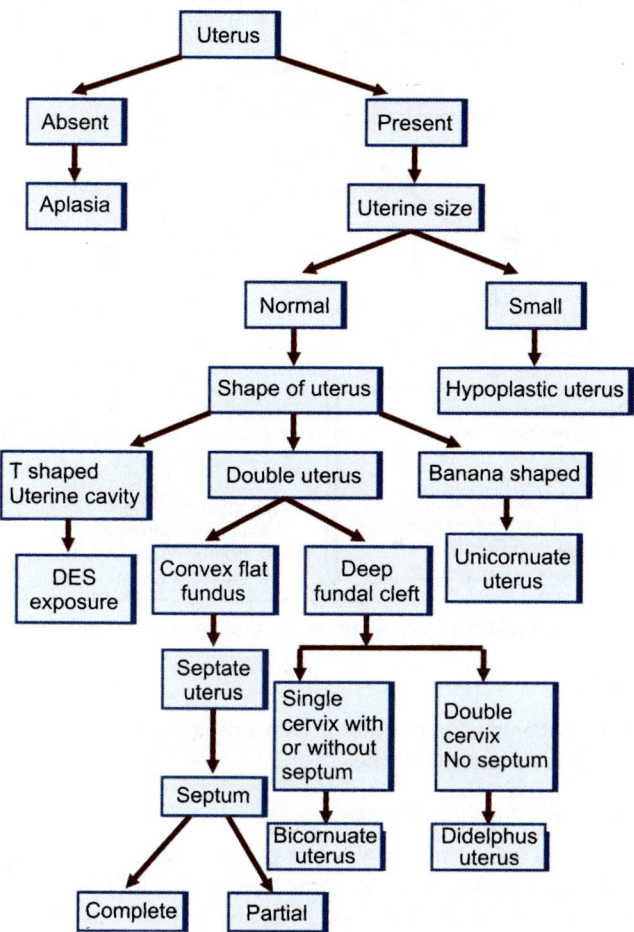

Fig. 5.12: Step by step approach to diagnosis of uterine anomalies through imaging

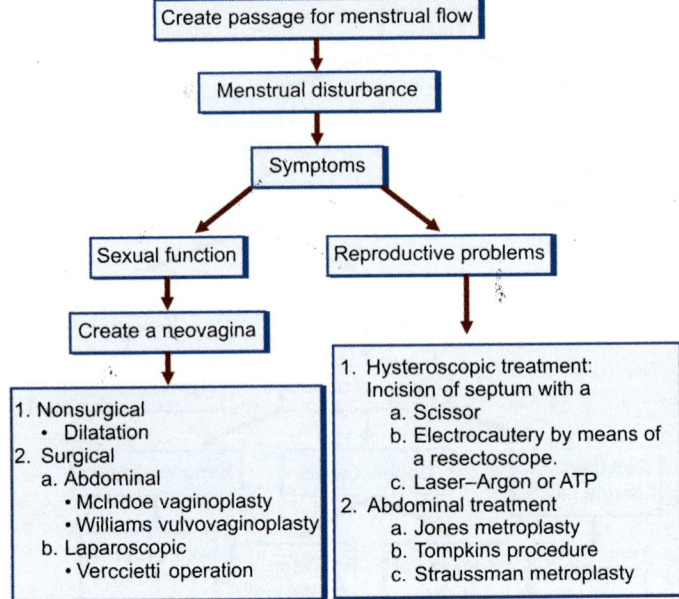

Fig. 5.13: Management of uterine anomalies

Class I

These patients usually present with primary amenorrhea with or without cryptomenorrhea.

Class Ia: Vaginal Atresia

It is characterized by an absence or hypoplasia of the uterus, proximal vagina, and, in some cases, the fallopian tubes occurring in 1:5000 neonates.[17] Vaginal agenesis can be partial or complete (as in MRKH syndrome).

Mutations in Mullerian inhibitory substance gene have been thought to be responsible for this disorder.[18] Urologic abnormalities are present in 15-40%, and skeletal anomalies in 12-50% of cases.

Diagnosis of Vaginal Agenesis

1. Primary amenorrhea
2. Secondary sexual characteristics are normal
3. The vagina may be completely absent, a short vaginal pouch, or a short vaginal dimple 1-2 cm superior to the hymenal ring may be seen.
4. Uterus is not palpable on rectal examination.
5. Imaging techniques confirm the absence of uterus.

Intravenous pyelography (IVP) and renal sonography to exclude anomalies of the urinary tract is a must.

Treatment

Principles of treatment: The treatment depends on the condition of the tubes and uterus and the degree of vaginal agenesis (Table 5.4).

Table 5.4: Treatment principles for vaginal agenesis
• Uterus and tubes diseased ⟶ Hysterectomy and neovaginostomy
• Vaginal agenesis less (short distance between lower blind pouch and upper vagina) ⟶ Give incision
• Vaginal agenesis more (long distance between lower blind pouch and upper vagina) ⟶ neovaginostomy: – Williams vulvovaginoplasty   – McIndoe procedure.

Treatment for infertility: Besides inability to have sexual intercourse, these young women are usually infertile, resulting in psychological pain and self-esteem issues, hence require counseling. Oocyte retrieval from their normal ovaries would give them a chance for a child with surrogacy when uterus and tubes are malformed.

Non-surgical Treatment

The nonsurgical approach consists of use of graduated dilators and may take several months or a few years before a functional vagina is formed. Hence, surgery is preferred as it is the most effective method of treatment for vaginal agenesis.

Surgical Treatment

High transverse vaginal septum

When distance between the lower blind pouch and upper vagina is small an incision can be given.

Step I: The neovaginal space is dissected until the septum is reached. (Fig. 5.14A)

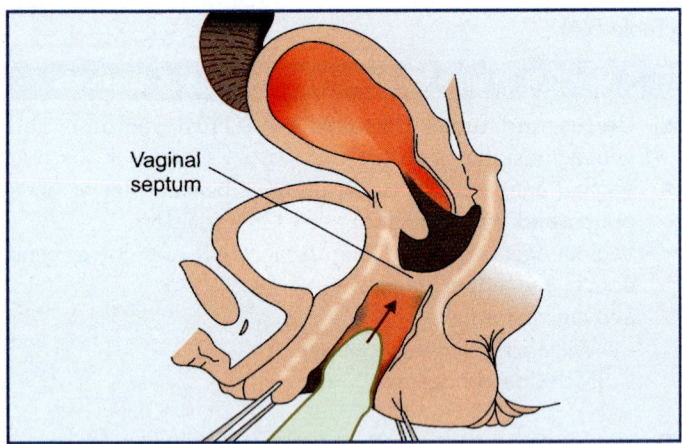

Fig. 5.14A: Dissection of space to reach septum

Step II: Needling is done to aspirate blood from hematocolpus assessing the thickness of the septum (Fig. 5.14B).

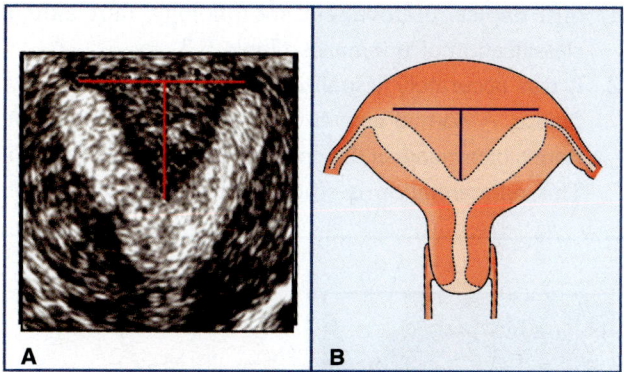

Figs 5.8A and B: Subseptate uterus – Fundal
indentation an acute angle at the center

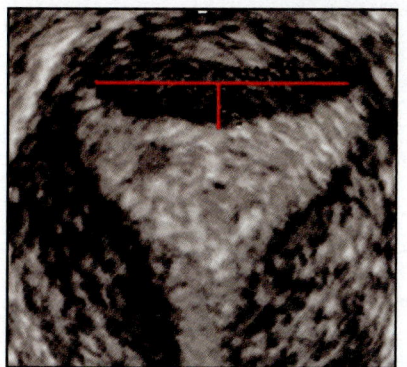

Fig. 5.9: Arcuate uterus with fundal
indentation at obtuse angle at the center

5. **Intravenous pylography (IVP):** A thorough evaluation of
   the urinary system is a must as anomalies of this system
   often coexist with uterine anomalies.

6. **Magnetic resonance imaging (MRI):** MRI may be the
   optimal imaging technique available for diagnosis of
   congenital Mullerian anomalies as:

1. MRI depicts uterovaginal morphology, thus aiding in classification of anomalies (Table 5.3).
2. It can accurately visualize the external contour of the fundus. A normal convex fundus differentiates a septate from a bicornuate or didelphic uterus (Figs 5.10 and 5.11). This differentiation is crucial in treatment, as a septate

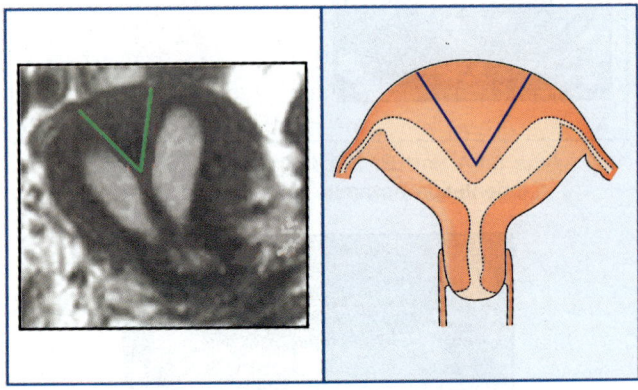

Fig. 5.10: Septate uterus with intercornual distance < 60 degrees

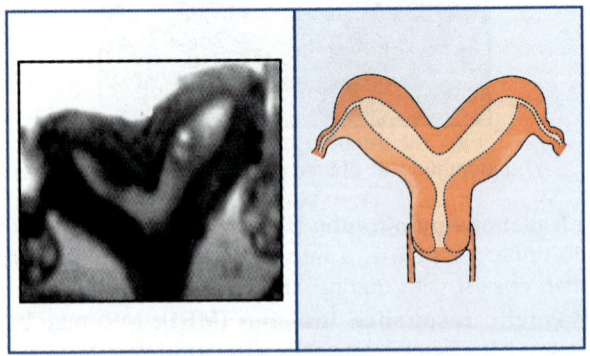

Fig. 5.11: Bicornuate uterus with fundal cleft > 1 cm

uterus requires septectomy, while a bicornuate or didelphic uterus does not usually require any surgical treatment.[16]

3. Avoids purely diagnostic surgery by accurately diagnosing Mullerian abnormalities that are not amenable to surgery.

4. A functioning communicating rudimentary horn can be diagnosed when the endometrial cavity is visualized on MRI.

5. Prediction of the composition of a uterine septum through recognition of its signal pattern and thickness, allows better treatment planning as a fibrous uterine septum is amenable to hysteroscopic resection but a uterine septum containing myometrium because of its vascularity necessitates a transabdominal metroplasty to ensure adequate hemostasis.

6. It also allows concurrent visualization of the urinary system.

MRI findings of the septate uterus, reveal a persistent longitudinal septum partially dividing the uterine cavity with intercornual angle less than 75° (Fig. 5.10). With bicornuate uterus the fundal cleft is more than 1 cm (Fig. 5.11). MRI is typically the most accurate in diagnosis and classification of the anomaly, followed by 3 D and transvaginal ultrasound and hysterosalpingogram (HSG).

The following parameters are recorded in MR images: (Table 5.3).

1. Uterine size

2. External fundal contour

3. Intercornual distance

4. Zonal anatomy

5. Presence of uterine or vaginal septa.

Table 5.3: Findings in uterine anomalies

Anomaly	Uterine size	External fundal contour	Intercornua distance	Zonall Anatomy	Uterine septum
Hypo-plastic	Small	Normal	< 2cm	Poorly differentiated	Absent
Septate	Normal	Convex, flat or < 1 cm Indentation	< 60 degrees	Muscular septum – Isointense and Thick	Complete–Reaches internal os
				Fibrous septum–Low intensity and Thin	Partial–Above internal os
Didelphus	Two uterine bodies with two cervix	Two separate hemiuterus	> 4 cm	Preserved in both the uteri	Absent
Bicornuate	Two uterine bodies and single cervix	Fundal cleft > 1cm	> 4 cm	Tissue separating two horns isointense with myo-metrium	Lower end may have a septum
Unicornuate	Banana shape	Hemiuterus	-	Preserved	

Diagnosis of uterine anomalies by MRI can be done in a stepwise manner (Fig. 5.12).

MANAGEMENT

Management of these conditions typically relates to 3 issues: menstrual problems, fertility problems, and sexual function problems. (Fig. 5.13) The presence and severity of these areas along with the type of anomaly present will help decide the appropriate management.

It is important to discuss with the patient her needs before embarking on any treatment. Often patients with this condition who present with infertility have other causes of infertility like endometriosis, anovulation or male factors. Hence, all other factors of infertility must be ruled out.

The mere presence of an abnormality does not necessitate treatment unless the patient is symptomatic as a result of it.

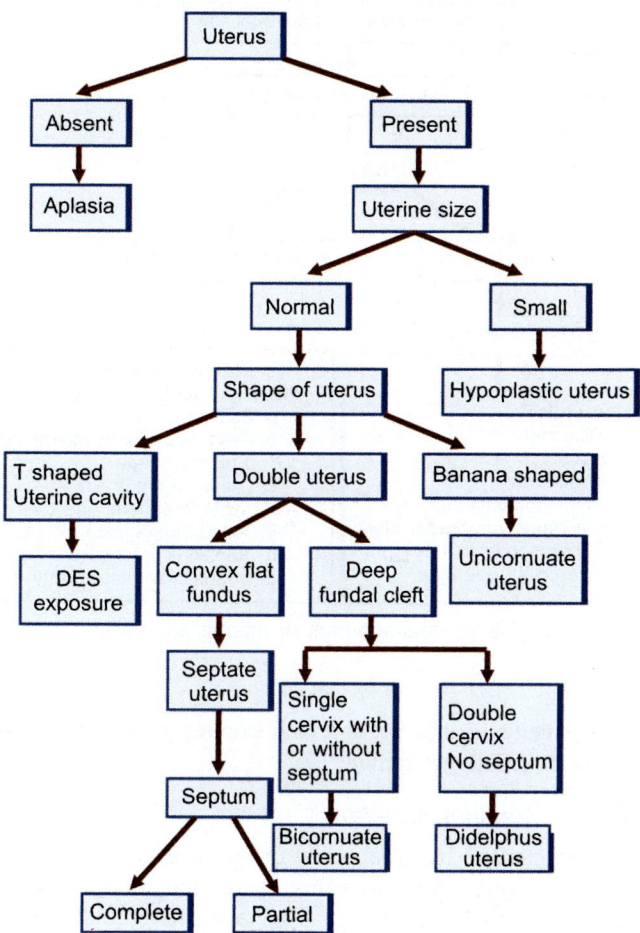

Fig. 5.12: Step by step approach to diagnosis of uterine anomalies through imaging

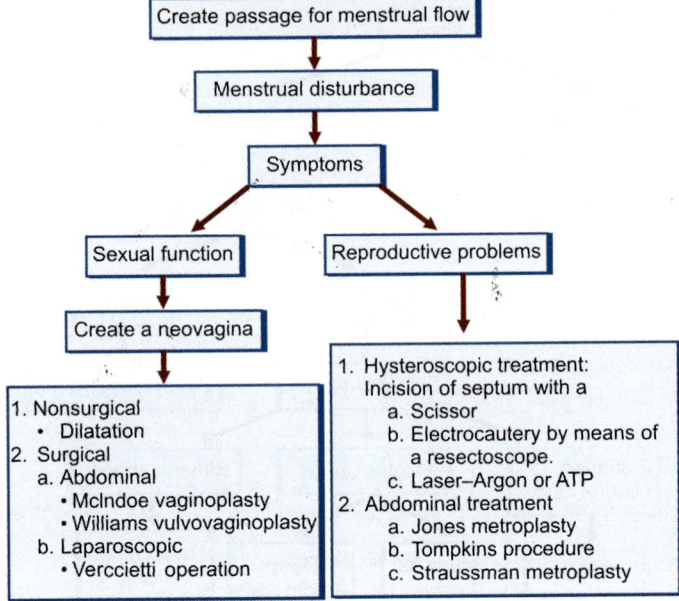

Fig. 5.13: Management of uterine anomalies

Class I

These patients usually present with primary amenorrhea with or without cryptomenorrhea.

Class Ia: Vaginal Atresia

It is characterized by an absence or hypoplasia of the uterus, proximal vagina, and, in some cases, the fallopian tubes occurring in 1:5000 neonates.[17] Vaginal agenesis can be partial or complete (as in MRKH syndrome).

Mutations in Mullerian inhibitory substance gene have been thought to be responsible for this disorder.[18] Urologic abnormalities are present in 15-40%, and skeletal anomalies in 12-50% of cases.

Diagnosis of Vaginal Agenesis

1. Primary amenorrhea
2. Secondary sexual characteristics are normal
3. The vagina may be completely absent, a short vaginal pouch, or a short vaginal dimple 1-2 cm superior to the hymenal ring may be seen.
4. Uterus is not palpable on rectal examination.
5. Imaging techniques confirm the absence of uterus.

Intravenous pyelography (IVP) and renal sonography to exclude anomalies of the urinary tract is a must.

Treatment

Principles of treatment: The treatment depends on the condition of the tubes and uterus and the degree of vaginal agenesis (Table 5.4).

Table 5.4: Treatment principles for vaginal agenesis
• Uterus and tubes diseased ⟶ Hysterectomy and neovaginostomy
• Vaginal agenesis less (short distance between lower blind pouch and upper vagina) ⟶ Give incision
• Vaginal agenesis more (long distance between lower blind pouch and upper vagina) ⟶ neovaginostomy: – Williams vulvovaginoplasty   – McIndoe procedure.

Treatment for infertility: Besides inability to have sexual intercourse, these young women are usually infertile, resulting in psychological pain and self-esteem issues, hence require counseling. Oocyte retrieval from their normal ovaries would give them a chance for a child with surrogacy when uterus and tubes are malformed.

Non-surgical Treatment

The nonsurgical approach consists of use of graduated dilators and may take several months or a few years before a functional vagina is formed. Hence, surgery is preferred as it is the most effective method of treatment for vaginal agenesis.

Surgical Treatment

High transverse vaginal septum

When distance between the lower blind pouch and upper vagina is small an incision can be given.

Step I: The neovaginal space is dissected until the septum is reached. (Fig. 5.14A)

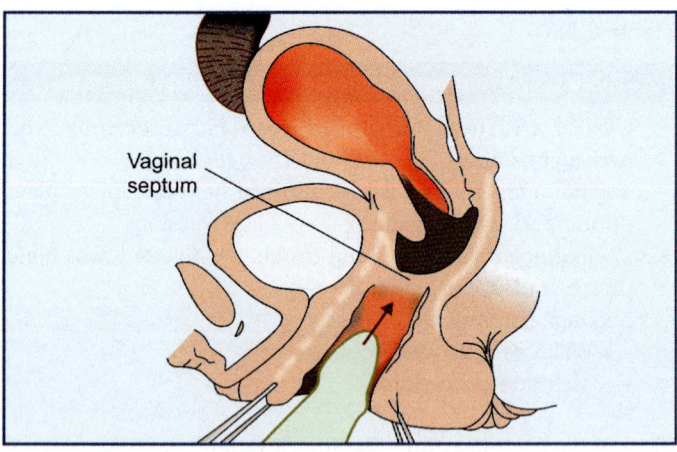

Fig. 5.14A: Dissection of space to reach septum

Step II: Needling is done to aspirate blood from hematocolpus assessing the thickness of the septum (Fig. 5.14B).

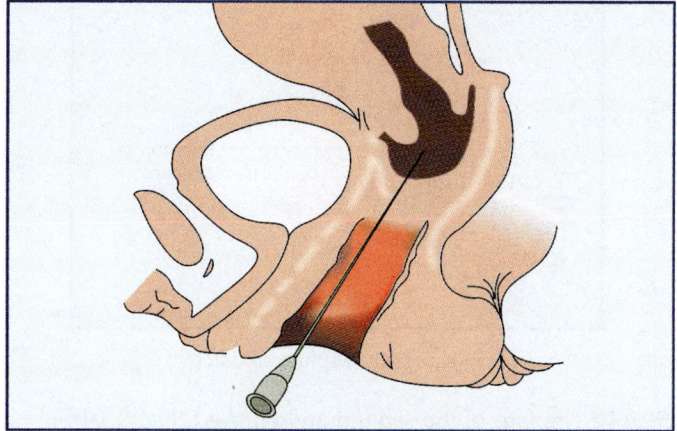

Fig. 5.14B: Needling of space above septum

Step III: Transverse incision is given on the septum after ensuring the extent of the bladder and rectum (Fig. 5.14C)

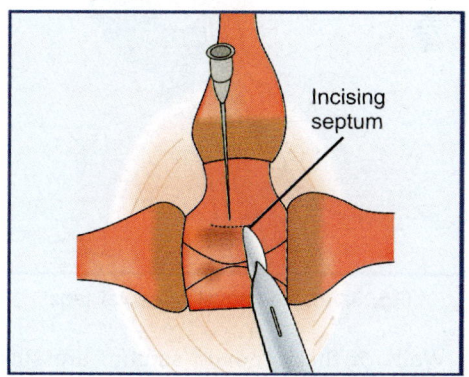

Incising septum

Fig. 5.14C: Incision on septum

Step IV: Excision of the septum is done (Fig. 5.14D)

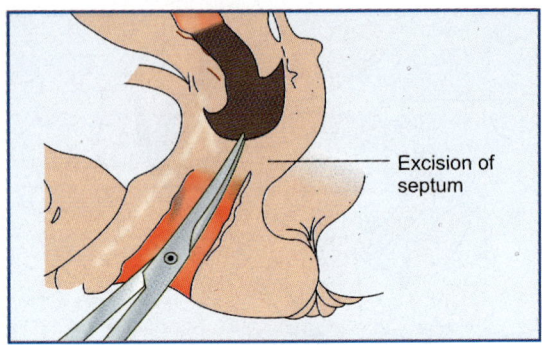

Fig. 5.14D: Septum excision

Step V: The tags of the septum are removed (Fig. 5.14E).

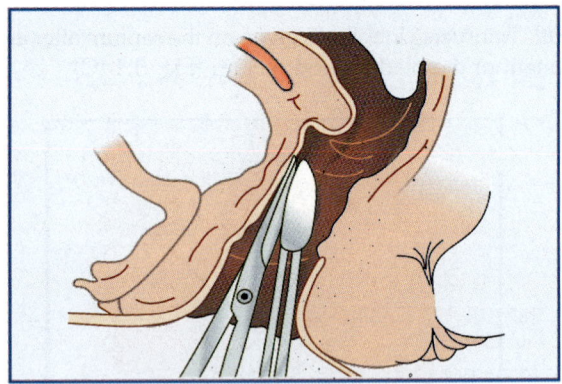

Fig. 5.14E: Removal of septal tags

Step VI: Walls of the removed septum are stitched with interrupted sutures (Fig. 5.14F).

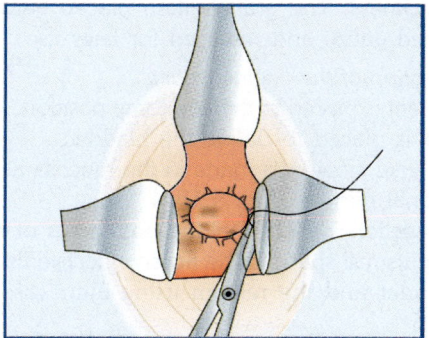

Fig. 5.14F: Suturing of edges of septum

A vaginal mould may be given to prevent stenosis and adhesion formation till epithelialisation takes place.

Time of surgery: It should be done when patient wishes to become sexually active.

Surgical Techniques for Vaginal Agenesis

Principle: Developing a space between the bladder and the rectum to create a neovagina which is covered by a graft.

Grafts: Full-thickness skin grafts have the advantage of less graft contracture and stenosis but a lower success rate and patient satisfaction compared with that of split-thickness grafts. Human amnion, not stripped from the chorion, transposition flaps and autologous buccal mucosa have been used as a graft for vaginoplasties. The use of artificial dermis and absorbable adhesion barriers show promise as exogenous graft sources in vaginal recon-struction.[19, 20]

McIndoe Vaginoplasty

Technique

Step I: Creating a split-thickness graft
- The graft is taken from the buttock or outer thigh and excised to a depth of 0.045 cm (0.018 in.) approximately 8 × 10 cms. A single layer is removed avoiding any variation in

graft thickness. The graft is then placed between saline-moistened gauze and reserved for later use.

Step II: Creation of the vaginal space
- The patient is placed in the lithotomy position, and a Foleys catheter is placed to define the bladder.
- A transverse incision is made in the mucosa at the apex of the vaginal dimple. (Fig. 5.15A)
- The dissection is started along both sides of the midline, creating a small space in the fibroconnective tissue between the bladder and the rectum using blunt dissection (Fig. 5.15B).

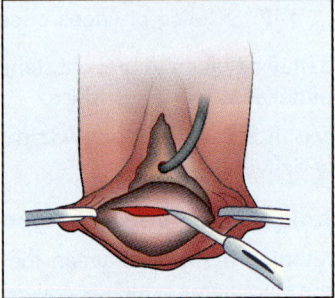

Fig. 5.15A: Transverse incision on vaginal mucosa

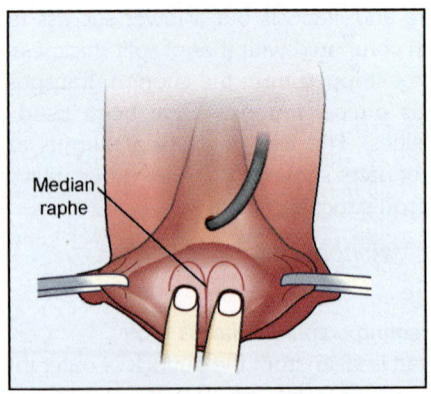

Fig. 5.15B: Dissection to create space between bladder and rectum

- The median raphe is divided with scissors, joining the spaces.
- The dissection is continued up to the peritoneum. (Fig 5.15C)
- Meticulous hemostasis is needed as graft may separate from its bed because of bleeding resulting in failure.

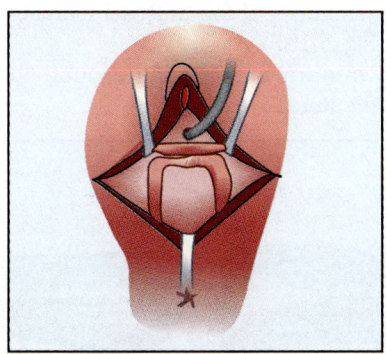

Fig. 5.15C: Dissection continued till peritoneum

Step III: Making a prosthesis
- The stent can be made from sterilized foam-rubber according to the size of the patient's vagina.
- The prosthetic material is covered by the placement of condoms over the surface which is tied at the open end. (Fig. 5.15D).

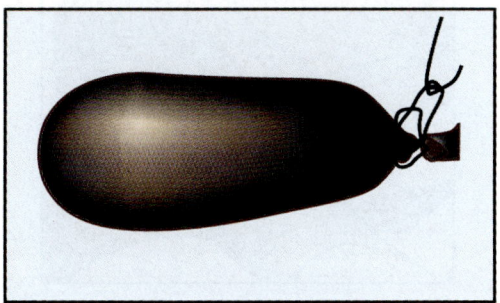

Fig. 5.15D: A condom is placed and tied over the rubber foam made according to the size of the vagina

Step IV: Attachment of graft attachment

o   The skin graft, with dermal aspect outside, is sutured over the stent, with 5-0 synthetic absorbable sutures. (Fig 5.15E)

o   The graft-covered prosthesis is carefully inserted into the vaginal canal. The edges of the graft are sutured to the previously cut edges of the mucosal margins of the vaginal introitus. (Fig 5.15F)

o   The labia minora are sutured around the stent using nonreactive sutures.

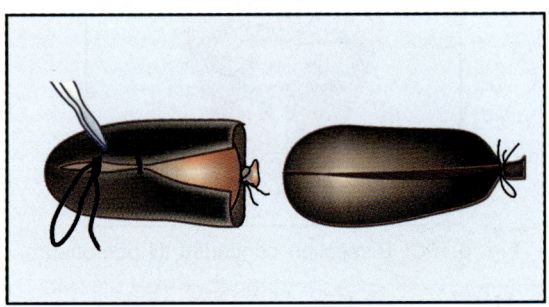

Fig. 5.15E: Suturing graft over vaginal mould

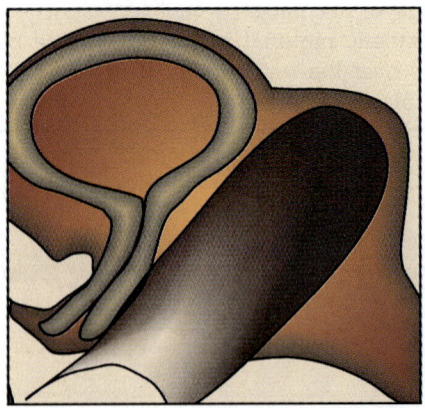

Fig. 5.15F: Graft edges sutured to vaginal margins

Postoperative care: One week after surgery, the labial sutures are removed, and the stent is removed with the patient under mild sedation. The neovagina is inspected to determine whether the graft has taken satisfactorily. A new foam covered with a condom is reinserted. Patient is educated on removal and reinsertion of mould after cleaning with povidone-iodine solution, covered with a fresh condom, lubricated, and reintroduced into the neovagina. Later a silicone form that is inserted at night for the next 12 months replaces the original stent. In most cases, the vagina is functional 6-10 weeks after surgery.

Surgical Complications
1. Postoperative fistula (4% risk)
2. Enterocele – Rarely an enterocele can occur.[3]
3. Infection,
4. Hemorrhage
5. Graft failure - Contracture of the graft and the development of excess granulation tissue can occur.

Results
Patient satisfaction is high. Although most patients cannot obtain full fertility, except through surrogates, they can have normal sexual relations.

William's Vulvovaginoplasty

Indications
It is indicated in patients who have
1. Previously failed vaginoplasty
2. Previous radical pelvic surgery.

Principle: It uses full-thickness skin flaps from the labia majora to create a vaginal pouch. Unlike the McIndoe procedure, vaginal dilation is required for only 3-4 weeks.

Technique

Step I: Horseshoe shaped incision is given on the vulva to extend across the perineum medially upto the external urethral meatus (Fig. 5.16A).

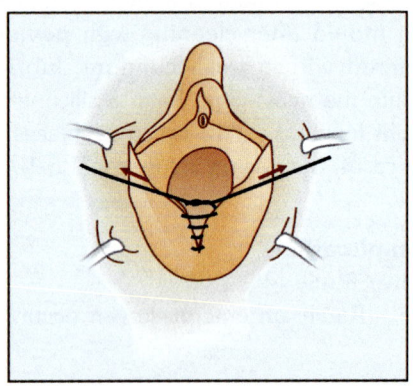

Fig. 5.16A: Horseshoe shaped incision on the vulva and inner skin margins are sutured

Step II: Inner skin margins are sutured (Fig. 5.16A)

Step III: Second suture layer approximates subcutaneous fat and muscle (Fig. 5.16B).

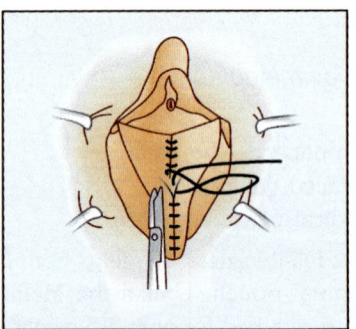

Fig. 5.16B: Inner skin margins are sutured followed by suturing of subcutaneous fat and muscle

Step IV: External skin margins are approximated with interrupted sutures (Fig. 5.16C).

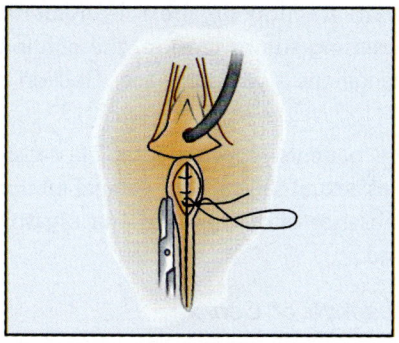

Fig. 5.16C: Suturing of external skin margins with interrupted sutures

Advantages

1. Simple procedure
2. Local complications are less
3. Absence of postoperative pain
4. Early recovery
5. Higher success rate of primary and repeat procedure
6. Elimination of need for dilatation, after 3-4 weeks hence easy postoperative care easy
7. Ideal for patients who do not have regular intercourse

Disadvantages

1. Technique cannot be used in patients with poorly developed labia
2. The vagina created by this approach is not anatomically similar to a normal vagina
3. Urine may momentarily collect in the pouch

Laparoscopic Procedure—Vercchietti Operation

Technique

A specifically designed traction device is placed on the outer surface of the abdomen and sutures attached to the device connect to an elliptically shaped plastic bead located at the introital area passing through the abdominal cavity. The device permits upward traction on the retrohymenal tissues. By gradually increasing suture tension, the continuous pressure creates and lengthens a vaginal space. Traction is required for one week.

Results: 89% patients reported complete satisfaction, where factors, such as sexual satisfaction, vaginal lubrication, and the presence or absence of dyspareunia and orgasm achievement were evaluated.[21]

Class Ib: Absence of Cervix

It is a relatively infrequent Mullerian anomaly. It usually occurs in the absence of either a portion or the entire vagina. A fistulous tract might be created from vagina to uterus inserting a T tube to maintain egress of blood. Often hysterectomy is done due to need for repeated reoperations.

Diagnosis: Patients usually present with cryptomenorrhea. Ultrasonography and MRI help in diagnosis. The differential diagnosis is with high transverse vaginal septum where there would be a collection of menstrual blood in the upper vagina.

Types of Cervical Anomalies

1. Cervical aplasia: Absence of uterine cervix. The lower uterine segment narrows to terminate in a peritoneal sleeve at a point well above the normal communication with vaginal apex (Fig. 5.17A).

2. Intact cervical body with obstruction of cervical os (the cervix is well formed, but a portion of the endocervical lumen is obliterated (Fig. 5.17B).

3. Cervical body consists of a fibrous band of variable length and diameter (endocervical glands may be noted on histopathologic examination (Fig. 5.17C).

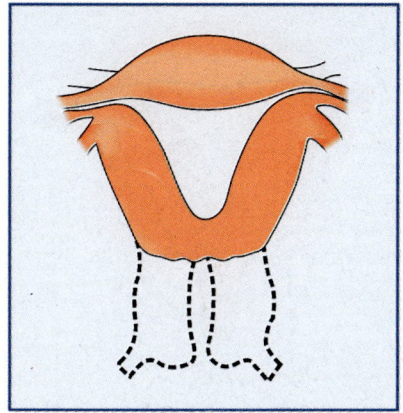

Fig. 5.17A: Complete absence of cervix

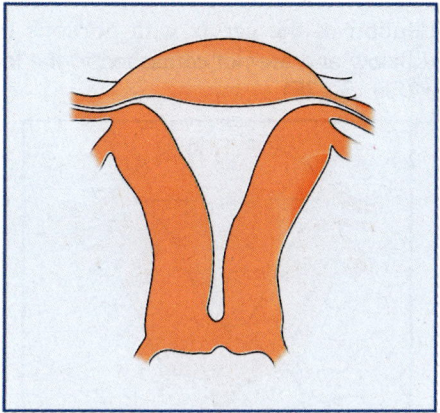

Fig. 5.17B: Intact cervical body with obstruction of cervical os

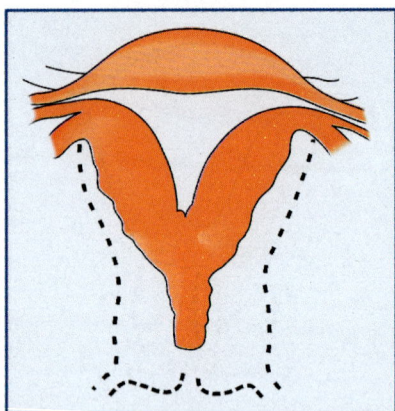

Fig. 5.17C: Cervical body consists of a fibrous band

4. Stricture on the midportion of the cervix (which is hypoplastic with a bulbous tip and no identifiable cervical lumen (Fig. 5.17D).
5. Fragmentation of the cervix with portions that can be palpated below and are not connected to the lower uterine segment (Fig. 5.17E).

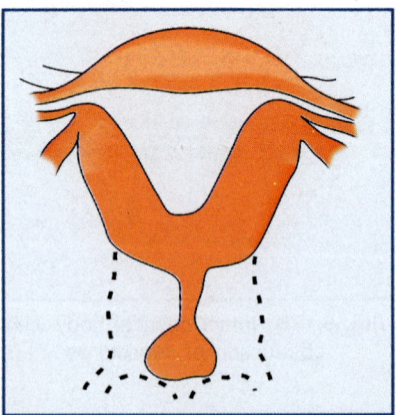

Fig. 5.17D: Stricture on the midportion of the cervix

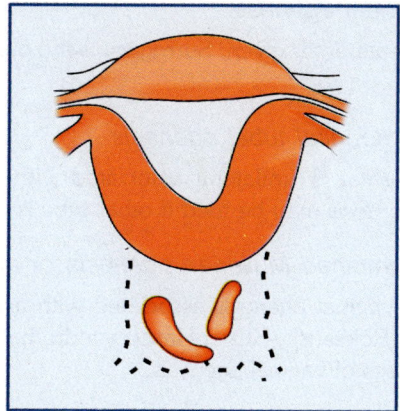

Fig. 5.17E: Fragmentation of the cervix

Treatment

Many methods have been tried.

Creation of passage with stent: A passage is created through the dense fibrous tissue between the uterine cavity and vagina with placement of a stent to keep it open.

Disadvantages
1. No cervical mucus formed as absence of endocervical glands which is necessary for sperm transport.
2. Restenosis of tract because of fibrous tissue.
3. Recurrent and severe pelvic infection which may require hysterectomy.

Hysterectomy with ovarian conservation: Many recommend hysterectomy.

Indications:
1. As first line of treatment eliminating problems like cryptomenorrhea, sepsis, endometriosis and multiple operations.
2. Fragmented cervix
3. Recurrent and severe pelvic infection after stenting.

Class Ic: Fundal agenesis

No surgical treatment is given. Surrogacy is the only option for fertility.

Class Id: Congenital tubal agenesis

Usually segmental or unilateral associated with unicornuate uterus. Anastomosis may be tried if other tube is damaged.

Class Ie: Combined Mullerian agenesis or aplasia

It consists of vaginal agenesis associated with a rudimentary uterus.(Mayer-Rokitansky-Kuster-Hauser syndrome) It represents 80 to 90% cases of vaginal agenesis.

Class II: Unicornuate uterus

The unicornuate uterus is formed when normal differen-tiation of only one Mullerian duct occurs and there is complete or partial arrest in development of the other horn. Unicornuate uterus constitutes 2.4-13% of all Mullerian anomalies.[22] Incidence of unicornuate uterus was 0.06%.[8] (Table 5.5)

Class	Rudimentary horn	Incidence
	**Table 5.5:** Incidence of subtypes of unicornuate uterus with rudimentary horn[23]
IIa	Contains functioning endometrium which may communicate externally	10%
IIb	Contains functioning endometrium which does not communicate externally	22%
IIc	Rudimentary horn has no cavity	33%
IId	Absence of rudimentary horn.	35%

Complications of functioning horn: Functioning endometrium which is non communicating is associated with increased morbidity and mortality.

Complications seen are:

1. Hematometra

2. Endometriosis
3. Ectopic pregnancy.

Endometriosis usually resolves after excision of the horn.

Urological anomalies: Associated urologic anomalies are frequent (44%), (especially in the presence of an obstructed horn) and include

1. Ipsilateral renal agenesis (67%),
2. Horseshoe kidneys, and
3. Ipsilateral pelvic kidney (15%).[24]

Infertility: Fecundity in these patients is impaired as ovulation occurring in the abnormal side is less likely to result in fertilization.

Reproductive outcomes: Unicornuate uterus is associated with the lowest reproductive outcome among all Mullerian anomalies except septum.[25]

Common obstetric problems seen are[9]

1. Abortion
2. Preterm delivery: It is seen in 10-20% patients.[26]
3. Cervical incompentence
4. Intrauterine growth restrictions
5. Mapresentation
6. Increased operative delivery
7. Complication involving accessory horn: Ectopic pregnancy, missed abortion and uterine rupture.

Unicornuate uteri is associated with a 40% fetal survival. This may be due to the small size of the uterus which does not allow enough space for adequate fetal growth or abnormal blood flow to uterus resulting in insufficient blood flow to the baby and intrauterine growth retardation.[27] Pregnancy in a noncommunicating horn is rare and is thought to be due to transperitoneal sperm migration into the fallopian tube of the rudimentary horn. The accessory horn may be excised prior to pregnancy as a preventive measure.

Treatment

Surgery is done only if endometrium is present in the accessory horn, with laparoscopic hemihysterectomy of the rudimentary horn being the treatment of choice. Removal of non functioning rudimentary horn is not indicated in infertile patients because most patients conceive without difficulty. Reconstruction metroplasty is not indicated in unicornuate uterus.

Surgical Technique for Rudimentary Horn Excision

The uterine artery which courses inferior to the fibromuscular band connecting the two horns is coagulated after dissecting the band. When the horn is attached to the unicornuate uterus, the uterine artery courses inferior to the horn and lateral to the unicornuate uterus.

When horns externally separate: The pedicle of the rudimentary horn is coagulated and divided using bipolar coagulation. The fallopian tube is removed after cutting and cauterizing the mesosalpinx. The vesicouterine space is dissected and the bladder attachments are coagulated and cut. The tube and rudimentary horn are removed.

When horns are not externally separated: The myometrium is resected at the junction of the horns by using bipolar coagulation followed by mechanical or laser cutting. A large rudimentary horn may need morcellation. In one study 6 out of 8 patients conceived after excision of the horn.[27]

If a pregnancy occurs in a noncommunicating horn, removal of the pregnant horn is advocated. Increased pedicle vascularity may cause difficulty. The pregnancies may be medically treated with methotrexate before horn excision.[28]

Class III: Didelphys Uterus

A doubled uterus results from the complete failure of the two Mullerian ducts to fuse together and is characterized by 2 hemiuteri, 2 endocervical canals with cervices fused at the lower uterine segment. Each hemiuteri is associated with one fallopian tube. Approximately 11% of uterine malformations are didelphys uterus.[2] The ones with unilateral obstruction are symptomatic as hemato-metrocolpos, hematometra, and hematosalpinx may develop.

Reproductive outcomes: Didelphys uteri have the best pregnancy outcomes of the uterine anomalies. This may be because they have better blood flow. There is a 35% spontaneous abortion rate, a 19% preterm delivery rate and a 60% live birth rate. Because of an acceptable fetal salvage rate and the difficulty of uteroplasty surgical therapy is rarely performed.

Renal agenesis most commonly occurs in association with uterine didelphys than with any other type of Mullerian anomaly with an incidence of 20%.[29,30]

Treatment

Nonobstructive: Metroplasty

When the vagina is not obstructed, indications for surgical correction are limited, with dyspareunia being the most notable. Decision to perform metroplasty should be indivisualized as only selected patients with a long history of recurrent spontaneous abortions or preterm births may benefit from metroplasty. The results may be disappointing. If needed the procedure of choice is the Strassmann metroplasty. This method unifies the uterine cavities at the fundus, while the cervices are left intact.

Stassart and associates (1992) reported favorable obstetrical outcomes after surgery. Cervical unification is technically difficult and can result in cervical incompetence or stenosis.[31]

Obstructive: Two surgical options exist

1. Full excision and marsupialization of vaginal septum
2. Hemihysterectomy with or without salpingectomy–It is not preferred in infertile patients.

Bicornuate Uterus: Class IV

Bicornuate uterus results from a failure of fusion between two normally developed Mullerian ducts at the fundus.

1. *Complete*: (Class IV a) which results in a two separate single horn uterine bodies sharing one cervix.
   - Bicornuate bicollis: It is a variant of bicornuate uterus in which the anomaly is combined with a muscular uterine septum that extends to the external os.
   - Bicornuate unicollis uterus: Complete uterine septa that extend to the internal are known as bicornuate unicollis uterus.
2. *Partial:* (Class IV b) Fusion between the Mullerian ducts occur at the lower part of uterus and cervix but not the fundus resulting in a single uterine cavity at the lower part and a single cervix.
3. *Arcuate uterus:* An arcuate uterus is considered a milder form of bicornuate uterus; it has a convex or flat external fundal contour and mild impression on the endometrial cavity.

Reproductive outcomes: Abortion rate was 35% which increased to 61% if septate uterus was present.[32] Pregnancies in women with a bicornuate uterus have a 15 -25% rate of preterm delivery. The incidence of preterm delivery is higher (66%) in women with a complete bicornuate uterus. As with unicornuate uteri, the preterm delivery rate may be increased by the small uterine cavity size and by a high incidence of cervical incompetence. Approximately 60% of patients can expect to deliver a viable infant, though they may present with late abortion or premature labor.[25]

Obstetric outcomes in bicornuate and septate uterus are related to length of unified cavity below the septum rather than the length of the septum.

Fertility: Ability to conceive is usually not impaired. In large study of infertile women, the incidence of bicornuate uterus was not significantly different from that of the fertile control group, suggesting that these patients usually have no difficulty becoming pregnant.[8]

> It is important to distinguish bicornuate uterus from septate uterus because bicornuate uterus does not usually require surgery and is associated with minimal reproductive problems, while the septate uterus can be surgically corrected and has a high association with reproductive failure.

Treatment

Metroplasty should be reserved for women who have experienced recurrent spontaneous abortions, midtrimester loss, premature birth, and in whom no other etiologic factor has been identified. Straussman procedure is the surgical treatment of choice for unifying the bicornuate uterus. It has the advantage of not requiring excision of uterine tissue and thus not reducing the potential uterine space.[33] Surgical reconstruction should be applied only to the corpus, leaving the septum intact in the lower segment. Transcervical lysis is not recommended because it can result in uterine perforation.

Subsequent pregnancy: The patient must use barrier contraception for 6 months, after which conception can be attempted.[3]

Results: Transabdominal metroplasty improves the reproductive performance of women who had recurrent spontaneous abortions or premature deliveries before surgery, with 86% viable births.[34]

Septate Uterus: Class V

Septate uterus is the most common structural abnormality of all Mullerian duct defects. It is found in 1.9 to 3% of the female population.[35] It is composed of poorly vascularized fibromuscular tissue and results from incomplete resorption of the medial septum after complete fusion of the Mullerian ducts has occurred. This may be complete or partial.

Fertility: Fertility does not appear to be substantially compromised in patients with a septate uterus.

Reproductive outcome: This anomaly is associated with the poorest reproductive outcomes of all the Mullerian duct anomalies. The complications seen during pregnancy are:

1. *Abortion*: Abortion may occur upto 60% if septum is complete. It may be due to the decreased functional uterine volume or inadequate blood supply to the relative avascular septum if implantation occurs there.
2. Intrauterine death
3. Intrauterine growth restriction
4. Preterm labor
5. Abnormal presentation
6. Dystocia
7. Infertility: It is an uncommon complication

The septum has a lower blood flow and placental implantation on the septum may be responsible for the higher incidence of intrauterine growth restriction and fetal loss seen in women with septate uteri. A live birth rate of 62% in women with septate uteri has been reported.[8] The outcome depends on the length of the common uterine cavity and not the length of the septum.

Urinary tract anomalies are usually not associated with septate uterus.

Surgical Techniques

Hysteroscopic resection of septum is preferred but if septum is thick and broad, metroplasty may be required

The decision to perform surgical correction of the septum should be based on poor reproductive performance rather than the mere presence of a septate uterus.

Hysteroscopic Resection of Septum

The surgical procedure of choice is transcervical lysis of the uterine septum combined with concurrent laparoscopy to reduce the risk of uterine perforation during septal incision (see Chapter 7).

Complete septate uterus: Foleys catheter is placed in one cavity of a complete septate uterus (Fig. 5.18A). The resectoscope is placed in the other cavity and the septum is incised till the bulb of the Foleys is visualized or both the internal os are visualized (Figs 5.18B and C).

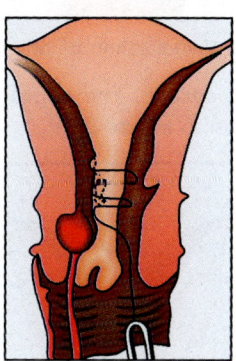

Fig. 5.18A: Foley's catheter introduced in one cavity while resectoscope incises septum

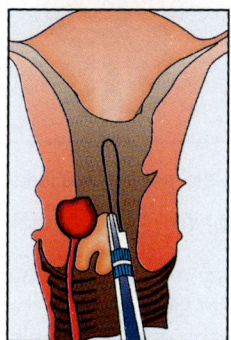

Fig. 5.18B: Resection of septum till bulb of Foley's visualized

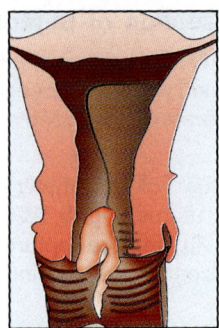

Fig. 5.18C: Visualization of two internal OS

Septum with single cervix: The septum is incised with a resectoscope as shown in Figure 5.19.

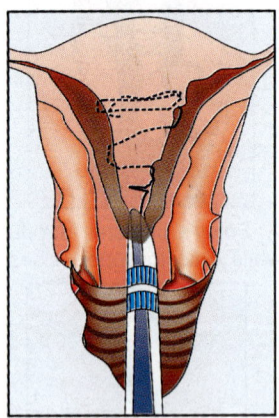

Fig. 5.19: Incomplete septum excised with resectoscope

METROPLASTY

Abdominal metroplasty may be done by any three techniques
1. Wedge Metroplasty of Jones
2. Medial bivalve technique of Tompkins
3. Straussman Metroplasty

The line of surgical incision in the 3 procedures are shown in Figure 5.20. The wedge incision for Jones metroplasty done for subseptate uterus (Fig. 5.20A). The line of incision used for Straussman to repair a bicornuate uterus runs from fundus to fundus and is a transverse line unlike Jones and Tompkins (Fig. 5.20B). The line of incision used during Tomkins metroplasty is carried through the midseptal area into the endometrial cavity (Fig. 5.20C).

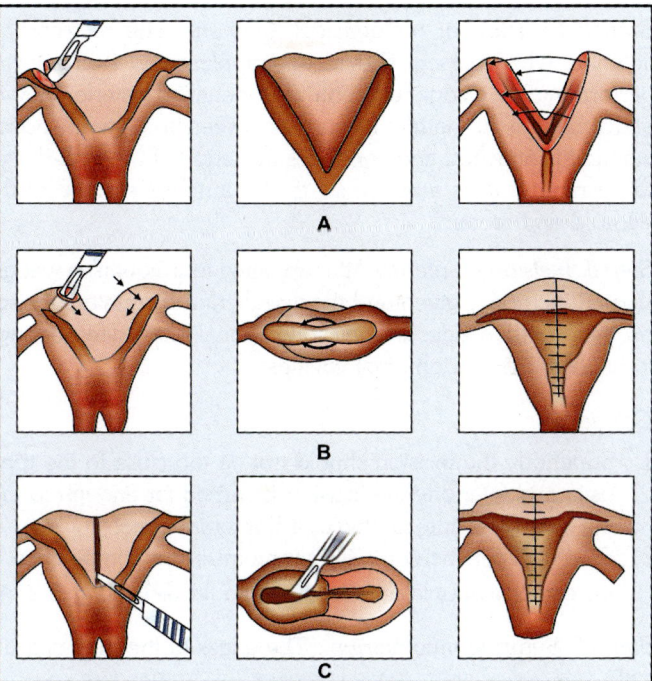

Figs 5.20 A to C: Line of surgical incision during Jones (A) Straussman (B) and Tompkins metroplasty (C)

Control of bleeding during the procedure is achieved either by placing a tourniquet at the lower uterine junction and another at the infundibulopelvic ligament or by injecting vasopressin diluted with saline.

Straussman's Metroplasty

It is not indicated in a septate uterus but it is the procedure of choice for unification of the two uterine cavities in bicornuate or didelphys uterus.

Pregnancy loss decreased from 53 to 4% after metroplasty.[36]

Step I: Excision of rectovesical ligament: The rectovesical ligament when present should be completely excised prior to performing the wedge resection. It is identified anteriorly by its attachment to the bladder It courses between both uterine horns, where it is attached and continues posteriorly in the cul-de-sac to terminate at its attachment to the anterior surface of the sigmoid and rectum.

Step II: Incision on uterus: After applying tourniquets, a wedge-shaped incision is given and the two uterine cornua are incised on their median sides in their longitudinal axes, deep enough to expose their endometrial cavities.

Caution

1. Superiorly the incision should not be too close to the tubal ostia and inferiorly the incision is carried far enough to join the two sides into a single endometrial canal.
2. Since deeper incision will compromise the competence of the cervix, a double cervical canal should be left (Fig. 5.21A).

Step III: Suturing myometrium: The edges of the myometrium will evert. Apposition of the opposing myometrium is achieved using interrupted figure of 8 sutures along the posterior and anterior uterine walls forming a united uterine cavity (Figs 5.21B to D).

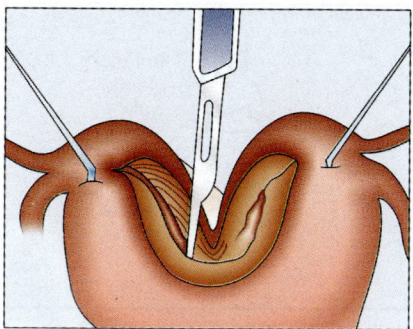

Fig. 5.21A: Incision on the uterus

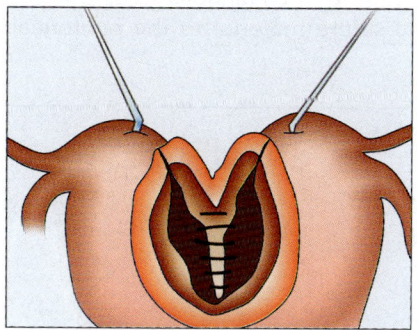

Fig. 5.21B: Suturing posterior myometrium

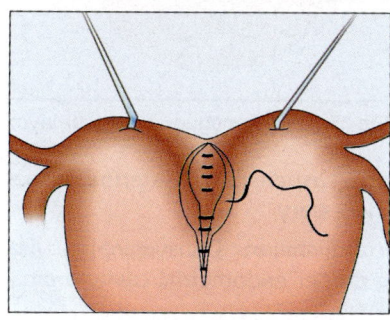

Fig. 5.21C: Suturing anterior myometrium

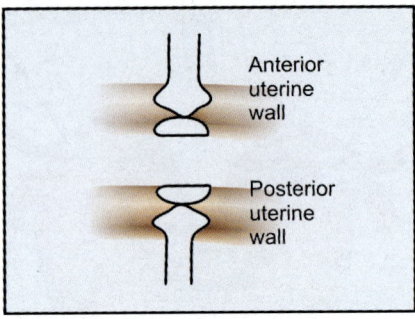

Fig. 5.21D: Figure of 8 stitches put in the myometrium

The second layer is continuous subserosal sutures, without exposing any suture material to the peritoneal cavity (Fig. 5.21E).

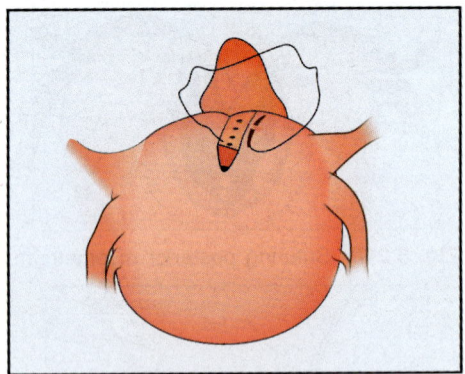

Fig. 5.21E: Continuous serosal layer

Step IV: Uterine suspension: A uterine suspension can be performed as necessary

Step V: Cervical dilatation: Transvaginal cervical dilatation is done, assuring proper endometrial cavity drainage

Modified Jones Metroplasty

Abdomen is opened by Pfanenstein incision. The septate uterus may demonstrate a median raphe across the fundus. A silk suture may be placed on this as a marker.

Step I: Outlining incision is to be made into each uterine cavity (Fig. 5.22A).

Step II: Incision is extended as a wedge beginning at the fundus.

Caution: Incision should be one cm away from the tubes and directed toward the apex of the wedge to avoid transecting the tube across its interstitial transit in the myometrium (Fig. 5.22B).

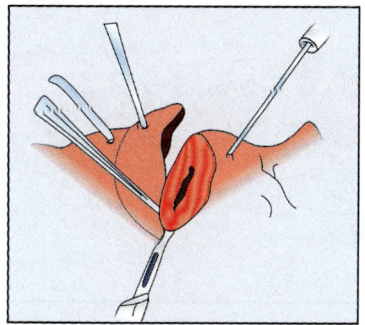

Fig. 5.22A: Outlining incision

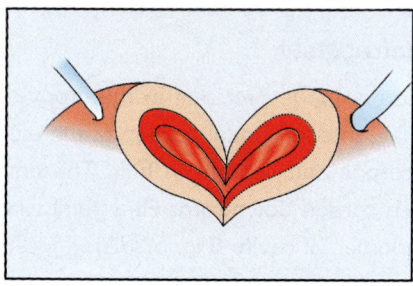

Fig. 5.22B: Incision extended as a wedge

Step III: After the wedge is removed the uterus is closed in three layers. Inner layer includes one third of the thickness of the myometrium as endometrium is too delicate to hold the suture. The inner sutures are placed in such a way that the knot is tied in the endometrial cavity (Fig. 5.22C). After the first few stitches are placed, the second layer is started as it reduces tension. Third layer is the serosal layer of interrupted stitches of non reactive material similar to that in Straussman metroplasty. (Fig. 5.21E).

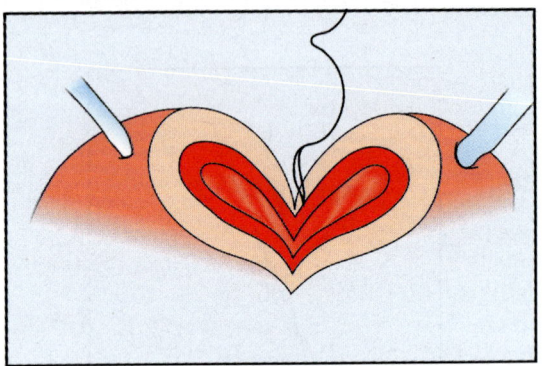

Fig. 5.22C: Inner layer sutured with interrupted sutures

Tomkins Metroplasty

Step I: Incision is made precisely in the groove that can be palpated on the anterior fundal portion of the uterus, dividing the uterine corpus and septum in half. The anterior fundal incision is then carried downwards till a point where the knife enters the endometrial cavity (Fig. 5.23A).

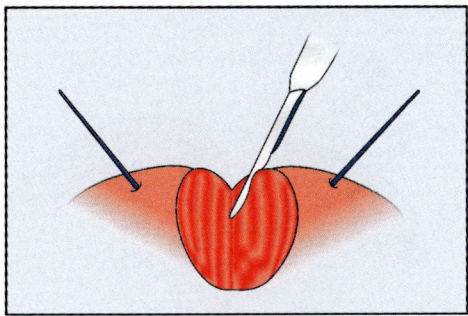

Fig. 5.23A: Longitudinal incision dividing
the corpus and septum

Step II: Each lateral septal half is incised to within 1 cm of the tube without removing any septal tissue .Each horn is thus converted into a semicylinder (Fig. 5.23B).

Step III: The myometrium is then reapproximated taking care not to place the sutures too close to the interstitial portion of the tube (Fig. 5.23C). Serosal stitches are applied as in Straussman's Metroplasty (Fig. 5.21E). It is important here to avoid traumatizing the myometrium and also avoid taking the endometrium with myometrium where ever possible.

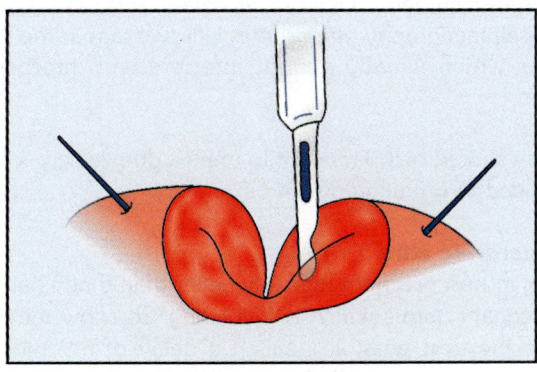

Fig. 5.23B: Incision of septum

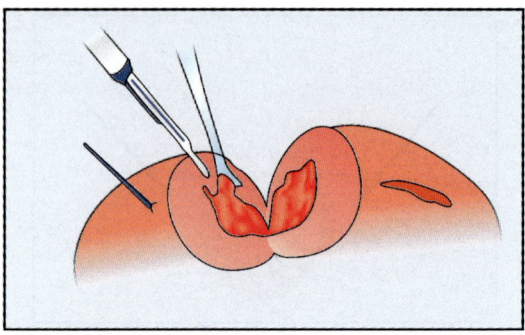

Fig. 5.23C: Reapproxmation of myometrium

Advantages
1. Simpler than Jones metroplasty
2. Conserves all myometrial tissue, leaving uterotubal junction in a more normal and lateral position
3. Provides better results than Jones metroplasty
   Many also include modified uterine suspension or plication of the round ligament to provide uterine support

Result: The final size of the cavity seems to be unimportant for reproductive capability and it is often smaller than normal. The uterine symmetry is a more important factor. Post operative hysterosalpingography often shows left over tags in the form of dogears which usually do not interfere with reproductive function.

There should be no attempt to unify a double cervix as it will lead to an incompetent os.

Postoperative care
Healing in non pregnant uterus is better than that what occurs in a pregnant uterus which is involuting. To allow the uterine incision the best possible healing a delay of 6-9 months in pregnancy is recommended.

Contraception: It is inadvisable to prescribe oral contraceptives because of their progestational effect on the myometrium and the possibility that healing under this circumstance would be similar to postpartum healing and lead to adhesion formation. Hence, barrier method with condom is recommended.

Mode of Delivery After Metroplasty

Patient should have cesarean section after metroplasty. However successful vaginal deliveries have been reported as the scar has excellent healing.

Class VI: Arcuate

This type of uterus is essentially normal in shape with a small, midline indentation in the uterine fundus which results from failure to completely dissolve the median septurn. This is given a distinct classification because it does not seem to have any negative effects on pregnancy.

Class VII: DES related

The daughters of mothers exposed to diethylstilbestrol (DES) during pregnancy are predisposed to uterine abnormalities. Two-thirds have abnormalities including a small, incompletely formed uterus ("hypoplastic"), a T-shaped cavity and 50% have cervical defects. There was a higher rate of primary infertility among exposed women (16% vs 6%).[37]

Treatment: Metroplasty is recommended for patients with T shaped uterus who have not achieved a successful pregnancy outcome. Using a slight modification of Straussman procedure, the center part of the crossbar of the T is unroofed and uterus is reunited in the midline, creating a symmetrical I shaped cavity. Lateral metroplasty may be required and has been done hysteroscopically.

Congenital uterine anomalies are often present in the infertile women but may not be the cause of infertility. These should only be treated if no other cause can be determined. They are, however an important cause of recurrent pregnancy loss.

REFERENCES

1. Greiss FC, Mauzy CH, Genital anomalies in women: an evaluation of diagnosis, incidence and obstetric performance. Am J Obstet Gynecol 1961; 82: 330.
2. Nahum GG. Uterine anomalies: how common are they, and what is their distribution among subtypes? J Reprod Med 1998; 43:877-87.
3. Rock JA: Surgery for anomalies of the Mullerian ducts. In: Tompson JD, Rock JA, eds. TeLind's Operative Gynecology. 9th ed. Philadelphia, Pa: JB Lippincott Williams and Wilkins; 2003; 705.
4. Chang AS, Siegel CL, Moley KH, Ratts VS, Odem RR. Septate uterus with cervical duplication and longitudinal vaginal septum: a report of five new cases. Fertil Steril. 2004; 81(4):1133-6.
5. Pavone ME, King JA, Vlahos N. Septate uterus with cervical duplication and a longitudinal vaginal septum: a Mullerian anomaly without a classification. Fertil Steril. 2006; 85(2):494.
6. Nickerson CW. Infertility and uterine contour. Am J Obstet Gynecol 1977; 129: 268.
7. Sorensen SS. Minor Mullerian anomalies and oligomenorrhea in infertile women: a new syndrome. Am J Obstet Gynecol 1981; 140: 6.
8. Raga F, Bauset C, Remohi J, Bonilla-Musoles F, Simon C, Pellicer A. Reproductive impact of congenital Mullerian anomalies Hum Reprod. 1997; 12(10):2277-81.
9. Michalas SP. Outcome of pregnancy in females with uterine malformations. Int J Gynecol Obstet 1991; 35: 215-9.
10. Stein AL, March CM. Pregnancy outcome in females with Mullerian duct anomalies. Journal of Reproductive Medicine 1999; 35(4): 411-4.
11. Heinonen PK. Clinical implications of unicornuate uterus with rudimentary horn. Int J Gynecol Obstet 1983; 21:145-50.
12. Sheth SS, Sonkawde R. Uterine septum misdiagnosed on hysterosalpingogram. Int J Gynaecol Obstet 2000; 69(3): 261-3.

13. Wu MH, Hsu CC, Huang KE. Detection of congenital Mullerian duct anomalies using three-dimensional ultrasound. J Clin Ultrasound 1997; 25(9):487-92.

14. Raga, F, Bonilla-Musoles, F, Osborne, N, Casañ, E, Klein, O, Bonilla, F Congenital Müllerian anomalies: a review of currently available imaging modalities. Ultrasound Rev Obstet Gynecol 2002; 2:56-67.

15. Forstner R, Hricak H. Congenital malformations of uterus and vagina. Radiologe 1994; 34(7):397-404.

16. Marten K, Vosshenrich R, Funke M, et al. MRI in the evaluation of Mullerian duct anomalies. Clin Imaging 2003; 27(5):346-50.

17. ACOG: American College of Obstetrics and Gynecology committee opinion. Nonsurgical diagnosis and management of vaginal agenesis. Number 274, July 2002. Committee on Adolescent Health Care. American College of Obstetrics and Gynecology. Int J Gynaecol Obstet 2002; 79(2):167-70.

18. Lindenman E, Shepard MK, Pescovitz OH. Mullerian agenesis: an update. Obstet Gynecol 1997; 90(2):307-12.

19. Noguchi S, Nakatsuka M, Sugiyama Y, et al. Use of artificial dermis and recombinant basic fibroblast growth factor for creating a neovagina in a patient with Mayer-Rokitansky-Kuster-Hauser syndrome. Hum Reprod 2004; 19(7):1629-32.

20. Motoyama S, Laoag-Fernandez JB, Mochizuki S, et al. Vaginoplasty with Interceed absorbable adhesion barrier for complete squamous epithelialization in vaginal agenesis. Am J Obstet Gynecol 2003; 188(5):1260-4.

21. Brun JL, Belleannee G, Grafeille N, et al. Long-term results after neovagina creation in Mayer-Rokitanski-Kuster-Hauser syndrome by Vecchietti's operation. Eur J Obstet Gynecol Reprod Biol 2002; 103(2):168-72.

22. Grimbizis GF, Camus M, Tarlatzis BC, et al. Clinical implications of uterine malformations and hysteroscopic treatment results. Hum Reprod Update 2001; 7(2):161-74.

23. Brody JM, Koelliker SL, Frishman GN. Unicornuate uterus: imaging appearance, associated anomalies and clinical implications. Am J Roentgenol 1998; 171:1341-7.

24. Rock JA, Schlaff WD. The obstetric consequences of uterovaginal anomalies. Fertil Steril 1985; 43(5):681-92.

25. Rock JA, Jones HW Jr. The clinical management of the double uterus. Fertil Steril 1977; 28(8):798-806.

26. The American Fertility Society. "The AFS classifications of adnexal adhesions, distal tube occlusion, tubal occlusion secondary to tubal ligation, tubal pregnancies, Mullerian anomalies and interuterine adhesions." Fertility and Sterility 1988; 49:944.

27. Donnez J, Nisolle M. Endoscopic laser treatment of uterine malformations. Hum Reprod 1997; 12(7):1381-7.

28. Cutner A, Saridogan E, Hart R, et al. Laparoscopic management of pregnancies occurring in non-communicating accessory uterine horns. Eur J Obstet Gynecol Reprod Biol 2004; 113(1):106-9.

29. Golan A, Langer R, Bukovsky I, Caspi E. Congenital anomalies of the Mullerian system. Fertil Steril 1989; 51(5):747-55.

30. Hinckley MD, Milki AA. Management of uterus didelphys, obstructed hemivagina and ipsilateral renal agenesis. A case report. J Reprod Med 2003; 48(8):649-51.

31. Stassart JP, Nagel TC, Prem KA, Phipps WR. Uterus didelphys, obstructed hemivagina, and ipsilateral renal agenesis: the University of Minnesota experience. Fertil Steril 1992; 57(4):756-61.

32. Buttram VC Jr, Reiter RC. Uterine anomalies. In surgical treatment of the infertile female. Baltimore: William and Wilkin 1985; 149-99.

33. Straussman EO: Fertility and unification of double uterus. Fertil Steril 1966; 17(2):165-76.

34. Lolis DE, Paschopoulos M, Makrydimas G, et. Reproductive outcome after Strassmann metroplasty in women with a bicornuate uterus. J Reprod Med 2005; 50(5):297-301.

35. Simon C, Martinez L, Pardo F, Tortajada M, Pellicer A. Mullerian defects in women with normal reproductive outcome. Fertil Steril 1991; 56:1192-3.

36. Musich JR, Behrman SJ. Obstetric outcome before and after metroplasty in females with uterine anomalies. Obstet and Gynecol 1978; 52(1):63-5.

37. Herbst AL, Hubby MM, Azizi F, Makii MM. Reproductive and gynecological surgical experience in diethylstilbestrol exposed daughters. Am J Obstet Gynecol 1981;141:1019- 28.

CHAPTER 6

Intrauterine Adhesions

Surveen Ghumman

The exact incidence of infertility caused by endometrium and structural abnormalities is unknown but it is thought to be 5 to 10%. Intrauterine adhesions are found frequently in patients with reproductive problems and after various types of uterine trauma. They are seen in 15 to 32% infertile patients more so in secondary infertility.

Adhesions are avascular strands of fibrous tissue with varying amount of white cell infiltration but can consist of inactive endometrium or myometrium. They usually connect the uterine walls anteroposteriorly but also may be seen as transverse bands. Shelf like protrusion from one wall is also known. Three types of adhesions have been described on histopathology: endometrial (65%), fibrous (25%) and muscular (10%), according to whether the cellular makeup of adhesion is endometrial, fibroblasts or myometrial. Vascular dense myometrial adhesions occur most often after myomectomy, intrauterine laser surgery or electrosurgical procedure. The evolution of adhesions following curettage involves a change in adhesions from thin endometrial strands to thick fibrous bands. The postulated mechanism for progression of adhesions is that adhesions limit uterine muscular activity and thereby cause reduced perfusion of estrogen to the endometrium, leading to atrophy.

ETIOLOGY

1. *Endometrial trauma* (Table 6.1)
   - Postpartum curettage or curettage for missed or incomplete abortion or hydatiform mole –The frequency of intrauterine adhesions following postpartum curettage varies greatly depending on the time during peurperium when curettage is performed. While the first 48 hours are a time of relative resistance to post-curettage adhesion formation , the uterus is especially vulnerable during the second to fourth week.[1] The reason for this has been postulated that:

i. The softness of the gravid uterus permits injury to the basalis layer of the endometrium.

ii. Damage to the basalis layer hinders endometrial regeneration and thus permits adherence to the opposing walls.

iii. The post-abortal or postpartum uterus undergoes titanic contractions which maintain the walls in apposition.

iv. The cleavage between the superficial and basal layers occurs more easily in pregnancy thus permitting surface denudation.

- Post-surgical adhesions: Cesarean section, myomectomy, hysterotomy, metroplasty
- Caustic abortifacients
- Uterine packing

2. *Infections:* Infection like tuberculosis or schistosomiasis can cause intrauterine adhesions.

3. *Pelvic irradiation*

4. *Estrogen deficient states*: Estrogen deficient states like lactation or hypogonadotropic gonadism where endometrial proliferation is delayed.

5. *Poor uterine blood flow*: Poor uterine blood flow leading to deficient endometrial nutrition and reduced steroid stimulation may promote adhesions formation.

6. *Missed abortion*: Retained placental remnants in missed abortion may induce fibroblastic activity and collagen formation before endometrial regeneration has taken place.

Table 6.1: Frequency of intrauterine adhesions after curettage for different indications

Indication	Percentage
Incomplete abortion[1]	6.4
Elective abortion[2]	22.9
Any postpartum hemorrhage[2]	3.7
Late postpartum hemorrhage[2]	23.4
Missed abortion[1]	30.9

It was hypothesized that sustained myometrial contractions could cause narrowing of the isthmus resulting in adhesions between the apposing endometrial surfaces. Trauma to the basal layer of endometrium results in granulation tissue that persists for several days. If granulation tissue from opposing walls is joined forming a bridge of tissue this may become infiltrated by myometrium and covered by endometrium.

Presenting Symptoms

1. *Menstrual complaints:* Menstrual complaints may be oligomenorrhea, amenorrhea, cryptomenorrhea. The menstrual pattern correlates well with extent of intrauterine adhesions and may be present in 60% of patients. Secondary amenorrhea can be due to complete obliteration of the uterine cavity or stenosis or atresia of internal os. Oligomenorrhea may be due to reduction in endometrial bleeding area and possible atrophic changes and unresponsiveness of the endometrium.
2. *Infertility:* It may be caused due to occlusion of tubal ostia or cervical canal which impede sperm migration or due to unsuitable endometrial environment for the blastocyst implantation.
3. *Recurrent abortion, preterm delivery or intrauterine death:* They may occur due to reduced uterine cavity, deficient endometrium, myometrial fibrosis and reduced uterine blood flow.
4. *Placental abnormalities:* Placental abnormalities like placenta previa, placenta accreta, increta and percreta may be occur. Placental adherence can be due to a defective basalis layer that allows invasion of trophoblasts into the myometrium.

Signs

1. Failure to bleed after estrogen progestogen withdrawal.
2. Inability to pass the uterine sound due to endocervical canal scarring or uterine cavity obliteration.
3. Presence of fibrosis in an endometrial biopsy.

Investigation

1. *Ultrasonography:* Thin cavity lining or calcification is suggestive of scarring. A well developed endometrial stripe is reason to recommend further surgery. The sensitivity of sonohysterography and hysterosalpingography in the diagnosis of intrauterine adhesions was high. Sonohysterography showed complete correlation with hysterosalpingography[3] (Fig. 6.1).

2. *Hysterosalpingography (HSG):* HSG is an excellent screening procedure where if findings are normal, hysteroscopy need not be performed. HSG is considered a relatively inexpensive procedure which provides important information of endocervical canal, uterine cavity and the fallopian tube. Single or multiple lacunar shaped filling defects are seen within the endometrial cavity. The defects are irregular, angular and often have faceted margins. The adhesions may obliterate the cavity or present as a fuzzy margin at the edge of the endometrial cavity (Fig. 6.2). These may be centrally or peripherally located, are irregular in shape and must present on each film to enable differentiation from polyp. In some patients the cavity may be obliterated

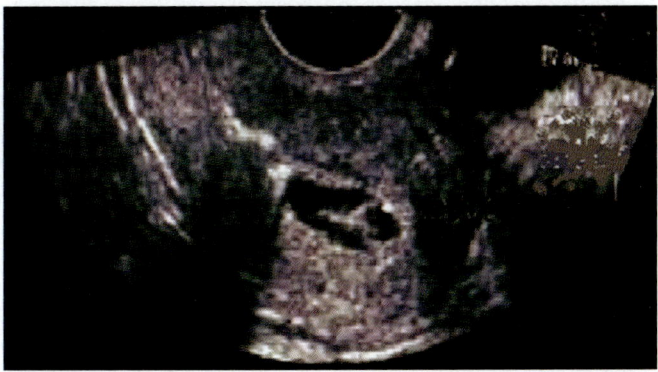

Fig. 6.1: Sonohysterography showing intrauterine adhesions

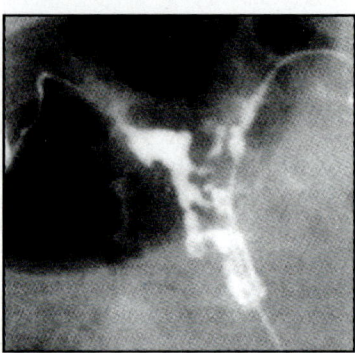

Fig. 6.2: Intrauterine adhesions showing irregular cavity

completely (Fig. 6.3). The degree of severity can be classified according to HSG findings (Table 6.2). Technical problems such as patulous cervix may prevent adequate uterine distension falsely suggesting presence of intrauterine adhesions in a normal cavity. Contrast should be instilled slowly with visualization of cavity under fluoroscopy with image intensification. Only 2 ml of dye should be instilled so as not to obscure the view. If adhesions are quite extensive extravasations of contrast material may occur. There is a good correlation between the extent of intrauterine adhesions as judged by HSG and the amount detected by hysteroscopy.

Table 6.2: Intrauterine synechiae classification by hysterosalpingography according to Toaff and Ballas[4]

Grade	HSG finding
Grade I	Small defect well inside the uterus
Grade II	Medium sized defect occupying one-fifth of the uterine cavity
Grade III	Several defects involving one-third of the cavity, which is asymmetric because of marginal adhesions
Grade IV	Intrauterine adhesions showing irregular cavity

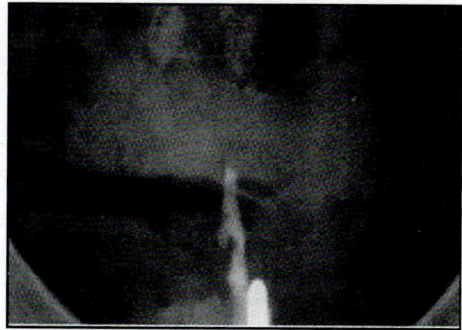

Fig. 6.3: Contracted uterine cavity due to adhesions

3. *Magnetic resonance imaging (MRI):* MRI may have a role supplementary to conventional studies in the evaluation of intrauterine synechiae. MRI is a sensitive method to diagnose a variety of gynecologic conditions. Uterine anatomy may be accurately imaged with MRI providing a noninvasive method to assess both myometrial and endometrial architecture.[5]

4. *Hysteroscopy:* The definitive diagnosis of intrauterine adhesions can only be made on hysteroscopy. A classification based on direct inspection of adhesions is developed to record extent and location of disease (Tables 6.3 and 6.4).

On making a comparison between hysteroscopy and hysterosalpingography, hysteroscopy gives a more definitive and accurate diagnosis because of direct visualization (Table 6.5).

TREATMENT OF INTRAUTERINE ADHESIONS

Transhysteroscopic Lysis of Synechiae (see Chapter 7)

Transhysteroscopic lysis of synechiae under direct visualization is the preferred therapeutic modality. Treatment consists of lysis of adhesion under direct vision by hysteroscope.

Table 6.3: Classification of intrauterine adhesions by hysteroscopic findings[6]

Class	Findings
Severe	• More than three fourths of the cavity involved • Agglutination of the walls or thick bands • Ostial area and upper cavity occluded
Moderate	• One-fourth to three-fourths of uterine cavity involved • No agglutination of the walls, adhesions only • Ostial areas and upper fundus only partially occluded
Minimal	• Less than one-fourth of uterine cavity involved • Thin or flimsy adhesions • Ostial areas and upper fundus minimally involved or clear

Treatment Objective

1. Restore uterine architecture to normal by lysis of adhesions under direct vision.
2. To prevent readherence of the uterine wall with use of intrauterine splint.
3. To provide stimulation of endometrial growth over the freshly dissected surfaces with use of postoperative high dose estrogen for a period of two months
4. To verify that the uterine cavity is normal prior to permitting the patient to attempt to conceive with a follow-up hysteroscopy.

Time of surgery: It is done in the follicular phase if patient is menstruating as endometrium is thin and field of vision is much clearer inside the uterus.

Anesthesia: Minimal disease can be done under local anesthesia utilizing a paracervical block and a narcotic administered intravenously. In case of severe disease general anesthesia is given as one may require simultaneous laparoscopy.

Table 6.4: American Fertility Society Classification of intrauterine adhesions

Patients name _____ Date _____

Age ___ G ___ P ___ Sp Ab ___ VTP ____ Ectopic ____ Infertile ___

Other specific history (i.e. surgery, infection, etc) _____

_____

HSG ____ Sonography ____ Photography ____ Laparoscopy ____
Laparotomy ____

Extent of cavity involved	< 1/3	1/3 – 2/3	>2/3
	1	2	4
Type of adhesion	Filmy	Filmy and dense	Dense
	1	2	4
Menstrual pattern	Normal	Hypomenorrhea	Amenorrhea
	1	2	4

Prognostic classification	HSG score	Hysteroscopy score	Additional findings
Stage I (Mild) 1-4	_____	_____	_____
Stage II (Moderate) 5-8	_____	_____	_____
Stage III (Severe) 9-12	_____	_____	_____

All adhesions should be considered dense   DRAWING
Treatment (Surgical procedures) _____

_____

_____

_____

Prognosis for conception and subsequent viable infant
_____ Excellent (>75%)
_____ Good (50 – 75%)
_____ Fair (25 – 50%)
_____ Poor (< 25%)

Physician's judgment based upon tubal patency
Recommended follow-up treatment ____

_____

HSG finding

Hysteroscopy finding

	Hysteroscopy	Hysterosalpingography
	Table 6.5: Comparison of hysteroscopy and hysterosalpingography	
Visualization	Direct	Indirect
Diagnosis	Definitive	Presumptive
Localization	Accurate	Fair
Morbidity	Low	Low
Cost	Moderate	Low
Role	Diagnosis/treatment	Diagnosis
Other data	None	Tubal status

Technique: A 7 to 9 mm hysteroscope is used. The resectoscope features a 90° wire loop attached to an electric generator. A right angled point electrode, Collins electrical knife or a twizzle may be used. The line of the incision is always in the horizontal axis of the uterus, keeping one cm away from the tubal ostia as the uppermost limit of hystero-adhesiolysis. Lateral incisions may be made if necessary. If on advancing the hysteroscope no landmarks are seen in the uterine cavity a concurrent laparoscopy is performed. If the cutting bipolar electrode tends to cut inside the myometrium the light from the microhysteroscope will shine through the serosa and can be seen laparoscopically. Hence, plane of instruments is changed before perforation takes place. Flexible or semi-rigid scissors can be used to divide each adhesive band in its center. Adhesions should not be excised. Incision is begun inferiorly and carried cephalad. The central incision should be approached first regardless of density. Once the outline of the uterine cavity can be delineated, marginal and sidewall adhesions are be approached. Stabilizing the endoscopic camera in left hand and rotating the operating microscope with right hand giving small incision without damaging the myometrium is the key to success.

Indications of laparoscopy during hysteroscopic resection:
1. Difficulty in negotiating internal OS
2. Extensive adhesions where lysis may be difficult
3. Non-visualization of any landmarks within the uterine cavity.

Sometimes more than one surgery is needed to resect all the adhesions.

Endometrial polyps up to 1.5 cm, pedunculated submucous myomas up to 1.0 cm as well as adhesions obliterating no more than 1/3rd of uterine cavity can be managed as "see and treat" procedures with a high compliance of the patients without preoperative analgesia or anesthesia.

Adhesions should be incised not resected as there are more chances of repeat adhesion forming after resection.

Other methods include electrosurgical or Nd:YAG laser. Coagulating current which causes charring and adhesion formation is not appropriate. Scars are avascular and if dissection is in the proper plane, bleeding does not occur. Since the use of laser or resectoscope show no advantage over scissors they are not preferred in the treatment of intrauterine adhesions.

Hysterotomy may be necessary in patients with extensive adhesions involving the endocervical canal and the lower uterine segment thus preventing access to the fundus. Presurgical sonography is essential to verify that some normal endometrium is present. It allows the surgeon to plan the site of entry into the uterus. The adhesions in the lower uterine segment and endocervical canal are disrupted from above with a dilator and a small Foley's catheter is passed into the uterus. The stem of the catheter is passed into the vagina to splint the endocervical canal.

The nature of intrauterine synechiae associated with tuberculosis is invariably dense and cohesive. Finding the appropriate cleavage plane during hysteroscopic lysis may prove to be technically difficult with unavoidable myometrial damage. In addition, accidental uterine perforation may occur.

Caution: GnRH analogues are not used prior to surgery as they would lead to a hypoestrogenic state where reformation of adhesions might take place.

Postoperative Care

1. *Foley's catheter or intrauterine contraceptive device (IUD) insertion*: Postoperatively an IUD is inserted in the uterine cavity and retained for two months to keep the raw dissected surfaces separated during the initial healing phase and prevent adhesion formation. The rate of reformation of adhesions decreased from 50% to 10% on placement of IUD.[7] The T shaped IUDs may have too small a surface area to prevent adhesion reformation and those containing copper may induce excessive inflammatory reaction. So copper must be removed or a loop IUD is recommended. A Foley's catheter 8F with a 3 ml balloon or a special silastic balloon can be used. The balloon is inflated and catheter kept in place for 7 days with antibiotic coverage. In comparison to IUD group the Foley's catheter group showed better results in terms of restoration of normal menses, (81.4 vs. 62.7%) and the conception rate (33.9 vs. 22.5%). The need for repeated treatment was also significantly less in the Foley's catheter group. The Foley's catheter, thus is a safer and more effective adjunctive method of treatment of intrauterine adhesions compared with the IUD.[8]

2. *Estrogens*: Conjugated estrogens are given in the dose of 2.5 mg twice daily for 60 days adding medroxy progesterone acetate 10 mg in the last 5 days. High dose sequential estrogen progestin treatment maximally stimulates the endometrium so that the scarred surfaces are re-epithelialized. Following withdrawal bleeding the IUD is removed.

3. *Repeat hysteroscopy*: The adequacy of therapy should be assessed accurately by repeat hysteroscopy or HSG following steroid induced withdrawal bleeding. Importance

of postoperative study to verify normalcy of the cavity prior to permitting conception cannot be overemphasized. Complications like placenta accrete were absent in cases where complete resolution of adhesions had taken place. There was an incidence of 5% to 35% of these complications where the cavity had not been assessed.

Hence hysteroscopy is useful to establish diagnosis, assess the severity of the lesion and enable complete lysis. This safer and more accurate technique, results in a gestational outcome that surpasses what was achieved by earlier therapeutic regimes and should replace all other treatment modalities like D and C for management of intrauterine adhesions.

Results

In terms of outcome of improvement in periods, pregnancy and reduction in abortion rate, the prognostic score depends on
- Actual amount of healthy endometrial lining.
- Success in restoring anatomic cavity volume to normal.
- Quality of endometrial lining, thin, thick, infected, shaggy or unhealthy.
- Other associated factors detected on laparoscopy.
1. Normal menstruation was resumed in 80% of cases with hypomenorrhea.
2. Follow-up hysteroscopy showed normal findings in 90% cases.
3. Pregnancy rate after hysteroscopic treatment of intrauterine adhesions: Pregnancy rates vary from 28.7 to 53.6%.[9] The initial severity of the adhesions appears to correlate best with the reproductive outcome.[10] Pregnancy index rate after the procedure was 43.8%, and the live birth rate was 32.8%. In patients 35 years of age or younger, 20 of 30 (66.6%) conceived compared with 8 of 34 (23.5%) in patients older

than 35 years. Age is an important predictive factor of success. The subsequent pregnancies also showed an increased risk of abnormal placentation.[11]

4. *Reformation:* In tuberculosis adhesion reformation rate of 50% has been reported.[10] The recurrence rate for severe adhesions was 48.9% and decreased to 35% after repeated treatment.[12]

Abdominal Metroplasty

Only in severe cases where uterine cavity is inaccessible by hysteroscope abdominal metroplasty may need to be done.

Anticipation and suspicion are critical aspects to any discussion on intrauterine adhesions. Infertility, recurrent abortions or menstrual aberration after any uterine trauma should cause the physician to suspect the presence of intrauterine adhesions. Primary prevention is only possible through avoidance of forced intrauterine interventions, especially in post-gravid uterus. HSG and hysteroscopy are the ideal methods for making a diagnosis of intrauterine adhesions. The safest, least traumatic and most precise treatment is hysteroscopic lysis. The addition of intrauterine splint and high dose estrogen therapy completes the therapeutic approach.

ENDOMETRIAL RECEPTIVITY

Endometrial receptivity can be defined as the histological and molecular changes occurring in a temporal and spatial manner in the endometrium so as to facilitate embryonic implantation. Under the influence of estrogen and progesterone, the endometrium undergoes these important changes so as to make it receptive to the implanting embryo. The ability of the decidua to respond optimally to the invading trophoblasts is determined by endocrine and endorgan interactions that long proceed ovulation. There are many causes of poor endometrial response.

Causes of Poor Endometrial Response

There can be many causes:
1. Postpartum endometritis
2. Uterine synechiea
3. D and C
4. Genital tuberculosis
5. Multiple leiomyoma
6. Squamous metaplasia of endometrium
7. Hyperprolactinemia
8. Elderly patient
9. With drugs like clomiphene

Tests to Assess Uterine Receptivity (see Chapter 1)

Treatment of Poor Uterine Receptivity

A step-wise protocol is followed for management of patients with persistently poor endometrial receptivity (Fig. 6.4).

Estrogens

Where endometrial response is suboptimal treatment is given by supplementing estrogen.
1. *Ethinyl estradiol* 0.05 mg/day from day 7 to 12.
2. *Premarin* 0.325 mg/day from day 7 to 12.
3. *Estradiol valerate* 2-8 mg from day 7 for 5 days or till plasma estradiol is 400-700 pg/ml.
4. *Vaginal estradiol* 0.1mg twice a day can be given from day 8.[12]

Change of Drug

Letrozole: If patients is on clomiphene one can change to letrozole which does not have an antiestrogenic effect on the endometrium because of its short half life and absence of estrogen receptor depletion.

Tamoxifen: It causes a raised estrogen levels due to multifollicular development and a direct action on the ovaries to enhance estrogen production, hence leading to a favorable response on the cervical mucus and endometrium. It is an alternative to clomiphene where there is persistently poor endometrial response.

Drugs to Improve the Endometrial Blood Flow

1. *Low dose aspirin*—Asprin 75 mg/day has also shown favorable results.
2. *Sildenafil*—Sildenafil in a dose of 25 mg four times a day intravaginally for 3-10 days has helped to improve endometrial receptivity. It should be used with caution as it has side effects like headache, hypertension and occasional death.[13]
3. *Nitroglycerine*—Nitroglycerine because of it vasodilating effect, is given in a dose of 800 ug sublingually 3 min before embryo transfer in IVF or 5 mg daily patch on day of ET and then daily.
4. *L-arginine*—L-arginine NO is formed from L-Arginine and leads to increased vascularity of ovarian follicle and better blood flow.

Immunosuppression

Treatment regimes involving administration of IVIG (intravenous immunoglobulin) and LITT (leukocyte immunotherapy)—whereby injecting paternal/donor leucocytes into the mother an attempt is made to alter the maternal immune response, thus making it favorable for implantation. Currently there is no consensus of opinion on either of these treatments.

Reducing Uterine Contractility

1. *Ritodrine*—Administration of this drug has shown better pregnancy rate in randomised controlled trials.
2. *Piroxicam*—10 mg of piroxicam given 1-2 hours before embryo transfer shows improvement in pregnancy rate.

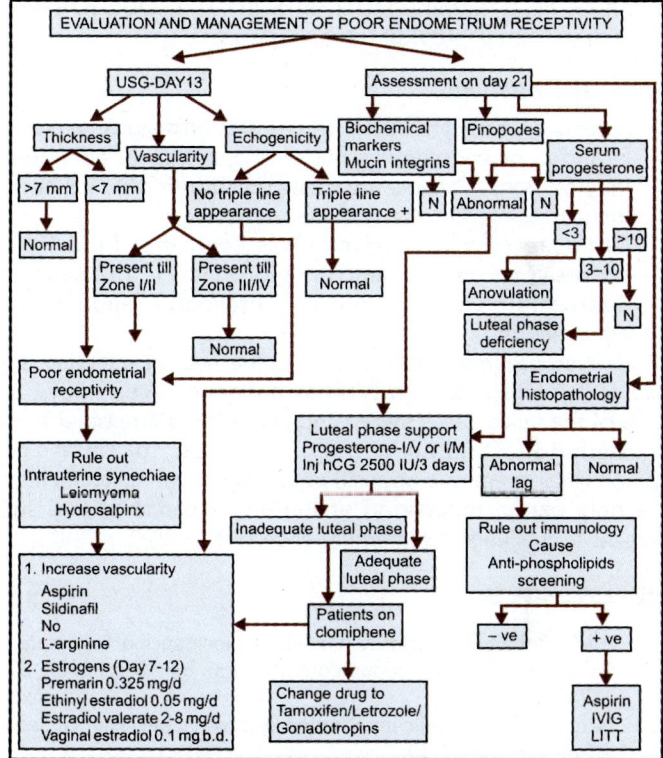

Fig. 6.4: Evaluation and management of poor
endometrium receptivity

Luteal Phase Support

1. *Progesterone:* Micronised progesterone can be given orally,
   per vaginum or per rectal in a dose of 200-400 mg in 2
   divided doses . However, the intramuscular route is preferred
   as progesterone levels are more sustained, in a dose of
   50-100 mg daily. Dyhydrogesterone can also be given in
   a dose of 20-30 mg/day.

2. *HCG:* HCG administration in a dose of 2500 IU every 3 days would provide luteal support.

Surgical Treatment

1. *Lysis of uterine synechiea:* In cases of adhesions following D and C or endometritis hysteroscopic lysis of adhesions may be done. Patients are treated with estrogens following this to regenerate the endometrium.
2. *Drainage of hydrosalpinx:* It is seen that fluid from hydrosalpinx impairs implantation. Hence, drainage of hydrosalpix can be done by ultrasound guidance or laparoscopically.

Despite progress and research in the field of infertility the rate of live birth rate with IVF has not gone beyond 30%. In 75% of the failed cases there is no cause for failure other than implantation forming a major obstacle to ART. The complexities of embryo apposition to invasion of the epithelium are only partly understood at the molecular level and still present a challenge to infertility specialist.

REFERENCES

1. Adoni A, Palti Z, Milwidsky A, et al. The incidence of intrauterine adhesions following spontaneous abortion. Int J Fertil 1982; 27: 117-8.
2. Bergman P. Traumatic intrauterine lesions . Acta Obstet Gynecol Scand 1961; 40: 1-39.
3. Bruno Salle, MD, Pascal Gaucherand, MD, Pierre de Saint Hilaire, MD, Rene Charles Rudigoz, MD Transvaginal sonohysterographic evaluation of intrauterine adhesions. Journal of Ultrasound 1999; 27:131-4.
4. Toaff R, Ballas S Traumatic hypomenorrhea-amenorrhea (Asherman's syndrome) Fertil Steril 1978;30:379.
5. Letterie GS, Haggerty MF. Magnetic resonance imaging of intrauterine synechiae. Gynecol Obstet Invest. 1994;37(1):66-8
6. March CM, Israel R, March AD. Hysteroscopic management of intrauterine adhesions. Am J Obstet Gynecol 1978; 30:653.
7. Polishuk WZ, Adoni A, Aviad I. Intrauterine device in treatment of traumatic intrauterine adhesions. Fertil Steril 1969;20:241 – 9.

8. Orhue AA, Aziken ME, Igbefoh JO. A comparison of two adjunctive treatments for intrauterine adhesions following lysis. Int J Gynaecol Obstet 2003 Jul;82(1):49-56

9. Pace S, Stentella P, Catania R, Palazzetti PL, Frega A. Endoscopic treatment of intrauterine adhesions. Clin Exp Obstet Gynecol 2003;30(1):26-8.

10. Pabuccu R, Atay V, Orhon E, Urman B, Ergun A. Hysteroscopic treatment of intrauterine adhesions is safe and effective in the restoration of normal menstruation and fertility. Fertil Steril. 1997;68(6):1141-3.

11. Fernandez H, Al-Najjar F, Chauveaud-Lambling A, Frydman R, Gervaise A. Fertility after treatment of Asherman's syndrome stage 3 and 4. J Minim Invasive Gynecol 2006;13(5):398-402.

12. Valle R, Sciarra J. Intrauterine adhesions: Hysteroscopic diagnosis, classification, treatment and reproductive outcome. Am J Obstet Gynecol 1988, 158, 1459–70.

13. Sher G, Fisch JD. Effect of vaginal sildenafil on the outcome of in vitro fertilization (IVF) after multiple IVF failures attributed to poor endometrial development Fertil Steril 2002;78 (5):1073-6.

CHAPTER 7

Hysteroscopic Infertility Surgery

Punita Bhardwaj

Intrauterine lesion can affect implantation in infertile women
The lesions most responsible are:
1. Intrauterine adhesions
2. Intrauterine septum
3. Submucus myoma or fibroid polyp

INTRAUTERINE ADHESIONS

Asherman's syndrome is the total or partial occlusion of the
endometrial cavity by adhesions. Ninety percent cases occur
following a pregnancy related curettage.

Incidence: Actual incidence of intrauterine adhesions is not
known as it is likely that some patients are asymptomatic and
have normal fertility and reproductive performance.

Antecedent factors: Antecedent factors responsible for
development of intrauterine adhesions are D & C after first
trimester abortion, PPH or hydatiform mole, Cesarean section,
metroplasty, myomectomy, infection such as endometrial
tuberculosis (Netter's syndrome), septic abortion and pelvic
radiation. If curettage is performed between 2nd and 4th weeks
following delivery or if curettage is performed because of missed
abortion the risk of IUA is extremely high as they are estrogen
deficient.

Symptoms: The symptoms would vary depending on the
degree of uterine cavity occlusion and type of adhesions. Patients
may present with amenorrhea, hypomenorrhea, oligomenorrhea dysmenorrhea, infertility, pregnancy wastage
including both 1st and 2nd trimester abortions, intrauterine
growth retardation, intrauterine fetal demise, errors of placental
implantation such as placenta accreta, increta and percreta.

Diagnosis: Definitive diagnosis is made by direct inspection
of the uterine cavity. Hysteroscopy and HSG should be
considered complementary rather than competing techniques.

One great value of hysteroscopy is that it allows classification
of intrauterine adhesions. Sonohysterography showed good
correlation with hysterosalpingography.[2]

MRI is also accurate in detecting intrauterine adhesions.[3]

Classification of Intrauterine adhesions: American Fertility Society classification of intrauterine adhesions has been discussed in Chapter.[6]

Technique *(see accompanying DVD ROM)*

Appropriate counseling is given and consent is taken. Hysteroscopy was performed in the follicular phase in the menstruating patients.

Anesthesia: General anesthesia was administered as they may require a laparoscopy to be done alongside.

Position: Patient positioned in the lithotomy position and draped in a sterile manner. The patient's thigh should be at a 90° angle to the pelvis in order to create enough space for the surgeon to manipulate the hysteroscope (provided simultaneous laparoscopy is not planned). The patient's perineum should be just past the edge of the table, with the coccyx and sacrum well supported on the flat surface of the table. The patient's legs should be supported in the leg stirrups to avoid any sudden movement which could cause nerve or muscle injury to the patient.

Cervical dilatation is done and hysteroscope introduced to the level of external os and advanced into the cavity. If cavity is not clearly delineated, laparoscopy is performed before proceeding further hysteroscopically. Pelvis is inspected and intensity of light source decreased. This is to guide the depth of adhesiolysis. Thinning of the myometrium allows the light from hysteroscope to shine brightly through the uterine serosa.

The cavity is inspected adhesions are identified and transected with scissors, knife or bipolar twizzle electrode. Bipolar twizzle electrode is the instrument of choice. The microhysteroscope does not require cervical dilatation (Non-electrolyte fluid media).

Adhesiolysis of dense circular intrauterine adhesions

Dense adhesions with circular fibrosis constricting the uterine wall may be seen in some cases (Fig 7.1). Laparoscopy is done along with hysteroscopic release of dense adhesions where there is danger of perforation (Fig. 7.2). Synechiae are released at the lateral walls (Figs 7.3 and 7.4). Gradual release of synechiae is done with short spurts of current being given as twizzle is touched to the tissue. Orientation to the cavity should remain the same throughout surgery with the camera remaining horizontal. Cavity after adhesiolysis is seen as in Figure 7.5.

Caution : Active electrode should always be in vision with movement towards the operator rather than away.

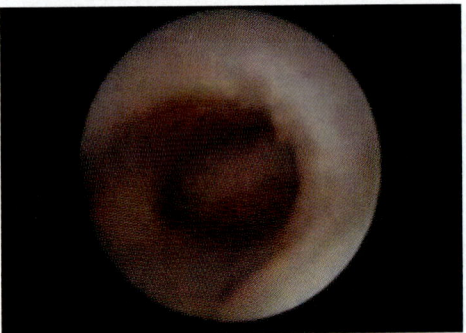

Fig. 7.1: Hysteroscopic view of circular fibrosis in the uterine cavity with constricting walls

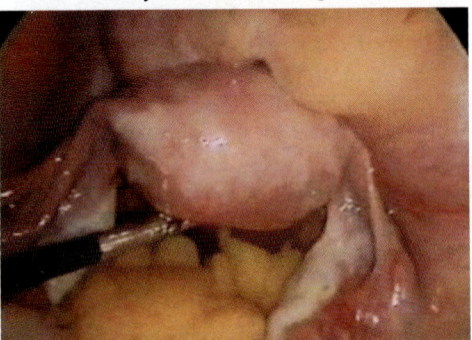

Fig. 7.2: Laparoscopy done with hysteroscopic resection in dense adhesions to avoid perforation

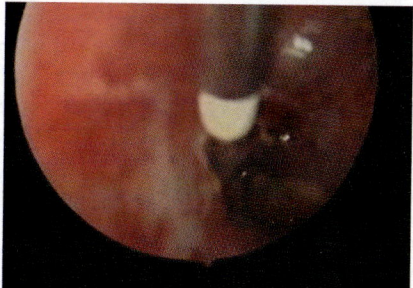

Fig. 7.3: Right lateral wall adhesions being released with the bipolar twizzle electrode

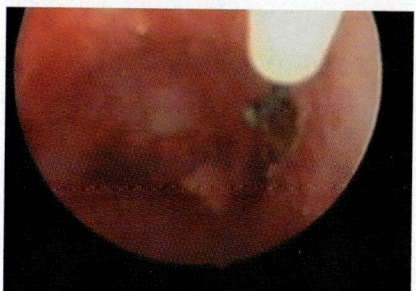

Fig. 7.4: Left lateral wall adhesions being released with the bipolar twizzle electrode

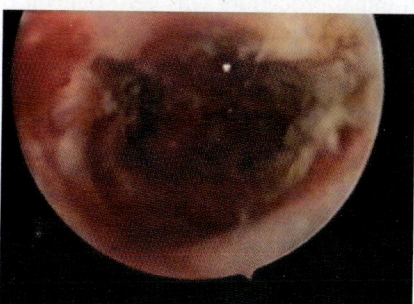

Fig. 7.5: Cavity after adhesiolysis

Intrauterine Mid Synechiae Adhesiolysis

Mid synechiae with bands extending from the anteroposterior walls is seen (Fig. 7.6). Both ostia should be visualized between adhesions if possible, (Fig. 7.7). Bipolar twizzle is used to release the synechiae in the center (Figs 7.8 and 7.9). Gradual release of synechiae is done with short bursts of energy given when twizzle touches the tissue. The uterine cavity regains its original dimension after adhesiolysis (Fig. 7.10).

Caution
1. Synechiolysis is done remaining at the center equidistant from the anterior and posterior walls to prevent perforation
2. Care should be taken not to injure the ostia or the lateral walls.

Methods to Prevent Readherence

Intrauterine device (IUD): An inert IUD is inserted and removed following withdrawal bleeding

Foley catheter: It is inserted into the uterine cavity for 5 days

Conjugated equine estrogen: 2.5 mg of conjugated equine estrogen are given daily for 60 days. Medroxy progesterone acetate 10 mg /day is added in the last 10 days.

Follow-up

Office hysteroscopy using CO_2 as distention media is done at follow-up. If initial procedure was very difficult or if persistent adhesions are suspected, follow-up is by hysteroscopy in an operating room. Some authors have reported normal findings on HSG studies in 90% of patients in follow-up. Prior to permission to conceive verification of normal uterine architecture is imperative.

Results: Hysteroscopic treatments results in an 88-98% return to normal cycles.[5] If no other infertility issues are present 79% of treated patients have normal pregnancies (75% of those with mild disease but only 31% with severe adhesions).[6,7]

Thus, hysteroscopy permits diagnoses, classification and therapy of intrauterine adhesions safely and accurately.

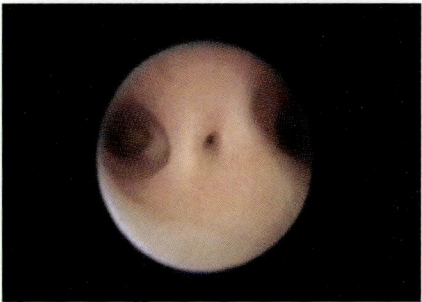

Fig. 7.6: Mid synecheia with thick band anteroposteriorly

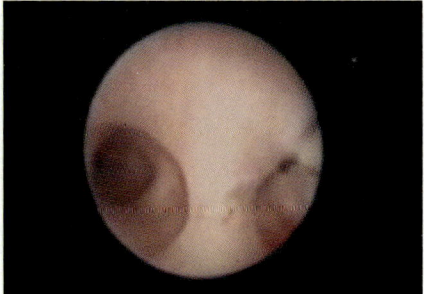

Fig. 7.7: Visualization of right ostia

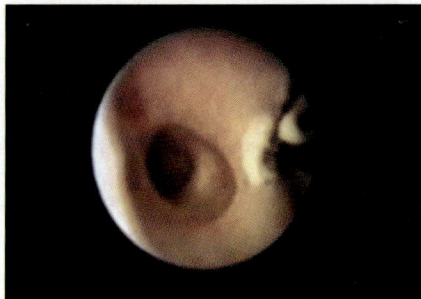

Fig. 7.8: Synechiae being released by bipolar twizzle at the middle

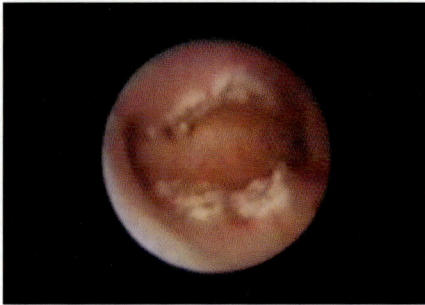

Fig. 7.9: Complete release of synechiae

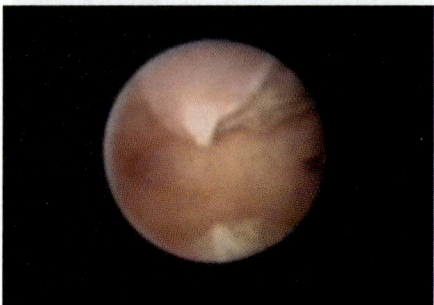

Fig. 7.10: Cavity after adhesiolysis

INTRAUTERINE SEPTA

Septate uterus is the most common structural abnormality of all Müllerian duct defects. It is found in 1.9 to 3% of the female population.[8] Septate uterus may be partial / complete.

Patients usually present with history of recurrent abortion. A complete infertility work-up is mandatory before surgical intervention for a uterine anomaly, so that other infertility factors can be ruled out. With the advent of operative hysteroscopy intrauterine septa are being diagnosed and treated hysteroscopically replacing other methods of therapy. Abdominal metroplasty is no longer done except in very thick septa.

Comparison of abdominal metroplasty and hysteroscopic incision of uterine septa

	Abdominal metroplasty	*Hysteroscopic incision*
Hospitalization	Yes	No
Surgery	Major	Minor
Avoid pregnancy	3-6 months	1 month
Delivery route	Cesarean section	Vaginal delivery

Prior to planning operative treatment laparoscopy is required to rule out bicornuate uterus which usually requires no treatment.

If septa is the only defect hysteroscopy is performed and incision accomplished easily with scissors, electro- surgically with knife or bipolar twizzle electrode to divide the septa in the center. Septa comprises of a fibroelastic band that retracts easily with only scanty bleeding.

Hysteroscopic Septal Excision

Hysteroscopic resection is the treatment of choice for septal resection.

Time: Hysteroscopic septal excision is carried out postmenstrually.

Technique

For transection of the septa a 120° scope is preferred. Three methods can be used.

1. First method uses the resectoscope with a loop electrode and blended current of 70-100 watts. The septum is transected until small areas of bleeding are seen which shows that myometrium has been reached. The intrauterine pressure should not be higher than mean areterial pressure as this may not allow bleeders to be seen easily.[9]

2. The second method uses a small scissors to transect the septa till small bleeding areas are seen The intrauterine pressure helps in expanding as it is cut.[10]

3. The third method uses a vaporizing electrode that can be used in isotonic sodium chloride solution.

The septum is removed rather than transected.

Narrow septa: For septa that are 3 cm or less wide at the top of the fundus, the incision is carried cephalad from the most inferior point of the septa and directed laterally as the most superior aspect of the uterus is approached.

Large wide septa: For patients with larger septa the incision is begun at the lower most portion of the septa and carried cephalad along one side until the margin is incised upto 0.5 cm from the junction with normal myometrium. The other lateral margin is incised alternately. Original very wide, V–shaped septum is converted to a broad notch between the tubal ostia. Finally the notch is incised beginning at one cornual recess and progressing to the other. Incision between muscle and septa junction causes a little bleeding, so this part of dissection is done at the end of the procedure so that blood loss is minimized and good view is maintained. The dissection is complete when the hysteroscope can move freely from one cornual recess to another without any obstruction. Both the ostia can be visualized even when the hysteroscope is in upper or middle fundus ; Laparoscopist observes that the entire uterus glows uniformly even when distal end of the hysteroscope is located in one cornual recess.

Postoperative Care

Conjugated estrogens 1.25 mg /d are prescribed for 25 days with MPA – 10 mg/ day the last 5 days of estrogen treatment.

Follow-up

Following first spontaneous bleed HSG/hysteroscopy is performed to verify that the cavity is normal.

Results: Reproductive success is significantly improved after hysteroscopic excision of the uterine septa to form a single cavity. There is significant improvement in the number of term deliveries from 4.3 to 81% after hysteroscopic.[10,11]

Performed with operative hysteroscopy, laparoscopy can also be used to improve the safety and efficiency of the procedure.

The value of hysteroscopic metroplasty had been proven in recurrent pregnancy loss. The role of metroplasty in primary infertility is controversial. It is an easy procedure with low morbidity potential and benefit of normal vaginal delivery.

SUBMUCOUS MYOMA AND POLYP (see Chapter 4)

COMPLICATIONS OF HYSTEROSCOPY

It is recommended that operative work is not carried out until the surgeon has become an expert in diagnostic hysteroscopy. An accepted rate for all complications during operative hysteroscopy is 3.8%.

Uterine Perforation

Perforation is the most common complication and complicates 1-2% of procedures. Approximately 50% occur during operator's first 3 cases.[12]

For any hysteroscopic procedure, the surgeon must have an understanding of uterine wall thickness. This allows the surgeon to manipulate the surgery based on the area of the uterus where he/she is operating (Table 7.1).

Table 7.1: Uterine wall thickness	
Location	*Range(mm)*
Anterior wall	17-25
Posterior wall	15-25
Fundus	15-22
Isthmus	8-12
Corpus	4-7

Perforation Occurs
- When dilating the cervix
- Introducing the hysteroscope
- During operative procedure
- During retrieval of tissue

Perforation occurs most easily at the cornual region which is the most difficult to resect and only 5 mm thick.

The depth of thermal damage is based on multiple factors, including degree of endometrial thinning, speed, pressure and duration of contact during motion and power setting Deaths have occurred resulting from trauma to intra-abdominal organs, infection and hemorrhage.

Diagnosis: Diagnosis is made on the basis of clinical suspicion and the following signs:

- Visualization of peritoneum or bowel
- Sudden loss of vision
- Rapid inflow of fluid distention media
- Abdominal distention.

Cervical laceration can occur during hysteroscopy. Prior cervical preparation with PGE2 helps in preventing it. Laminaria tent can be inserted when anticipating difficult cervical dilatation.

Management

1. *Observation:* Careful observation of the patient may be all that is required when uterine perforation occurs while dilating the cervix, introducing the hystero-scope and during retrieval of tissue. Perforation at the start of the procedure should be managed conser-vatively with surgery scheduled for sometime in the future. Positive findings on abdominal examination should be treated with suspicion, as perforation is not always recognized at the time of surgery.

2. *Laparoscopy:* If clinical signs of ongoing hemorrhage are detected then laparoscopy should be performed to define and treat the injury. Laparoscopy should also be performed when perforation occurs with the active electrode. The great danger at laparoscopy is of missing diathermy bowel injury with the patient presenting some days later with peritonitis. Laparotomy or even hysterectomy may be required in occasional cases.

3. *Laparotomy:* Laparotomy may be necessary to adequately assess and repair injury to major blood vessels bowel or urinary tract. It may be needed if bowel perforation is suspected but cannot be located at laparoscopy.

Hazards of Liquid Distention Media

Electolyte free solution is used in electrosurgery. Glycine, sorbitol, dextran 70 and dextrose 5% have all been used. These fluids do not conduct electric current and allow for better visualization when bleeding occurs.

Glycine 1.5% : Glycine 1.5% is most commonly used.It provides optically clear view, it is hypo-osmolar, has toxic metabolites and a depressant effect on the myocardium.

Dextran 70: Dextran 70 is viscous and difficult to work with. Dextran caramelizes and damages instruments if not cleaned immediately. The complications encountered are:

1. *Anaphylactic shock:* It occurs even when small volumes of dextran are intravasated.

2. *DIC:* As dextran reduce the number of clotting factors and decreases platelet adhesiveness.[13]

3. *Circulatory over load:* Dextran 70 is a volume expander with a high risk of pulmonary edema. With each 100 ml of Dextran 70 absorbed, the intravascular volume is increased by 800 ml Normal saline or Hartmann's solution are safer as these are isoosmolar but volume overload can still occur. Liquid media are absorbed or intravasated from the uterine cavity into the uterine vasculature as blood vessels are transected during the operative procedure. Transtubal intraabdominal absorption is probably of less significance as intraabdominal aspiration of fluid at laparoscopy does not seem to prevent complication. Running fluid balance should be maintained as standard practice irrespective of the procedure being performed.

Symptom: Overload symptoms include hypertension bradycardia, nausea, vomiting, visual disturbance, headache, hypotension, agitation, lethargy, confusion. Seizures, coma and death may follow if the syndrome is not recognized and treated appropriately.

Acute hyponatremia is less well tolerated by the body and death can occur when serum sodium is at a level of 120 mmol/l (Table 7.2). Patients with mild hyponatremia can deteriorate rapidly, resulting in seizures followed by respiratory arrest in a matter of minutes. Therefore, prompt treatment for hyponatremia is essential.

Table 7.2 : Stages of hyponatremia		
Stage	*Sodium level*	*Symptoms*
Mild	130 to 135 mEq/L	Changes in mental status: apprehension, disorientation, irritability, twitching, nausea, vomiting, shortness of breath
Moderate	125 to 130 mEq/L	Signs of impending pulmonary edema: moist skin and mucous membranes, pitting edema, polyuria, dilute urine, pulmonary rales
Severe	120 to 125 mEq/L	Vital sign changes including hypotension and bradycardia, anemia, jaundice, cyanosis, further changes in mental status.
Hyponatremic encephalopathy	< 120 mEq/L	Congestive heart failure, lethargy, confusion, muscular twitching, focal weakness, convulsions.
	< 115 mEq/L	Coma, death

Management: Obtaining sodium levels every 30 min while the patient is in the recovery room is recommended. If the patient's sodium is less than 125 mosm, forced diuresis with lasix 40 mg IV, fluid restriction and administration of 3% sodium chloride at a rate to correct hyponatremia by 1.5-2 mosmol/L/h is required. Central pontine myclinolysis is a danger if hyponatremia is corrected too rapidly (See Table 7.3).

Fit young women may easily absorb 1.5 l of glycine / normal saline but women with cardiovascular disease may become compromised.

Glycine can cause elevated blood ammonia levels. Glycine when absorbed in excess causes intravascular volume expansion and, dilutional effects. This is known as TURP syndrome. Glycine should be used with caution in patients with impaired liver or renal function tests.

Prevention: This complications usually occur in the immediate postoperative period. Prevention may be accomplished by:

- Using appropriate distention media and delivery systems
- Keeping operating time to a minimum
- Avoiding entering the vascular channels
- Keeping fluid pressures below 80 mmHg and gas pressure below 100 mmHg
- Meticulous accountancy of fluid balance. The procedure must be abandoned if the deficit rises to 2 litres or there is evidence of venous congestion.

Table 7.3: Management of fluid overload[14]

Deficit(ml)	Management
< 500	Continue surgery
500-1000	Continue surgery
1000-1500	Expedite procedure. Check urea and electrolytes. Give frusemide intravenously ? Catheterize
1500-2000	As above. Give frusemide 40 mg intravenously Terminate procedure?
>2000	As above. Terminate procedure

Gas Embolism

Insufflating machines for laparoscopy must never be used. Air and other gases if used for operative hysteroscopy can cause fatal air embolism. This is a rare complication.

Precaution: When performing hysteroscopic surgery and changing from one electrode to another, the entire resectoscope should be removed, rather than leaving the sheath in situ and just removing the handpiece.

Hemorrhage

Hemorrhage can be encountered during hysteroscopy Check the hemostasis at the end of the procedure. The distention pressure can be lowered to visualize bleeding vessels. If a high pressure is used, then there is a net inflow into these vessels.[15]

Management

1. *Coagulation:* If a bleeder is noted coagulate while in view with a roller ball electrode.
2. *Foley's catheter:* Foley's catheter balloon can be inserted into the uterus and distended with 2 to 3 cc of water for tamponade. This can be removed 24 hours later.
3. *Vasopressin and misoprostol:* Vasopressin and misoprostol are alternate medications that can help with vasoconstriction and uterine contractions.
4. *Hysterectomy:* Rarely a hysterectomy is required for intractable hemorrhage as a last resort.

Infection

Post-operative infection after operative hysterscopy is uncommon but cases of tubo-ovarian abscess have been reported. Patients with history of pelvic inflammatory disease are more at risk. Cystitis and endometritis are the more common infections associated with hysteroscopic procedures. When infection does occur it should be managed along conventional lines.

Hematometra and Cyclical Pain

Cyclical pain is reported in upto 25% of patients with intrauterine adhesions following surgery. Overdilatation of cervix, to Hegar16 at the end of the procedure can help to reduce the incidence of this complication. Hematometra should be excluded with ultrasound. When no hematometra is found simple analgesics would suffice.

REFERENCES

1. Adoni A, Palti Z, Milwidsky A, et al. The incidence of intrauterine adhesions following spontaneous abortion. Int J Fertil 1982;27:117-8.
2. Bruno Salle, Pascal Gaucherand, Pierre de Saint Hilaire, Rene Charles Rudigoz. Transvaginal sonohysterographic evaluation of intrauterine adhesions Journal of Ultrasound 1999;27: 131-4.
3. Letterie GS, Haggerty MF. Magnetic resonance imaging of intrauterine synechiae. Gynecol Obstet Invest 1994;37(1): 66-8.
4. Pace S, Stentella P, Catania R, Palazzetti PL, Frega A. Endoscopic treatment of intrauterine adhesions. Clin Exp Obstet Gynecol 2003;30(1):26-8.
5. March CM, Israel R, March AD. Hysteroscopic management of intrauterine adhesions. Am J Obstet Gynecol 1978;130:653-4.
6. Pabuccu R, Atay V, Orhon E, Urman B, Ergun A. Hysteroscopic treatment of intrauterine adhesions is safe and effective in the restoration of normal menstruation and fertility. Fertil Steril 1997;68(6):1141-3.
7. Fernandez H, Al-Najjar F, Chauveaud-Lambling A, Frydman R, Gervaise A. Fertility after treatment of Asherman's syndrome stage 3 and 4. J Minim Invasive Gynecol 2006; 13(5):398-402.
8. Simon C, Martinez L, Pardo F, Tortajada M, Pellicer A. Müllerian defects in women with normal reproductive outcome. Fertil Steril 1991; 56: 1192-3.
9. Cararach M, Penella J, Ubeda A, Labastida R. Hysteroscopic incision of the septate uterus: Scissors versus resectoscope. Human Reproduction 1994;9:87-9.
10. Valle RF. Hysteroscopic treatment of partial and complete uterine septum. Int J Fertil Menopausal Stud 1996;41:310-5.
11. Hickok, Lee R MD. Hysteroscopic treatment of uterine septum: A clinicians experience. Am J Obstet Gynecol 2000;182 (6): 1414-20.
12. Agostini A, Cravello L, Bretelle F, Shojal R, Roger V, Blanc B. Risk of uterine perforation during hysteroscopic surgery. J Am Assoc Gynecol Laparasc. 2002;9(3):264-7.

13. Jedeikin R, Olsfanger D, Kessler I. Diseminated intravascular coagulopathy and adult respiratory distress syndrome: life-threatening complications of hysteroscopy. Am J Obstet Gynecol 1990;162(1):44-5.
14. Loffer FD, Bradley LD, Brill AI. Hysteroscopic fluid monitoring guidelines. The adhoc committee on hysteroscopic training guidelines of the American Association of Gynecologic Laparoscopists. J Am Assoc Gynecol Laparosc 2000; 7(1): 167-8.
15. Bradley LD. Complications in hysteroscopy: Prevention, treatment and legal risk. Curr Opin Obstet Gynecol 2002;14(4):409-15.

CHAPTER 8

Tubal Reconstructive Surgery

Surveen Ghumman

Tubal infertility with or without associated peritoneal pathology accounts for up to 35% of all cases of infertility. Reconstructive tubal surgery was at one time the only treatment option for infertile women with damaged fallopian tubes. Wider availability and better results of in vitro fertilization and assisted reproduction has provided such couples with another therapeutic alternative. It is imperative to provide accurate therapeutic and prognostic information to aid them in their decision. Age and cost must also be taken into consideration. It is seen that although excellent results are achieved after microsurgical reversal of sterilization, the pregnancy outcome after repair of post infectious tubal disease is not encouraging. Although anatomic reconstruction results in tubal patency in most instances, alteration of tubal function remains a stumbling block to a successful pregnancy.

Causes of Tubal Blockage

1. **Pelvic infections**: They can be ascending or proximal (appendicitis). They are asymptomatic in 15% of cases

   Chlamydial infection: It may be subclinical and destructive to the fallopian tube. Complete obstruction may not occur but fusion of fimbria and impairment of ciliary activity may occur and may compromise fertility by altered ovum transport. *Chlamydia* is responsible for 50% of cases of tubal infertility.

   Gonococcal infection: Gonococcal endosalpingitis produces tubal occlusion occurring along the entire length of the tube and may result in hydrosalpinx or tuboovarian inflammatory mass. It may be accompanied by secondary infection. The frequency of tubal obstruction was 2.6% with mild inflammatory changes, 13.1% with moderate changes and 28.6% with severe inflammatory changes.[1] *Tuberculosis:* It is an important cause of tubal factor infertility and may cause irreparable damage to the tubes.

2. **Pelvic surgery**: Pelvic surgeries, can cause peritubal adhesions. The most traumatizing operations are ovarian

cystectomies, myomectomies, ectopic pregnancy, bowel surgery, and appendicectomies.

3. **Endometriosis**: It causes peritubal adhesions.

Preoperative Evaluation

Before performing surgery for distal tubal disease, the surgeon must carefully evaluate each couple. The tests which are essential to rule out other causes of infertility are done:

1. Sperm status – Semen analysis
2. Ovulation documentation – Progesterone level, basal body temperature, endometrial biopsy, ultrasonography
3. Assessment of uterus – Ultrasound hysterosalpingogram, laparoscopy, hysteroscopy
4. Current pelvic inflammatory disease is ruled out
5. Assesment of tubes: A careful patient evaluation of the fallopian tubes is essential before a therapeutic decision is made (Table 8.1) (See Chapter 2).

Preoperative counseling It is a very important aspect of the treatment. The surgeon should explain the chances of success and subsequent ectopic pregnancy. Other options like IVF and adoption must be discussed with the couple. Counseling ensures that patients have a realistic expectation of a successful outcome.

Table 8.1: Preoperative assessment of tubal parameters

Preoperative assessment of tubal parameters
1. Peritubal adhesions
2. Tubal patency and fimbrial appearance.
3. Tubal dilatation
4. Tubal folds.
5. Tubal thickness

Investigations for tubal parameters
- History and examination
- Ultrasonography
- Hysterosonography
- Hysterosalpingography
- Falloposcopy
- Laparoscopy and chromotubation

The extent of tubal disease is classified as mild, moderate and severe (Table 8.2).

Table 8.2: Classification of extent of tubal disease[2]	
Extent of disease	Findings
Mild	• Absent or small (<15mm in diameter) hydrosalpinx
	• Inverted fimbriae easily recognized when patency achieved
	• No significant peritubal or periovarian adhesions
	• Rugal pattern on preoperative hysterogram
Moderate	• Hydrosalpinx 15 to 30 mm in diameter
	• Fragments of fimbriae not readily identified.
	• Periovarian or peritubal adhesions with fixation, a few cul de sac adhesions
	• Absence of rugal pattern on preoperative hysterogram
Severe	• Large hydrosalpinx > 30 mm in diameter
	• No fimbriae
	• Dense pelvic or adnexal adhesions with fixation to the ovary and tube to broad ligament, pelvic side wall, omentum or bowel.
	• Obliteration of cul-de-sac
	• Frozen pelvis (adhesion formation so dense that limits of organs are difficult to define)

Indications of primary management of tubal infertility by IVF or ICSI

1. Marked damage of tubes not amenable to surgery.
2. Absent tubes.
3. Double tubal block (cornual and fimbrial)
4. Failed surgical treatment.
5. Tubal defect complicated by other major infertility factors e.g. Oligospermia or intractable ovulation dysfunction

Tubal surgery for infertility must deal with four major areas of tubal diseases (Fig. 8.1). They are classified according to International Federation of Fertility and Sterility into eight categories (Table 8.3).

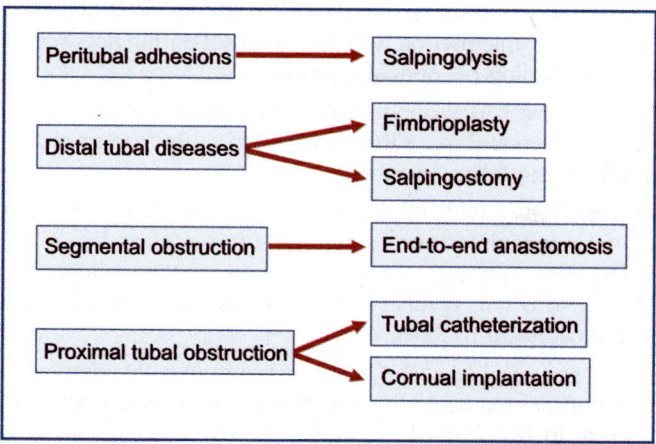

Fig. 8.1: Surgical options for four major areas of tubal disease

Tubal surgery may be done by laparotomy using microsurgical techniques or by laparoscopy.

Advantage of Laparoscopic Surgery

- Adequate exposure.
- Magnification.
- Minimal tissue handling.
- Strict attention to hemostasis.
- Prevention of tissue drying by maintaining a closed abdomen and continuous irrigation.
- Less risk of infection by using small incisions, a closed operating space, lack of retractors and packs and less likelihood of introduction of foreign bodies.

Microsurgical Approach to Fallopian Tube

Microsurgery represents the approach to gentle operative technique using fine, delicate needles and sutures, delicate instruments and continued irrigation of operative site with surgery performed under magnification provided by binocular lens, hood or microscope with a magnification ranging from 1 to 20 depending on optical system.

Magnification: It is thought that magnification greater than 6 is unnecessary and more than 4 is critical in the cornuoisthmic portion of the fallopian tube.

Sutures: Suture with minimal reactivity should be used for oviduct approximation. Fewer the sutures used lesser the foreign body reaction. Absorbable non reactive sutures 8-0 with a 4 to 6 mm reverse cutting needle have proven useful for microsurgical procedures.

Energy source: Laser may be used although the degree of tissue trauma and acute thermal damage as assessed by depth of injury in histological sections is similar in CO_2 laser and electrosurgery. Precise lysis of adhesions with minimal tissue damage results from laser therapy but there is no clear evidence to suggest decrease in adhesion formation or increased pregnancy rate.

It was seen that term pregnancy rates were doubled and patency rates definitely improved with microsurgery.[3] However a recent Cochrane review emphasized that there is no evidence of advantage or disadvantage of using microsurgery over standard techniques; laparoscopic approach over laparotomy; the use of CO_2 laser or electrocoagulation over thermo-coagulation.[4]

General Considerations for Tubal Microsurgery

1. Tubal lavage is performed during the procedure either by inserting an intrauterine catheter or a transuterine lavage using a 20 gauge needle.

Table 8.3: Classification of tubal procedures (According to International Federation of Fertility and Sterility)[5]

1. Lysis of periadnexal adhesions (salpingolysis – ovariolysis): Classified with adnexa of least pathology:
   - Minimal: 1 cm of tube or ovary involved
   - Moderate: partially surrounding tube or ovary
   - Severe: encapsulating peritubal and/or periovarian adhesions
2. Lysis of extra adnexal adhesions
   - Minimal
   - Moderate
   - Severe
3. Tubouterine implantation
   - Isthmic: implantation of isthmic segment
   - Ampullary: implantation of ampullary segment
   - Combination: different types of implantation on right and left tubes
4. Tubotubal anastomosis
   - Interstitial (intramural)- isthmic
   - Interstitial (intramural)-ampullary
   - Isthmic – isthmic
   - Isthmic – ampullary
   - Ampullary- ampullary
   - Ampullary – infundibular (fimbrial)
   - Combination of different type of anastomosis on right and left tube
5. Salpingostomy: Surgical creation of new tubal ostium
   - Terminal
   - Ampullary
   - Isthmic
   - Combination: different types of salpingostomy on right and left
6. Fimbrioplasty: Reconstruction of existent fimbriae
   - By deagglutination and dilatation
   - With serosal incision for completely occluded tube
   - Combination: different types of fimbrioplasty on right and left tubes
7. Other reconstruction tubal operations
8. Combination of different types of operations
   - Bipolar: for occlusion at both proximal and terminal ends of tube
   - Bilateral: different operations on right and left side

2. Heparinized ringer lactate solution (5000 U/L) is used for intraperitoneal irrigation.
3. The initial adhesiolysis may be performed at 2 to 3 X loupe magnification. If increased magnification is desired microscope may be used.
4. Since peritoneal defects heal from baseup and ischemia is a potent stimulation to postoperative adhesion formation the surgeon should peritonize with restraint and without tension.
5. Adhesions attached to the pelvic structures should be divided 1 to 2 mm from the involved structure to allow for retraction and lessen chances of injury to the structure if additional coagulation is required.
6. If ovary or tube is to be removed it should be done at the end of the surgery, after the other pelvic structures are repaired. This allows the surgeons to make a more informed judgment as to whether the organ in question should be removed.
7. Peritoneal platforms should be developed as one of the last steps of the procedure avoiding unnecessary stress to tissues making up the platforms.

Salpingolysis

Peritubal adhesions represent 5% of tubal factor infertility cases. The etiology of these adhesions could be pelvic surgery, pelvic inflammatory disease or endometriosis. Adhesions due to pelvic inflammation are broad or shallow, usually not too vascular and extend from one structure to another leaving a potential space between the involved structures, an aspect that facilitates adhesiolysis. Adhesions due to prior surgery are dense and cohesive with intimate conglutination of adjacent structures. Since the underlying stromal layer of the two structures coalesce the lysis is technically difficult with high recurrence rate.

Adhesions cause infertility by
- Destroying the tubo ovarian relationship
- Preventing ovum pickup.
- Affecting follicular development

Principles of Adhesiolysis

1. Adhesions are place under tension by holding up the structures with an atraumatic forceps before excising.
2. It is imperative to divide one layer at a time entering between the two layers to prevent trauma to underlying structures.
3. When microelectrode is used for this purpose the electrosurgical unit is put on blend setting which on cut mode combines coagulating with cutting current to provide hemostasis along with division.
4. Damage to the peritoneal or ovarian surface is avoided keeping the transaction line 1 mm away from the surface.
5. All broad adhesions (more than 5 to 6 mm) are excised and removed. Shallow adhesions are simply divided.

Steps of Adhesiolysis

Assessment of adhesions: The entire pelvis is surveyed and extent of adhesions assessed.

Adhesiolysis in pouch of Douglas: Adhesiolysis is begun from the cul-de-sac if adhesions are present there. Adhesions involving omentum, bowel and uterus may be divided electrosurgically using a fine needle monopolar insulated microelectrode or by laser, scissors or scalpel dissection. Bleeding is controlled by bipolar coagulation. Frequent irrigation must be done. Omentum may be folded back on itself (omentopexy) after it has been dissected. Once the rectosigmoid and omentum are dissected they are positioned away from the operative field.

Release of adnexa: Next the adnexa are released from the lateral pelvic wall. A Teflon rod may be placed beneath the adhesions to facilitate the dissection and to protect the ureter and major blood vessels. Adhesions that remain attached to the ovary are folded over a dissecting rod and excised (Figs 8.2A and B). Careful identification of fimbria ovarica should be done and avoidance of vascular compromise of fimbrial end should be ensured.

The uteroovarian ligament may be held to facilitate counter traction and expose the line of cleavage. During ovariolysis, it is important to preserve as much peritoneum as possible while freeing the ovary. Dissection starts high in the pelvis, just

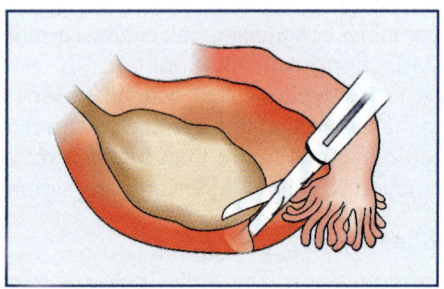

Fig. 8.2A: Adhesiolysis around the ovary

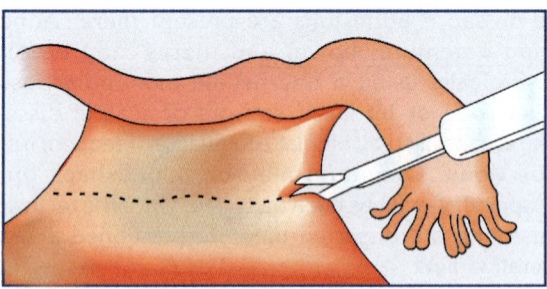

Fig. 8.2B: Salpingolysis

beneath the infundibulopelvic ligament. Scissors are used both bluntly and sharply to mobilize the ovary from the sidewall and continued in a methodical manner until the cul-de-sac is reached.

When open abdomen adhesiolysis is done the adhesions are divided at the distal end thus freeing the adnexa making elevation of adnexa possible. Adhesions are then excised from the tubal serosa or ovarian surface. With laparoscopic access the order is reversed and careful lysis should be carried out at the junction of the adhesions and adnexal structures.

Laparoscopic Approach: Lysis of adhesions is done by placement of adhesions on traction by elevating the uterus or by forceps or probe placed through another puncture site. The adhesions are incised parallel to the organ of interest and 1 mm away to prevent damaging its mesothelial envelope. Hydrodissection can delineate the extent of the adhesions and involvement of adnexa. For laser lysis of extensive adhesions, the laser beam should be small, spot sized and in super pulse mode. It should be applied to the edge of the adhesions with an arc like motion to vaporize the tissue. Reflective probes or irrigation solution can serve as a backstop for the carbon dioxide laser. Copious irrigation to remove dead or carbonized tissue should be performed (See Chapter 9 and accompanying DVD ROM).

Results: Pregnancy rates after salpingolysis range from 32 to 70%. The ectopic pregnancy rate was 5 to 8%. Salpingolysis by laparoscopy yielded 62% pregnancy rate[6] Fayez has reported a 67% pregnancy rate with laparoscopic salpingolysis in comparison to 30 to 60% intrauterine pregnancy rates reported after salpingolysis by laparotomy. [7] Lasers offered no added advantage.

Salpingoplasty

Salpingoplasty is a corrective procedure involving the distal part of the tube by either fimbrioplasty or neosalpingostomy (Fig. 8.3). In women with extensive tubal damage as evidenced by complete obliteration of tubal anatomy by adhesions or an attenuated tubal muscularis dilated beyond 3 cm and in patients with bipolar disease attempts at reconstructive surgery are deferred in favor of *in vitro* fertilization. Rates of implantation and live pregnancy are halved in the presence of hydrosalpinx due to intermittent drainage of fluid into the uterus. Thus distal tubal surgery like salpingectomy or salpingostomy to drain hydrosalpinx is recommended prior to attempting IVF to improve results.

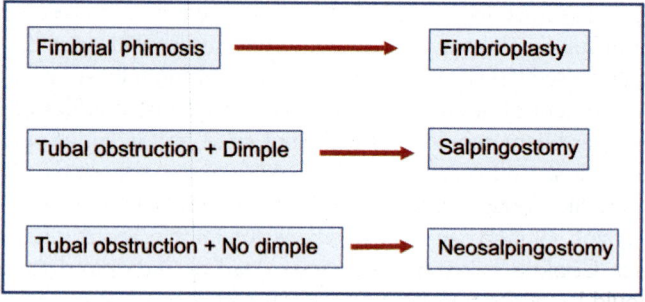

Fig. 8.3: Management of distal tubal diseases

Fimbrioplasty

Often the fimbrial end of the tube is altered after infection or pelvic surgery. A ring of scar tissue may compress the fimbriae folding them inwards. Fimbrioplasty is the reconstruction of the fimbriae or infundibulum in a tube that exhibits fimbrial agglutination or prefimbrial phimosis resulting in partial distal occlusion.

Steps

Introduction of forceps: Fimbrial agglutination can be dealt with by introducing a delicate forceps into the phimosis and opening it. If opening is not visible or covered with fibrous tissue the tube is distended with transcervical chromotubation. (Figs 8.4A to C). Small incision may also be necessary where it is covered with fibrous tissue.

Division of mucosal bridges: A careful search for mucosal bridges is made and these are either teased apart or coagulated with bipolar forceps and then divided.

Fimbrial eversion: A few sutures may be applied to maintain fimbrial eversion.

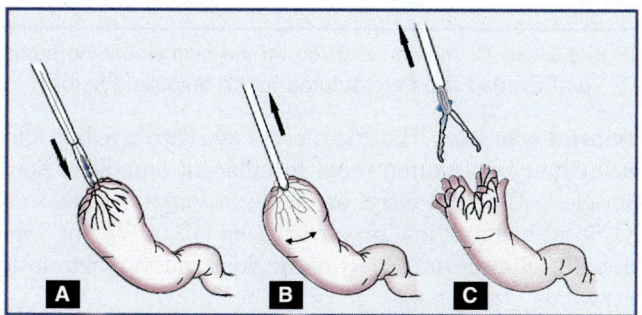

Figs 8.4A to C: Fimbrioplasty introducing a forceps into the phymosis and opening it

Prefimbrial Phimosis

It is located at the true abdominal ostia that are the apex of the infundibulum.

Steps

Incision on antimesenteric border: An incision is given on the anti mesosalpingeal border of the tube which commences on the infundibulum and continues past the stenotic area into the distal ampulla (Figs 8.5A to C). Either it is done electrosurgically or by scissors. Care is taken to prevent damage to the mucosa. The length and direction of the incision is planned to provide an ample ostium, yet maintain excellent perfusion and proper anatomy with minimal mucosal damage.

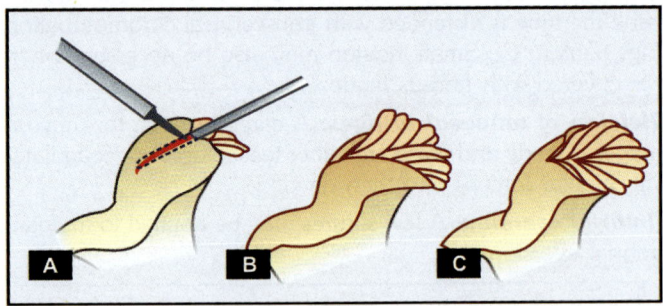

Figs 8.5A to C: Incision is given on the antimesenteric border and everted flaps are sutured to the ampullary serosa

Fimbrial eversion: The edges of the two flaps are then folded back either by securing them to adjacent ampullary serosa with No. 7-0 or 8-0 vicryl or by electrosurgery or defocused CO_2 laser beam of low power intensity (10-50 W/cm^2) which desiccates the serosal aspect of the flaps causing them to fold backwards (Table 8.4).

Laparoscopy: The procedure can be done laparoscopically with the same results (See Chapter 9 and accompanying DVD ROM).

Phimosis may be released by introduction of an alligator forceps which is opened inside the lumen and gradually withdrawn out with open jaws. Deagglutination is achieved by repeating this movement a few times in various directions. Also an incision can be given on the fibrous bands constricting the tubal ostia. Fimbrial eversion is done (Table 8.4).

Result: A wide variation in pregnancy rates is seen 30 to 70% with comparable rates in laparoscopic procedure.

Table 8.4: Techniques of fimbrial eversion

Fimbrial eversion can be maintained by four methods to prevent reocclusion

i. Bruhat technique: It uses a defocused CO_2 laser at low power ($500W/cm^2$) to desiccate the serosa which then everts the edges of the incised tube. It is fast but cannot be applied if the walls are thick.

ii. Endocoagulator or bipolar forceps with low power density can be used with a light brushing technique to obtain desiccation

iii. Intussusceptions Technique: The edges of the newly created ostium are then pulled proximally while the probe is used externally to prolapse the ampullary portion of the tube through the opening. The border of the incision acts as a restrictive collar to maintain eversion of the mucosa. This method is less successful if tubal wall is thick or ostial opening is large.

iv. Suturing of the margins of the tube to the serosa. This is the best technique if there are thick tubal walls.

Neosalpingostomy

It is the creation of a new stoma to establish tubal patency in a tube with completely occluded distal end. Neosalpingostomy is classified according to location at which the new stoma is formed as

- Terminal
- Ampullary
- Isthmic

Isthmic and ampullary salpingostomies are rarely done except in reversal of prior fimbriectomy.

Steps

Salpingolysis: Salpingolysis is done and the tuboovarian ligament is dissected free. Once tube is free it is easy to identify the site at which the neostomy should be performed.

Care should be taken to maintain fimbria in as normal a condition as possible by first identifying fimbriae ovarica.

Incision on distal end of tube: The distal end of the tube is stabilized and the tube is distended by injecting methylene blue through the fundus. The white avascular area at the tubal ostia may be identified and the scar incised by monopolar microelectrode or laser. The opening may be enlarged with hemostats. Normal looking fimbriae may protrude from the incision (Fig. 8.6A).

Widening incision: If no fimbriae are identified an initial incision is made at 6 O'clock in the direction of the fimbriae ovarica. It becomes possible to view the tube from within while placing additional incisions along its circumference. These incisions are made between endothelial folds over avascular areas avoiding vascular mucosal folds which will be shaped as fimbriae (Fig. 8.6B). Mucosal bridges should be divided.

Everting tubal edges: The edges created are grasped and rotated outward and secured to the tubomuscularis with 8-0 sutures or by desiccating the serosal surface (Table 8.4) (Fig. 8.6C).

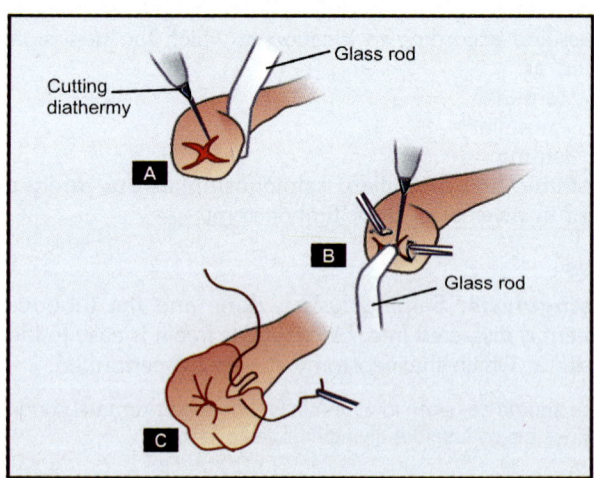

Figs 8.6A to C: Neosalpingostomy: Incisions are made over avascular fold; edges are everted and sutured on the tubal serosa

Tuboscopy: After completing salpingostomy it is desirable to inspect the interior of the tube with a tuboscope to get valuable prognostic information.

Thick Walled Hydrosalpinx

This requires a modification of this technique

Excision of serosa and muscularis: The fibrotic and thickened ampullary serosa and musculature is excised distally but not through the mucosa (Fig. 8.7A).

Incision on mucosa: Four incisions are made in the mucosa (Fig. 8.7B).

Eversion of flaps: The flaps are sutured to the corresponding sites (Fig. 8.7C).

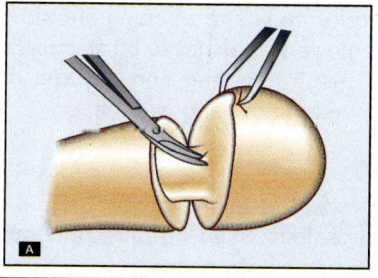

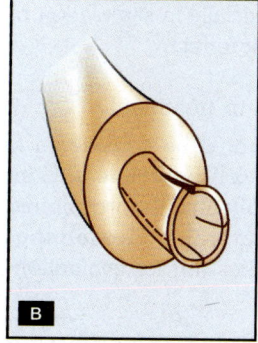
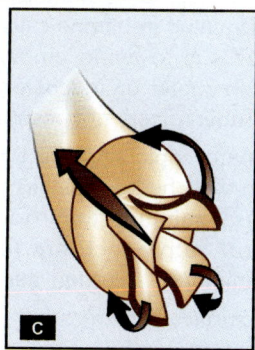

Figs 8.7 A to C: Neosalpingostomy in thick walled hydrosalpinx. A. Excision of ampullary serosa and muscularis B. Incision given on mucosa. C. Mucosal flaps everted and sutured

Alternative technique: Excise the distal portion of the thickened tube in full thickness and make four incisions, the edges of which are everted and fixed with fine sutures.

Laparoscopic neosalpingostomy: Laparoscopic salpingostomy has the advantage that it can be performed in the initial diagnostic laparoscopy, avoiding a second intervention and results in cost saving. It has pregnancy rates similar to laparotomy.

Steps are similar to abdominal surgery (see Chapter 9). The dimple or avascular area at the clubbed end of the fallopian tube is incised in a cruciate manner with scissors, needle point cautery or high power density laser along the avascular planes. In addition relaxing incisions to complete eversion of Fallopian tube may be performed. The opening should not be more than 12 mm. Hemostasis is achieved by electrosurgery or laser. Because gentle tissue handling and burying of the knot is desired intracorporeal knot tying is done.

Salpingectomy

Indication for removal of hydrosalpinx
1. Large hydrosalpinx seen on ultrasonography
2. Pyosalpinx or hematosalpinx
3. Draining in uterine cavity especially in stimulation phase. This is to avoid embryotoxic effect.
4. No rugae or mucosal folds
5. Tuberculosis not responsive to treatment.

Laparoscopic salpingectomy should be considered for all women with hydrosalpinges prior to IVF treatment. Currently unilateral salpingectomy for a unilateral hydrosalpinx and bilateral salpingectomy for bilateral hydrosalpinges is recommended, although this requires further evaluation.

Other surgical options:

Further randomized trials are required to assess other surgical treatments for hydrosalpinx, such as salpingostomy, tubal occlusion or needle drainage of a hydrosalpinx at oocyte retrieval. The role of surgery for tubal disease in the absence of a hydrosalpinx is unclear and merits further evaluation. [8]

Peritoneal Platform

It is created to prevent the ovary from adhering to the pelvic sidewall and posterior broad ligament. Using 2-0 or 3-0 synthetic absorbable, stitch is taken 5 mm below the inferior surface of lateral one third of the ovary. It is placed through the peritoneum piercing it with several shallow bites parallel to the inferior surface of the ovary. The suture is then placed in the uterine musculature approximately 1 cm inferior to the uterine insertion of the tuboovarian ligament and tied. The resulting peritoneal platform rotates the ovary away from the pelvic sidewall and posterior broad ligament (Fig. 8.8).

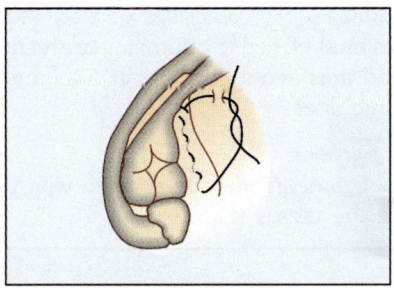

Fig. 8.8: Peritoneal platform created by placing several stitches in the peritoneum and uterine musculature which prevent the ovary from adhering to the lateral side walls

Caution
a. Care should be taken to locate the ureter and place sutures away from it.
b. The peritoneum should be pierced superficially when taking a suture to avoid piercing major blood vessels.
c. If uterine suspension is to be performed the surgeon should factor this in when placing the peritoneal platform sutures thus avoiding undesirable tissue tension.

Uterine Suspension

1. *Round ligament plication*

A uterus fixed in retroversion by adhesions may cause dyspareunia and may hamper ovum pickup. This is avoided by round ligament placation. The middle section of the round ligament is reversed and fixed at the respective uterine and internal ring insertion of the round ligament with permanent suture of 1-0 size. An additional suture is placed at the midpoint of the triplicated ligament to prevent separation of the round ligament bundles (Fig. 8.9).

Caution

    a. Care must be taken to avoid occluding the proximal part of the tube.

    b. Avoid piercing major blood vessels in the vicinity of the internal ring.

    c. All sutures must be tied to approximate and not overpower tissues and thus avoid postoperative adhesion formation at ischemic sites.

2. *Uterosacral plication*

The uterosacral ligaments may be plicated with each other to further antevert the uterus (Fig. 8.9).

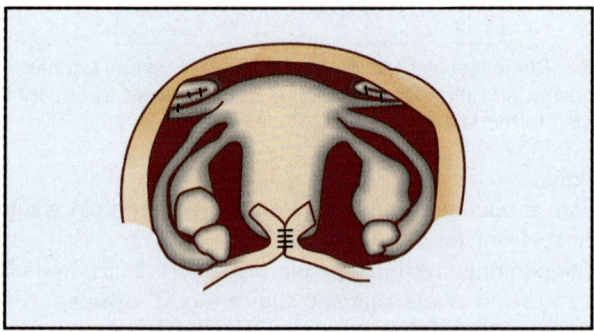

Fig. 8.9: Uterine suspension by round ligament and uterosacral plication

3. *Ventral suspension*

A synthetic absorbable suture of 1-0 material is placed as a horizontal mattress suture in the uterus at the top of the fundus. Each end of the suture is then passed through their respective peritoneum, rectus sheath and fascia. At the time of peritoneal closure the suture is tied bringing the uterus firmly against the inferior surface of the peritoneum. This procedure may cause significant patient discomfort and is no longer used.

Result

The patients with most favorable results have small hydrosalpinx, healthy mucosa, thin tubal walls and filmy adhesions.

Prognosis depends upon

- Condition of the fimbria once patency is established
- Extent and nature of peritubular adhesions
- Condition of muscularis or ciliary epithelium
- Size of the hydrosalpinx
- Age of the patient

The most important prognostic factor in tubal reconstructive surgery is tubal morphology.

If hydrosalpinx of more than 2.5 cm is present pregnancy rate decreases from 50 to 10%.[9] Pregnancy rates decrease from 61 to 7 % if rugae are absent on HSG. Distal tubal obstruction treated by microsurgical technique of neosalpingostomy had a success rate varying from 80% in mild disease to 16% in severe disease. Choice of technique such as microscopic neosalpingostomy or use of loupe has not shown to affect the pregnancy rates significantly.[10] However, microsurgery improved pregnancy rates in severe category by decreasing adhesion formation.

It was seen that 70% of patients had patent fallopian tubes on second look laparoscopy and very few adhesions. The relatively low term pregnancy rate implies persistent impairment of tubal function even after anatomic consideration.[11]

Comparison of results: Salpingolysis has the best results (64%) followed by fimbrioplasty (60%), and salpingostomy (31%).[12]

Repeat surgery: A second salpingostomy is not recommended if tubal block is found on HSG performed 9 to 12 months postoperatively as there is less than 10% success rate.[13]

Tubal Reanastomosis

Anastomosis is performed anywhere along the tube either to treat occlusions resulting from disease process or to reverse prior sterilization.

Preoperative assessment: A preoperative HSG should be done for assessment of any pathology in the uterine cavity and length of intramural portion of the tube in cornual block.

Microsurgical tubal reanastomosis for reversal of sterilization adheres to the principles of atraumatic accurate anastomosis and precise approximation of the tubal segment (Table 8.5). Depending on the tubal segment that is approximated tubotubal anastomosis can be

- Intramural – isthmic
- Intramural – ampullary
- Isthmic – isthmic
- Isthmic – ampullary
- Ampullary - ampullary
- Ampullary - infundibular

Table 8.5: Principles of microsurgery in tubal anastomosis

1. Always cut at a relatively avascular segment
2. Bipolar coagulation used to control bleeding tissue should be grasped between two electrodes without bringing the two electrodes together. If the electrodes are squeezed together, tissue will be crushed and extruded, causing current to bypass it, since the current will flow higher up on the forceps where the electrodes touch. Such torn crushed non coagulated vessels will bleed when the forceps are released. Hence, the tissue to be coagulated should be gently grasped making sure the electrodes are separated.
3. Power should be such that passage of current gradually coagulates. High power settings should be avoided, since they instantly carbonize the tissue, welding it to the electrodes and causing bleeding when the forceps are disengaged.
4. The greater the distance between the electrodes the higher the setting required to get a flow current. Also drier the tissue, the less conductive it is. Hence, it must be ensured not to grab an excessive amount of tissue and to keep the tissue moist.
5. If it is necessary to coagulate blood vessels close to the tissue that must be protected from thermal damage, the tissue should be irrigated while the vessel is being coagulated. The flow of the liquid acts as a heat sink. It is possible to form a pool of boiling liquid that will damage a wide area of tissue if flow of irrigating solution sufficient to carry away excess heat not maintained. Also too copious irrigation may prevent coagulation of the tissue by keeping the tissue cool.
6. Absolute hemostasis is not necessary as capillary oozing of cut edges is consistent with living tissue and ceases when edges are apposed.
7. During an anastomosis one should try and get equal and symmetric bites on both stumps.
8. To overcome tension separating two stumps the first part of the knot should be double throw.
9. Excessive mechanical manipulation and trauma sufficient to macerate and obliterate normal anatomy should be strictly avoided.

Isthmic – Isthmic Anastomosis

It shows good results as there is no luminal disparity.

Steps

- ***Excision of fibrous tissue:*** The fibrous band of tissue joining the proximal and distal segments of the fallopian tube is dissected from the fallopian tube till the proximal segment is reached. (Fig. 8.10A)
- ***Transection of proximal stump of tube:*** The proximal portion of the tube is distended with chromotubation to identify the distal tip which is picked up with atraumatic forceps. A small portion of the occluded tip is resected with straight scissor or a sharp microblade taking care to halt at the mesosalpinx in the immediate periphery of tubal muscularis to avoid damaging adjacent vascular arcade. Successive transaction of the tube at 1 to 2 mm intervals helps to identify the occlusion site.
- ***Transection of distal stump of tube:*** The proximal portion of the distal segment is resected in the same manner after distending it by descending hydropertubation. (Fig. 8.10B) Hemostasis is obtained by precise electrodessication of the more significant bleeders.
- ***Anastomosis of muscular layer:*** Anastomosis of the segment is carried out by taking 7-0 vicryl interrupted sutures in the muscularis placed at 12, 4 and 8 o'clock or 12, 3, 6, 9 o'clock. The stitches are taken from outside in on one side and inside out on the other side so, that the knots lie externally. The first suture is always placed. at the mesosalpingeal border. (6 o'clock) to ensure proper alignment of the two segments. The sutures are tied but not so tight so as to interfere with the vascular supply of the fallopian tube (Fig. 8.10C).

- *Application of serosal sutures:* An additional layer of interrupted sutures 7-0 or 8-0 vicryl will approximate the serosa (Fig. 8.10C).
- *Approximation of mesosalpinx:* The mesosalpinx is carefully approximated with an anchoring knot of 4-0 or 5-0 vicryl at the base of the proximal and distal segments to avoid tension at the anastomotic site. All knots should be placed anteriorly to avoid adhesions with the ovary (Fig. 8.10D).
- *Chromotubation:* It is done as a last step. There may be leakage from anastomotic site but it can be ignored as long as there is free spill from fimbrial end.

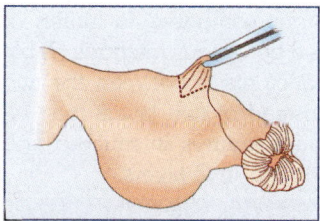

Fig. 8.10A: Fibrous band joining the two segments of the fallopian tube is dissected

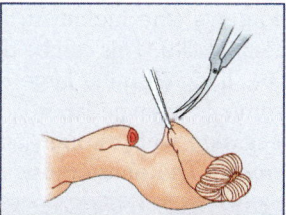

Fig. 8.10B: Proximal part of distal segment is resected with the scissors

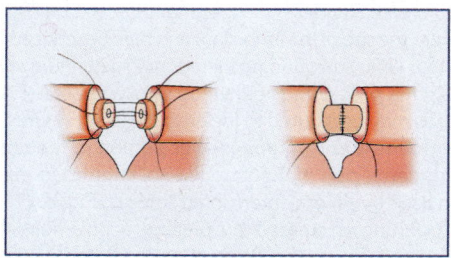

Fig. 8.10C: Interrupted sutures are placed in the muscularis at 6 o'clock, 9 o'clock, 12 o' clock and 3 o'clock. Serosa is sutured with interrupted stitches in the second layer

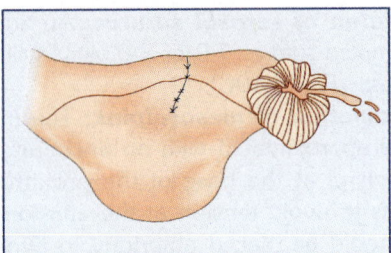

Fig. 8.10D: Mesosalpinx is sutured to avoid tension in the anastomosis and chromotubation

Isthmic Ampullary Anastomosis

The major difference in the procedure is that it is associated with a large discrepancy in the diameter of the two tubal segments (the lumen of the isthmus compared to lumen of the ampulla). This can be decreased by various methods (Table 8.6). If significantly large discrepancy exists between the two segments a single layer closure instead of two layers may be necessary with through and through sutures in mucosa and serosa. The anastomosis is performed in 2 layers.

Table 8.6: Methods to decrease the luminal disparity in tubal anastomosis
1. Proximal stump can be cut at a 30-degree angle (Fig. 8.11A).
2. Isthmic lumen is widened by a 2 to 3 mm slit, partially excising the corners to create a wider oval opening (Figs. 8.11A B).
3. Alternatively, the size of the ampullary end may be reduced by plicating the muscular layer surrounding the opening with interrupted sutures after which the prolapsing epithelium is invaginated (Fig. 8.11C).
4. The isthmus may be sutured to the ampulla using sutures that join its perimeter to the corresponding lower portion of the ampulla. The upper redundant part of the ampulla not sutured to the isthmus is closed on itself by several interrupted sutures (Fig. 8.11D).
5. A small opening is created by placing a fine needle from the angiocatheter through the fimbrial end, instead of resecting the proximal portion of the ampullary end

Contd...

Contd...

6. With the use of microscissors the serosa over the tip of the ampullary stump is incised in a circular manner to expose the muscularis of the occluded end where a small incision is made into the ampullary lumen to correspond to the lumen of the proximal tubal segment (Fig. 8.11E)

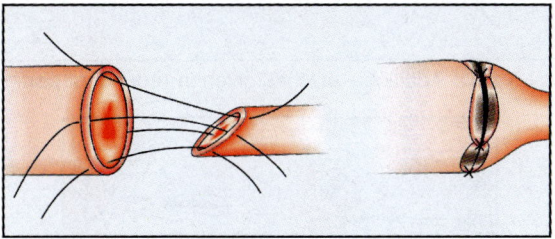

Fig. 8.11A: Isthmic portion cut at 30 degrees to increase diameter

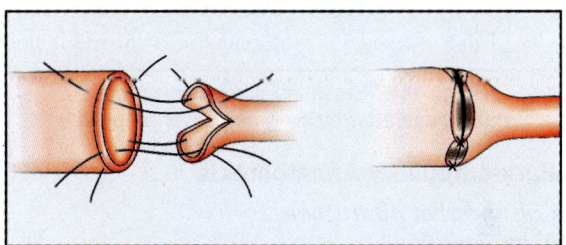

Fig. 8.11B: Incision given at isthmic end to increase the diameter

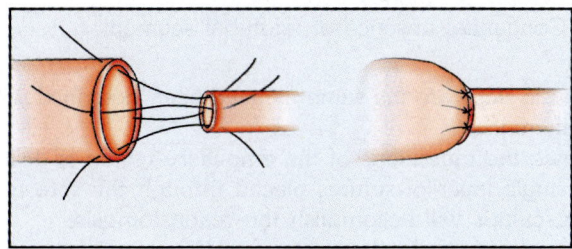

Fig. 8.11C: Additional plicating sutures given to invaginate prolapsing epithelium

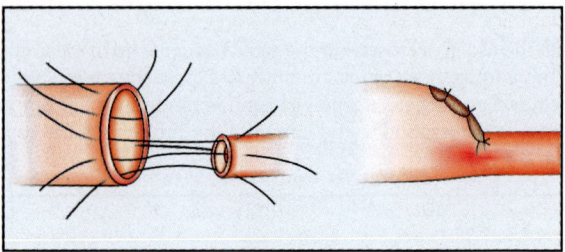

Fig. 8.11D: Additional stitches given in redundant portion

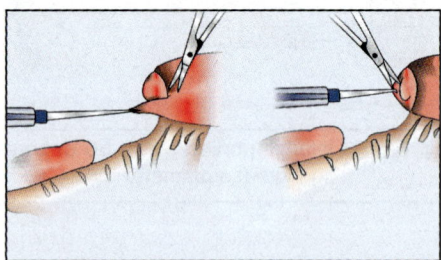

Fig. 8.11E: Small incision given on the muscularis after incising serosa of ampulla

Ampullary-ampullary Anastomosis

Causes of midtubal obstruction
1. Endometriosis
2. Sterilization
3. Ectopic pregnancy
4. Congenital absence of midtubal segment.

Steps
The basic steps are the same as have been described with a few differences
1. Since the muscularis of the ampullary region is delicate, a single layer of sutures placed through the serosa and muscularis will accomplish the reanastomosis.
2. The difficulty in these cases is the propensity of the ampullary epithelium to prolapse through the lumen. These

epithelial fronds should not be excised as suggested by some as it may lead to subsequent intraluminal adhesion formation at this site. They should be replaced with a micro-forceps while tying the sutures. Care should be taken not to include these epithelial fronds within the suture knot or between the segments that are being approximated.

3. Greater number of interrupted sutures may be required because of the large diameter.

While dissecting the ampulla the microelectrode is not used so as to avoid thermal damage to the mucosa through this very thin muscle layer.

Ampullary-infundibular Anastomosis

It is required when the distal ampullary portion of the tube has been excised by prior sterilization or removal of tubal gestation.

Steps:

The basic steps are the same for the anastomosis

- A probe with a conical tip is introduced into the infundibular segment.
- A circular incision is given with microscissors corresponding to the size of the ampullary segment.
- A two-layer anastomosis is performed.

Tubo-cornual Anastomosis for Proximal Disease

Occlusive diseases at uterocornual junction are:
- Obliterative fibrosis
- Chronic inflammation
- Salpingitis isthmica nodosa
- Intratubal endometriosis
- Ectopic gestation
- Tuberculosis
- Trauma due to previous sterilization, myomectomy, uterine suspension or other surgery

Tubal plugs, synechiae or spasm may cause it and are treatable by selective salpingography or tubal cannulation. The management strategy must take into account—

1. Condition of distal tube.
2. Extent and nature of pelvic adhesions.
3. Presence of associated pelvic disease.
4. Status of other fertility parameters like male factor infertility.

The selection of treatment must be individualized according to investigative findings, wishes of the patient and expertise of the surgeon. Traditional approach of uterotubal implantation has been replaced by anastomosis.

Intramural-isthmic Anastomosis

It is the anastomosis often required to treat cornual disease. Preoperative HSG shows length of proximal segment.

Steps

Infiltration with vasopressin: The cornual region is infiltrated with dilute vasopressin (20 units of vasopressin diluted in 100 ml of Ringer's lactate)

Transection of proximal segment: The tube is transected at mid isthmus. The tube is cut transversely avoiding damage to the nutrient vessel coursing beneath the tube and parallel to it. Depending on the extent of the intramural tube that is excised, and thus the site at which the anastomosis is formed tubocornual anastomosis may be juxtamural, intramural or juxtauterine (Fig. 8.12). If the whole intramural segment is involved it is removed and anastomosis is performed between the isthmus and the uterine tubal ostium.

Dissection of intramural portion of tube: It is essential that dissection of the intramural tube is done from the surrounding uterine musculature. It is done by a curved microscissors thus decreasing risk of creating a large defect at the cornua. The tube needs to be cored out. For this a 6-0 suture

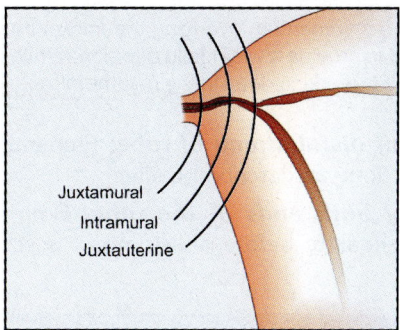

Fig. 8.12: Site of anastomosis depending on
the extent of intramural block

is placed through the lumen of the tube and gentle traction is
exerted. Dissection is continued just outside the circular muscle.
Each time the surgeon dissects 2 mm of the tube, the section
is transected and tube inspected under high magnification

Maintenance of hemostasis: The only vessels that require
bipolar coagulation and division are branches that penetrate
directly into the tube. Irrigation defines the vessels, allowing
coagulation to be done easily. The identification and
coagulation process begins superiorly to prevent blood from
obscuring open vessels positioned inferiorly. Tiny vessels situated
near the mucosa should not be coagulated as it may damage
the mucosa. If bleeding is brisk and the cut end of the vessel
is not seen, gentle pressure may cease the bleeding.
Occasionally, a large venous sinus is encountered. Since
coagulation would result in excessive damage while achieving
hemostasis, it is best to close the sinus with 8-0 suture.

***Chromotubation to establish patency of proximal
segment:*** After transecting the tube its patency is established
by transcervical chromotubation and normalcy of the cut
surface is evaluated under magnification.

Crescent of the myometrium overlying the intramural part of the tube is excised to provide a wider field of vision. While transecting the tube as one is working deep in the myometrium.

Preparation of distal stump of tube: Preparation of distal isthmic end is done as described earlier.

Inspection of both ends of the tube: Both ends of the tube must be healthy before anastomosis is started (Table 8.7).

Table 8.7: Ideal characteristics of intramural tube prepared for anastomosis should exhibit the following
1. On lavage the stream of methylene blue should be cylindrical with uninterrupted egress. If it is not so a monofilament suture or a stent is passed into the intramural tube and threaded gently into the uterine cavity.
2. Tubal mucosa should appear velvety and healthy
3. Tubal musculature should be well perfused
4. Myometrium surrounding the tube should be devoid of fibrosis or other pathological conditions.

Myometrial sutures: Sutures are taken as described before at 6, 3 and 9 o'clock and 12 o'clock (Fig. 8.13). If the cornual crater is deep and it is difficult to take sutures an incision is given at the cornua of the uterus. The edges of the incision are approximated at the end of the procedure.

Suturing of serosa and mesosalpinx: The serosal layer is approximated. Mesosalpinx is closed only anteriorly (Fig. 8.13).

Intramural Ampullary Anastomosis

The important difference in this is the luminal disparity. The ampullary stump is prepared as described before (Fig. 8.11E).

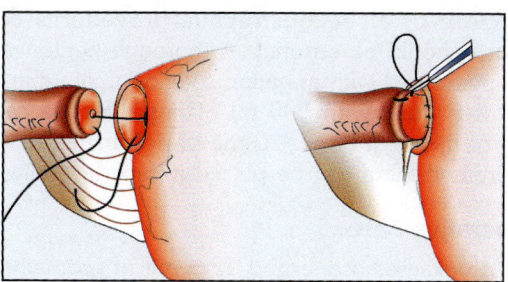

Fig. 8.13: Sutures are taken from muscularis of the isthmic end and intramural portion starting at 6 o'clock. The serosa is taken in the second layer

Advantages of microsurgical tubocornual anastomosis over tubouterine implantation:

- Maintains integrity of the uterine cornua
- Less disturbance of vascular tree.
- Preserves a longer tube
- Obviates need for cesarean section
- Yields better results.
- Preserves function of the uterotubal junction.
- Post implantation pelvic pain and irregular bleeding is absent. It occurs in one-third of patients undergoing implantation.

Checking luminal patency after anastomosis: Leakage at the anastomotic site is acceptable provided flow of dye from the distal end of the tube is observed and there is no tension at the anastomotic site. If the uterus is expanding with the dye and the proximal part of the tube is not, the surgeon may gently massage the myometrium in the vicinity of the cornua which sometimes results in release of the obstruction. If unsuccessful in establishing the flow in the proximal segment the surgeon may do nothing further provided the proximal segment was determined to be patent earlier, the surgeon is confident that the anastomosis is technically satisfactory and the preoperative HSG revealed a normal proximal segment.

At the close of all reconstructive procedures complete hemostasis should be ensured. A thorough peritoneal lavage may be performed with irrigation solution until returning fluid is clear. It is done with 500 ml of ringer lactate containing 500 mg of hydrocortisone. 20 mg of dexamethasone and 25 mg of promethazine can be placed intraperitoneally.

Postoperative Care

10 mg of dexamethasone and 12.5 mg of promethazine are continued parenterally every 4 hours for 7 doses. Prophylactic antibiotic are given.

Role of postoperative hydrotubation: The routine practice of hydrotubation or second-look laparoscopy following female pelvic reproductive surgery shows no added benefit.[14]

Follow-up

First check-up is at one month. If patient does not conceive an HSG can be done at 9 to 12 months and a follow-up laparoscopy at 18 months. Usually more than half the patients who conceive do so by 10 months.[15]

Results of Tubal Anastomosis

Various studies have shown a success rate varying from 32 to 88% (Table 8.8). Success of the procedure depends on
1. Tubal length (less than 4 cm has poor prognosis).
2. Site of reanastomosis: Isthmic area shows best results (Table 8.8).
3. Method of sterilization: If tubal ligation has been done by monopolar electrocautery it is associated with destruction of large amount of Fallopian tube. Electrocautery damage of oviduct cilium may extend upto 2 cm from site of cautery. However upto 50% may conceive after tubal cautery and reanastomosis.[16] Fallopes ring and silastic band sterilization are associated with 85% pregnancy rates after recanalization.

4. Associated pelvic pathology: Endometriosis or hydrosalpinx decreases success rate.
5. Time interval from sterilization to anastomosis (more than 4 years shows poor prognosis)
6. Tubal vascularity: Tubal vascularity decreases with time.
7. Presence of other infertility factors
8. Adherence to good surgical principles (Table 8.5).

Table 8.8: Success of reversal of sterilization at various sites [17]	
Site of anastomosis	Pregnancy rate (%)
Isthmic – Isthmic	88
Cornual – Isthmic	78
Isthmic – Ampullary	67
Ampullary – Ampullary	67
Cornual – Ampullary	53

Causes of Failure

1. Recurrence of adhesion especially the thick vascular ones.
2. Failure to excise microscopic disease in proximal segment of the tube including salpingitis isthmica nodosa, endometriosis, fibrosis and chronic salpingitis.
3. Postoperative infections
4. Inadequate tubal length
5. Faulty techniques
6. Disturbance in tubo-ovarian relationship.
7. Development of other causes of infertility like male factor.

Tubal Implantation

Repair of cornual obstruction is the most difficult and challenging of infertility surgery. Implantation should be reserved for those cases where anastomosis is not possible and patient is not willing to go for IVF ET.

Procedures

1. Cornual implantation
   - Closed
   - Open
2. Posterior wall implantation
   - Closed
   - Open

A portion of the tube is inserted into a site in the uterus which can be prepared by incision or excision or by use of a reamer or borer. It can be done blindly (closed) or visually (open) by incising the uterus and viewing the insertion and implantation. In the closed technique the approximation of the endosalpinx and endometrium is assumed rather than visualized.

Steps

1. ***Preparation of the proximal portion of the distal segment:*** Incisions are made till the patent part of the tube is reached. Lateral tubal incisions 1 cm long is made through the tube at 3 o'clock and 9 o'clock positions dividing the tube into mesenteric and antimesenteric half. In this manner a fishmouth is fashioned. Mesosalpinx is dissected back for 1 cm. A 2-0 absorbable *suture* is placed through each half of the fish mouth serosa through endosalpinx (Fig. 8.14).
3. ***Preparation of the uterine wall:*** Any defect at the cornua is closed. Vasopressin is injected in the region. A borer with a diameter of 1 cm is inserted into the serosa at the level of ovarian ligament with angulation to midline. The borer comes out within the core of myometrium. The implantation can also be done at the cornual end.
4. ***Implantation:*** The thread on the mesenteric half of the tube is passed through the new opening into the uterus

downward through the endometrium and myometrium and exiting at the serosa. The other end of the thread is similarly brought out 3 to 5 mm from the previous one. The same procedure is repeated with the antimesenteric end with the needle being directed upwards. The sutures are pulled to ease the fishmouth into the uterine cavity and tied, splaying the tube within the endometrial cavity. The serosa of the tube is apposed to the serosa of the uterus (Fig. 8.14).

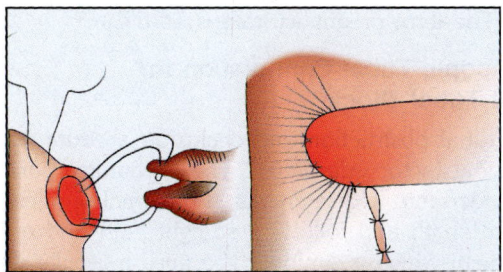

Fig. 8.14: Tubal implantation at the cornual end – Closed method

Open Method

The myometrium is incised and the endometrium is directly exposed for mucosa to mucosa placement of sutures (Fig. 8.15).

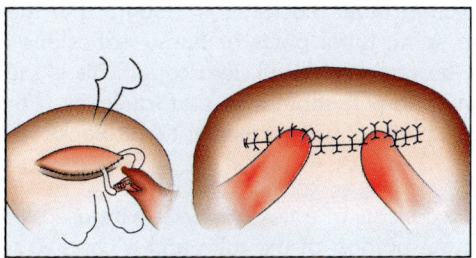

Fig. 8.15: Tubal implantation in the posterior wall – Open method

Complications

1. Bleeding from uterine wall
2. Infection
3. Delayed postoperative bleeding – seen with use of prosthesis.
4. Uterine rupture
5. Ectopic pregnancy 2 to 4%.
6. Post implantation pelvic pain and irregular vaginal bleeding: Occur in one-third of patients.

Results: The term pregnancy rate is 14-69%.[18]

Hysteroscopic Tubal Cannulation for Proximal Tubal Block

Proximal tubal obstruction and occlusion account for 10 to 25% of tubal factor infertility.[18] The intramural part of the tube is divided into two segments: A proximal segment which is 1 cm in length and follows a straight path and a 1.5 cm distal segment which is sinuous. The thick muscular wall and the convoluted intramural course make the uterotubal junction a likely site for blockage by uterine debris. Contrary to the belief that all proximal tubal obstructions are due to an inflammatory process or endometriosis only 7 out of 18 cases when surgically resected showed an organic pathology.[19] Since rest of the tubes showed only inflammation and fibrosis with no blockage a surgical correction was not warranted in most of the proximal tubal blocks. It is thought that these blocks are due to some tubal plugs or flimsy adhesions or polyps which can be removed by hysteroscope. This is the basis for tubal cannulation. It should be performed as a first line of treatment in patients with proximel tubal block[20] (Fig. 8.16).

Technique

It essentially consists of a flexible guide wire used to negotiate the intramural portion of the tube and a cannula to direct it towards the tubal ostium. A flexible or rigid hysteroscope is used.

Anesthesia: Hysteroscopic cannulation is done under general anesthesia if a simultaneous laparoscopy is required for chromotubation.

Tubal ostia are identified on hysteroscopy. The 7 Fr outflow catheter is now introduced through the opening channel and aligned towards the ostia. Terumo guide wire is then introduced through the outflow catheter. The hysteroscope and outflow catheter are positioned in such a way that if the guide wire is pushed it should enter the ostia. Often the end of the hysteroscope must be placed within 2 mm of the ostia in order to provide extra stability for the guide wire. The flexibility of the guide wire is altered by varying the length of the wire protruding from the outer catheter. The guide wire is now pushed into the ostia for 2 to 3 cm always keeping the outflow catheters almost in a straight line for easy sliding. It is not necessary to cannulate the ampullary portion of the tube because it can damage the delicate mucosa. Once the wire enters the ostia its position is documented by laparoscopy. The procedure is repeated on the other side. Hysteroscope is withdrawn and the chromopertubation done and observed through laparoscope to confirm results of cannulation. Angioplasty catheter can be used for cannulation. The balloon can be distended giving long lasting mechanical dilatation.

Complications:

1. Perforation: It is reported in 10%. It is left to heal sponta-neously.
2. Markedly distorted cavity makes the procedure difficult
3. Ectopic pregnancy: The chances of ectopic pregnancy increase in the presence of distal tubal disease.

The pregnancy rate per attempted cannulation was 19%. Ectopic pregnancy was seen in 5% and perforation in 1 to 2%. Reocclusion may be due to a significant pathology and procedure may have to be repeated.

Fluoroscopic Fallopian Tube Catheterization

Fallopian tube catheterization is an extension of hysterosalpingography. It is usually done 2 to 3 days after cessation of bleeding, on an outpatient basis.

Technique

Equipment: The diameter of the hysterocath is chosen to match the cervical size. The 5.5 catheter is introduced into the 9 French sheath. The adapter is tightened to stabilize the catheter within the hysterocath.

Contrast medium: The catheter is filled with half strength water soluble contrast medium. Half strength is used since it does not impede subsequent visualization of the catheters, full strength contrast material is used when injecting directly into the fallopian tube for better visualization.

Placing the Hysterocath: The hysterocup allows traction to be placed on the uterus by the vacuum cup and provides a sterile conduit through which catheter can be advanced.

Initial hysterosalpingography: First a hysterosalpingography is done to confirm obstruction.

Selective salpingography: If tubal obstruction is present the 5.5 French catheter is advanced into the tubal ostium. This is accomplished using a 0.035 inch J guide wire initially to maneuver the catheter into the corneal portion of the uterus. Once this is accomplished the 0.035 inch straight wire LT guide wire is used to lodge the catheter directly into the tubal ostium. Embedding the catheter into the myometrium results in painful extravasation and obscures anatomy. With the 5.5 French catheter successfully wedged in the tubal ostium full strength contrast medium is injected. Approximately 20% of the time this direct injection will open the tube. If it does not it will indicate the direction of the proximal portion of the tube and the exact site of obstruction.

When the resistance is encountered at the site of obstruction, short probing motions with the guide wire are used to overcome the obstruction. If this is unsuccessful, or the obstruction is located more distally or there is a bend in the fallopian tube the small catheter wire is exchanged for a softer tapered system. The catheter is advanced over the guide wire once recanalization is accomplished, dilating the tube. The guide wire is removed and contrast inserted. Same procedure may be carried out on the other side if needed.

HSG: Post procedure hysterosalpingogram is done.

Follow-up: Patient is told that she may have spotting for a few days. Intercourse need not be postponed.

Contraindications:
- Acute pelvic infection
- Iodinated contrast allergy
- Tubal obstruction after tubal anastomosis

Results: Approximately 90% of the tubes can be recanalised. In isolated proximal tubal obstruction with a pregnancy rate of 50%.

Proximal tubal block is a common cause of infertility and considering the simplicity, ease and lack of morbidity of the transcervical cannulation it should be tried as the first procedure for proximal tubal block.

Tubal Surgery vs ART

In vitro fertilization/embryo transfer (IVF/ART) results have shown significant improvements during the last decade with a success rate of 35% per cycle. Tubal surgery also shows good results. This rate, for those who are < 35 years of age at the time of reversal, is >70%, with most pregnancies occurring within 18 months after surgery. Those who are 35 years of age or more will have a 55% rate of intrauterine pregnancy (IUP). Satisfactory IUP rate (50%) after tubocornual

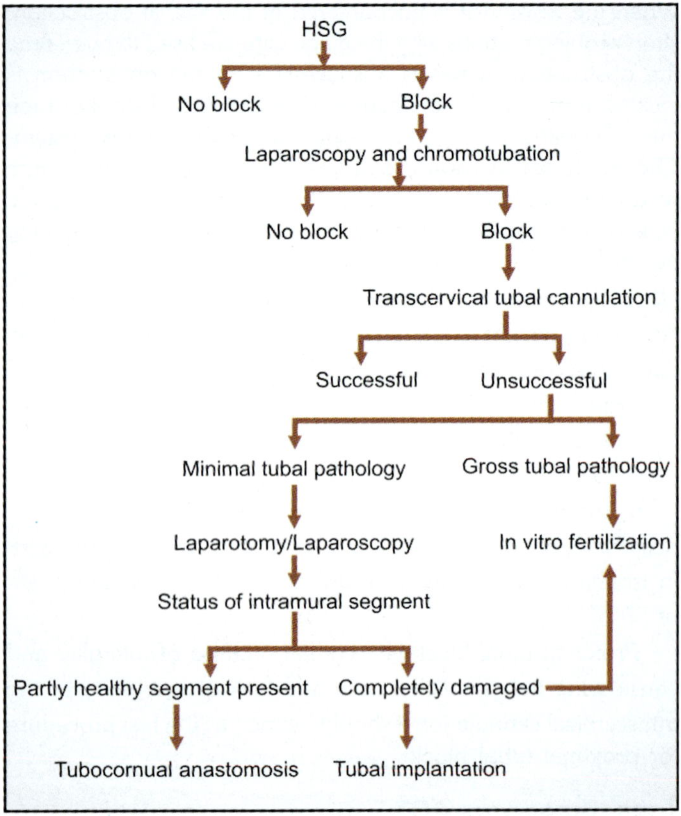

Fig. 8.16: Approach to patient with provisonal tubal obstriction

anastomosis for proximal tubal disease was noted. The IUP rates after salpingo-ovariolysis and fimbrioplasty are 60% and 50%, respectively.[21] Salpingostomy also provides a beneficial effect upon embryo implantation in both in vivo and in vitro attempts at conception. ART should be resorted to when the expected success rate with surgery is poor. The surgical feasibility should be based on objective proper evaluation of the tubal pathology.

Surgery in properly selected cases can give superior results to ART

The proper selection of patients is mandatory to obtain the optimal results. When adnexa are relatively free from adhesions and the tubes are not thickened or dilated salpingoplasty remains a reasonable alternative. However in patients with thickened and grossly dilated tubes or dense pelvic adhesion are better served with *in vitro* fertilization. Also we have to consider the fact that with surgery we get permanent cure with the chances of normal repeated conceptions while with ART it is only a single trial with conception effected only in the IVF centers

Surgery and ART are complementary approaches that can be used singly or in combination to improve the outcome for couples with tubal infertility. The evidence suggests surgical management of tubal infertility still has an important place in infertility treatment in the era of ART. Surgeons have to work closely with the ART specialist to give all infertile couples a chance to conceive.

REFERENCES

1. Westrom L. Effect of acute pelvic inflammatory disease on fertility. Am J Obstet Gynecol 1975; 121:707-16.
2. Rock JA, Katayama KP, Martin EJ Factors influencing the success of salpingostomy techniques for distal fimbrial obstruction. Obstet Gynecol 1978; 52:591-5.
3. Winston RML. Is microsurgery necessary for salpingostomy? The evaluation of results. Aust NZ Obstet Gynecol 1981: 21:143-7.
4. Ahmad G, Watson A, Vandekerckhove P, Lilford R. Techniques for pelvic surgery in subfertility. Cochrane Database Syst Rev 2006 19;(2):CD000221.
5. Gomel V Microsurgical reversal of female sterilization: a reappraisal Fertil Steril 1980;33:587-9

6. Gomel V, Yarali H. Infertility surgery: microsurgery. Curr Opin Obstet Gynecol 1992; 4:390-8.

7. Fayez JA. An assessment of the role of operative laparoscopy in tuboplasty. Fertil Steril 1983; 39: 476-82.

8. Johnson NP, Mak W, Sowter MC. Surgical treatment for tubal disease in women due to undergo in vitro fertilization Cochrane Database Syst Rev. 2004;(3):CD002125.

9. Gomel V. Salpingo-ovariolysis by laparoscopy in infertility. Fertil Steril 1983; 40:607-11.

10. Rock JA Bergquist CA, Kimbal AW Jr, et al. Comparison of operating microscope and loupe for microsurgical tubal anastomosis: a randomized clinical trial. Fertil Steril 1984; 41:229-31.

11. Verhoevan HC, et al. Surgical treatment for distal tube occlusion. J Reprod Med 1983; 28:293-8.

12. Donnez J, Casanas – Roux F. Prognostic factors of fimbrial microsurgery. Fertil Steril 1986; 46:200-2.

13. Lauretsen JG, Pagel JD, Vangsted P, Starup J. Results of repeated tuboplasties. Fertil Steril 1982; 37:68.

14. Johnson NP, Watson A. Cochrane review: Postoperative procedures for improving fertility following pelvic reproductive surgery. Human Reproduction Update 2000; 6(3):259-67.

15. Groff TR, Edelstein J A, Schenken RS. Hysterosalpingography in the preoperative evaluation of tubal anastomosis candidates. Fertil Steril 1990; 53:417.

16. Winston RML. Reversal of sterilization. Clin Obstet Gynecol 1980; 23:1261-8.

17. Henderson S. The reversibility of female sterilization with the use of microsurgery: a report on 102 patients with more than one year of followup. Am J Obstet Gynecol 1984; 149:57-69.

18. Musich J, Behrman S.Surgical management of tubal obstruction at the uterotubal junction. Fertil Steril 1983; 40:423-40.

19. Sulak PJ, Letterie GS, Coddington CC, Hayslip CC, Woodward JE Klein TA. Histology of proximal tubal occlusion Fertil Steril 1987; 48:437-40.

20. Kodaman, Pinar H, Arici, Aydi, Seli, Emre Evidence-based diagnosis and management of tubal factor infertility. Curr Opin Obstet Gynecol 2004;16(3):221-9.

21. Gomel V, McComb PF. Microsurgery for tubal infertility J Reprod Med. 2006; 51(3):177-84.

CHAPTER 9

Laparoscopic Surgery for Tubal and Peritubal Pathology in Infertility

Punita Bhardwaj

Many tubal and peritubal factors like, peritubal adhesions, proximal and distal tubal block, endometriosis and previous ectopic pregnancy could be responsible for infertility. Tubal causes account for 25% of infertility in women.[1]

Ectopic Pregnancy (EP)

Implantation of pregnancy outside the uterine cavity is an ectopic pregnancy, 95% of which occur in the fallopian tube, commonest being ampullary ectopic. Risk factors include, history of infertility, pelvic inflammatory disease, pelvic surgery (particularly tubal surgery), assisted conceptions and presence of an intrauterine device.

Clinical presentation: The woman classically presents with amenorrhea, abdominal pain and adnexal mass. There may be history of syncopal attacks (See Chapter 14).

Diagnosis: Definitive diagnosis of Ectopic pregnancy is based on clinical history, physical exam and laboratory and diagnostic image findings. With development of immunoassay utilizing monoclonal antibodies to Human chorionic gonadotrophin and high resolution ultrasound scanners ectopic pregnancy can be diagnosed early (See Chapter 14).[2]

Unruptured tubal pregnancy has a positive association with future fertility. Hence early diagnosis and conservative surgical management are therefore important.

Treatment: Treatment may vary according to a number of factors. There are three treatment options (For details See Chapter 14).
1. Conservative
2. Medical
3. Surgical

Laparoscopic Management of Ectopic Pregnancy

Laparoscopic surgery must be carried out by or under direct supervision of those fully trained in laparoscopic surgery. For all but the most experienced endoscopist hemodynamically unstable patient with ruptured ectopic pregnancy is best treated by laparotomy.

Apart from surgeons skill, the next most important pre-requisite for safe laparoscopic surgery is good equipment.

Equipment: Essential equipment includes a 10 mm 0° telescope, light source of 250 W or greater, TV camera and monitor, suction / irrigation probe, monopolar needle, point diathermy grasping forceps, bipolar coagulation forceps, scissors and pre-tied ligature loops.

Laparoscpic Management Consists of

- Laparoscopic – Injection of embryotoxic substances into Ectopic Pregnancy sac
- Linear salpingostomy
- Salpingectomy

Laparoscopic – Injection of Embryotoxic Substances into EP Sac

50 mg intratubal methotrexate injection into EP sac after aspiration has been advocated if there is no hemoperitoneum and ensuring that blood vessel is not penetrated. Direct injection is of particular use in cases of interstitial or cornual ectopic pregnancies where other forms of surgery are more difficult and bloody.[3]

The substances injected into the fallopion tubes or the ectopic pregnancy are:

- Methotrexate
- PGF2 Alpha
- Hypoosmolar glucose solution
- Potassium chloride (Robertsen *et al* 1987)

Contraindications to conservative laparoscopic surgery.
Absolute Contraindications

- Patient hemodynamically unstable
- General Contraindications to laparoscopy

- Hematosalpinx > 6 cm
- βHCG - > 20,000 IU/l

Relative Contraindications

- Marked obesity
- Hematosalpinx > 4 cm
- Acute and continuing hemorrhage
- Significant hemoperitoneum
- Dense pelvic adhesions
- Cornual pregnancy

These recommendations may be modified based on the clinical situation and the experience of the endoscopic surgeon. Excellent suction irrigation device is obligatory, fast flow insufflators to ensure adequate pneumo- peritoneum is a must. In cases where salpingostomy is not feasible or contraindicated, salpingectomy is carried out.

Technique

Salpingostomy

Infraumbilical incision for placement of laparoscope is used with a suprapubic / lower lateral second puncture site for introduction of probe to manipulate the pelvic organs. Second puncture is made 2-3 finger width above the symphysis pubis in the midline or similar distance above the anterior superior iliac spine lateral to inferior epigastric artery, the trocar being advanced under direct vision through the anterior peritoneum. Once within the peritoneal cavity status of all abdominal viscera is noted.

Tube is grasped distal to the site of planned salpingostomy incision and put on a stretch.

Dilute vasopressin solution (one ampoule of 20 units in 100 ml normal saline) is injected into the antimesenteric border of the tube overlying the ectopic gestation if the patient is not bleeding actively. Some surgeons also inject the mesosalpinx or cauterize vessels within the mesosalpinx.

An incision is made over the antimesenteric border of the ectopic with electrosurgery, scissors or laser. Incision covers 2/3rd of the length of ectopic gestation and is deep enough to expose the clots around ectopic gestation or allow extrusion of products of conception. Products are removed with an atraumatic grasping instrument gently. Irrigation under pressure or pressure applied externally may dislodge the products. The tube is grasped proximal and distal to the incision and gently palpated to search for remaining placental tissue. If found the tissue is grasped from existing incision or incision extended to allow easy removal of any remaining trophoblastic tissue.

All tissue coming from the ectopic site should be removed from the abdominal cavity to prevent reimplantation.[4] This can be done by

1. Removing piecemeal by 10 mm grasping forceps.
2. Through posterior colpotomy.
3. Placing in an endobag introduced through a 10 mm port.

Site of salpingostomy is copiously irrigated to ensure hemostasis. Bleeding points identified and desiccated with precise bipolar instrument. Salpingostomy incision is left to heal by secondary intention. Cases where suture closure of incision is done, postoperative adhesion and or obstruction rates are higher.

Thorough abdominal lavage is carried out and hemostasis ensured. A decrease of pneumoperitoneum pressures exposes bleeders that require attention. Ports are removed under vision. Gas is evacuated scope withdrawn under vision. All ports more than 7 mm are closed under vision.

Persistent Ectopic Pregnancy (PEP)

Removal of pregnancy is incomplete and residual trophoblast continues to survive. Diagnosis is made by a lack of fall, or rise in serum hCG level postoperatively. PEP can be treated by a reoperation or methotrexate.

Salpingectomy

The Ectopic sac is visualized on the tube (Fig. 9.1). The tube is stretched and bipolar coagulation is used to coagulate starting from the lateral end (Fig. 9.2). The mesosalpinx is coagulated close to the tube to interrupt the blood supply and then incised (Fig. 9.3). Finally medial end is stretched, coagulated and incised to remove entire tube (Fig. 9.4). Specimen is parked in the anterior fornix (Fig. 9.5). Cooling is done with saline (Fig. 9.6). A 10 mm tenaculum is used to pull out specimen. The tenaculum should have a good grip on the specimen and it should be removed longitudinally (Fig. 9.7). Lavage is done and salpingectomy site is inspected to ensure hemostasis before removing the laparoscope (Fig. 9.8).

Follow up: Serial β HCG to rule out persistent ectopic pregnancy done weekly till negative.

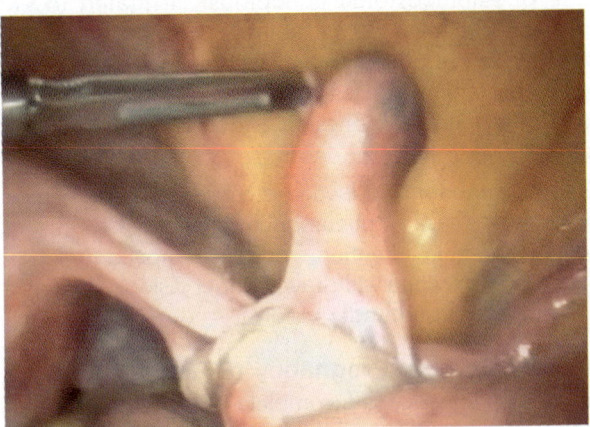

Fig. 9.1: Unruptured ectopic sac is visualized on the tube

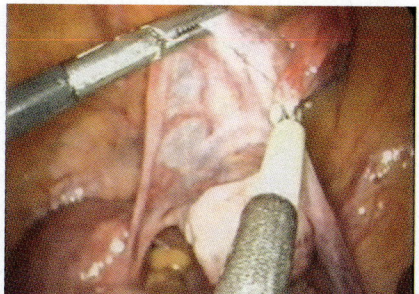

Fig. 9.2: Tube stretched, coagulation starting from lateral side

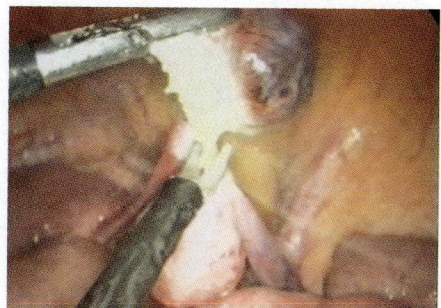

Fig. 9.3: Mesosalpinx is coagulated close to the tube and incised

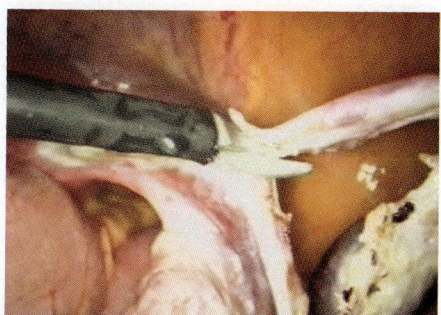

Fig. 9.4: The medial end of the tube is coagulated and incised to remove the tube

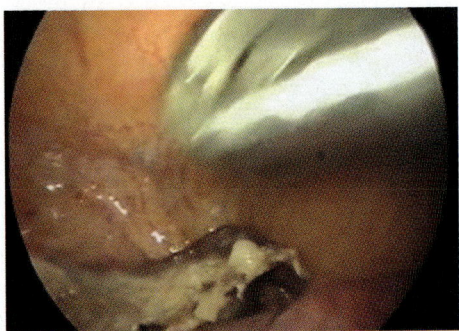

Fig. 9.5: Specimen parked in anterior fornix

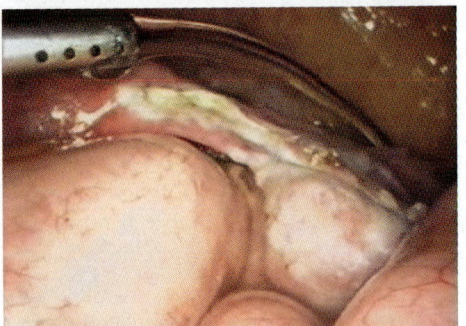

Fig. 9.6: Cooling done with saline

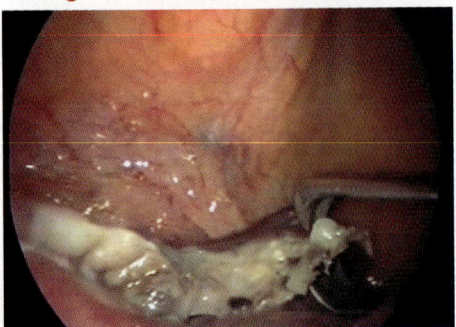

Fig. 9.7: Tenaculum used to pull out specimen

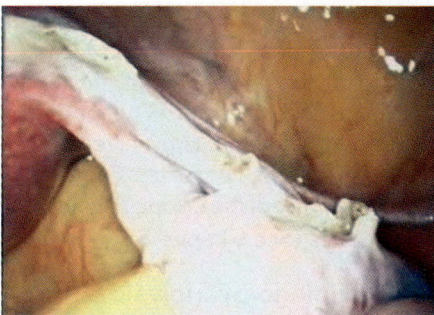

Fig. 9.8: Inspect salpingectomy site before closure

Laparoscopic Reconstructive Surgery for Tubal Disease

The tube is responsible for ovum pickup, it maintains sperm motility, furnishes the environment for fertilization and is responsible for embryo transport. Pelvic infection and surgery accounts for most of the tubal damage which results in infertility.

Tubal status can be assessed by HSG, sonohystero-salpingography and falloposcopy before a laparoscopy (See Chapter 2).

Endoscopic Microsurgical Principles

Microsurgical principles include techniques to minimize tissue injury by delicate handling of tissues, appropriate intraoperative irrigation to prevent drying, meticulous hemostasis and avoiding introduction of foreign body into the peritoneal cavity. Microsurgery demands precise alignment and apposition of tissue planes with appropriate use of fine instruments and suture material. Laparoscopic procedures fulfill all the above criteria and more.

Apart from providing magnification with direct illumination, the peritoneal cavity remains closed (though distended with carbon dioxide) and tissue drying can be prevented. The absence of abrasive abdominal pads and lack of exposure of peritoneal cavity to latex gloves and talcum powder prevents the introduction of foreign body. The pneumoperitonium pressure (approximately 12 mm Hg) decreases venous oozing and allows for spontaneous hemostasis.[5]

Reconstructive surgery of the fallopian tubes can be classified into various categories (See Chapter 8).

Laparoscopic Salpingo-ovariolysis

It is the treatment of choice for periadnexal adhesions.

Technique

Lysis of abdominal wall adhesions: Any adhesions of anterior abdominal wall are first dealt with (Fig. 9.9). Inspect all adhesions to ensure that there is no bowel from above downwards. Adhesions are cauterized by bipolar cautery close to the abdominal wall and cut (Figs. 9.10 to 9.12). Traction is given by the grasper.

Salpingo-ovariolysis: The tube may be embedded in a tuboovarian mass (Fig. 9.13). Adhesions are put at a stretch with right side bowel retractor and left side ureteric dissector (Figs 9.14 to 9.16). They are usually not too vascular and in joining one structure to another they leave a space which facilitates adhesiolysis. Broad adhesions are excised completely shallow ones are transected. Tissue planes are developed by entering the adhesions and spreading the jaws of the instrument or by using hydrodissection. They are divided one layer at a time, parallel to relevant viscus, avoiding damage to adjacent serosa or ovarian surface using micro electrode or scissors. (Fig. 9.17). It is important to use thermal energy judiciously in such cases. Bleeders along the incision line are desiccated using blend settings on the electro surgical unit. Bowel needs to be delineated before using any sharp instruments. Fimbria become visible as

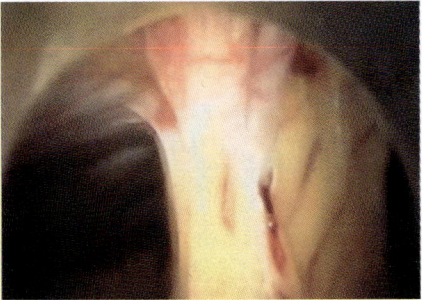

Fig. 9.9: Adhesions over the anterior abdominal wall

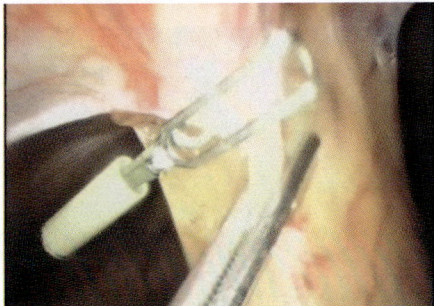

Fig. 9.10: Traction given by grasper and bipolar cautery used to coagulate

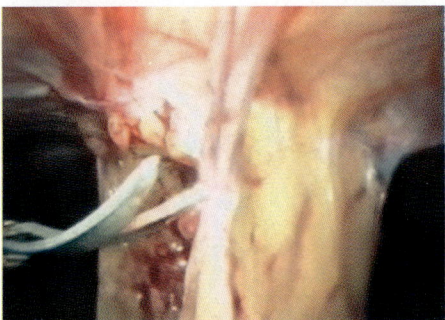

Fig. 9.11: Adhesions incised

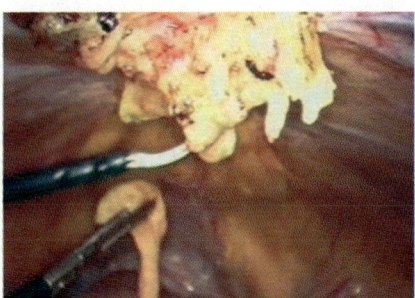

Fig. 9.12: Complete separation of adhesions close to the abdominal wall

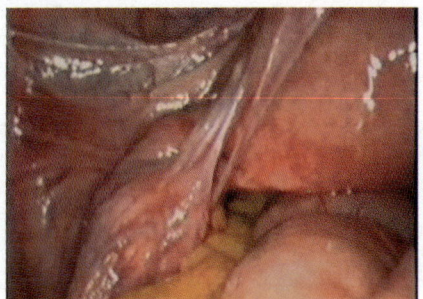

Fig. 9.13: Adhesions forming a right tubo-ovarian mass

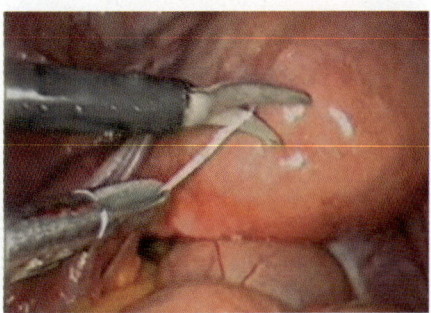

Fig. 9.14: Flimsy adhesions put at a stretch and cut

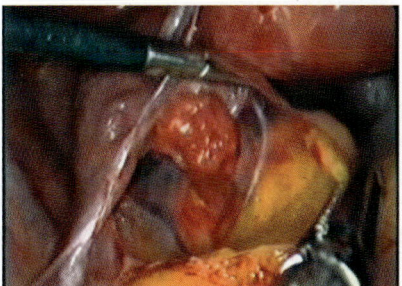

Fig. 9.15: Adhesions put at a stretch with right side bowel retractor and left side ureteric dissector

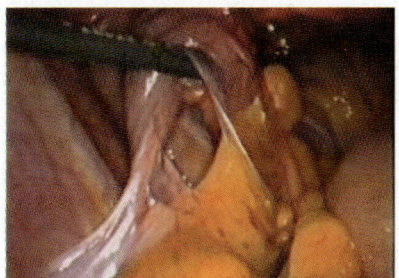

Fig. 9.16: Adhesions being released from epiploicae

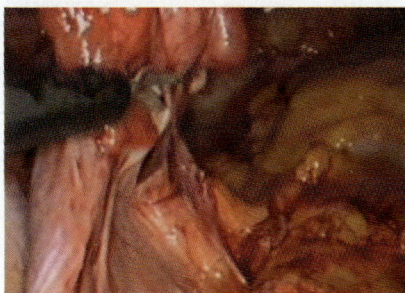

Fig. 9.17: All adhesions cut parallel to the viscous

adhesions get released (Fig. 9.18). Gradual release of adhesions is carried out. Adhesions may be released at cornual end in a similar manner (Fig. 9.19).

The ovary is released from the ovarian fossa (Fig. 9.20). Adhesions of the tube and ovary are released by sharp or blunt dissection (Fig. 9.21).

Chromotubation is done to see the spill of the dye (Fig. 9.22). Peritoneal irrigation and lavage is done at the end of the procedure (Fig. 9.23).

Fimbrioplasty

Fimbrial phimosis is often present with a tubo-ovarian mass (Fig. 9.24). Periadnexal adhesions are treated first to release the tube (Fig. 9.25). Adhesions are released from the ovary (Fig. 9.26). Usually there is a small distal opening which becomes apparent after distending the tube with chromopertubation. This is accessed by a dissector (Fig. 9.27). The fibrous band enclosing the fimbria is incised from all sides (Figs 9.28 and 9.29). The dissector is introduced and withdrawn with open prongs to widen opening (Fig. 9.30). The phimotic fimbrial end may be

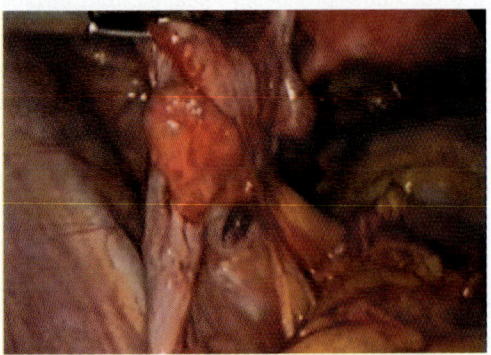

Fig. 9.18: Fimbria visible as adhesions get released

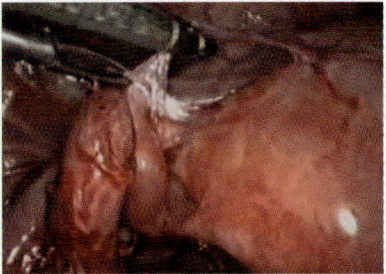

Fig. 9.19: Adhesions at the cornual end being released

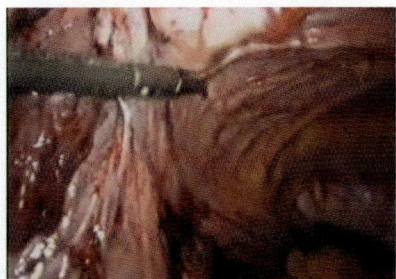

Fig. 9.20: Ovary being released from the ovarian fossa

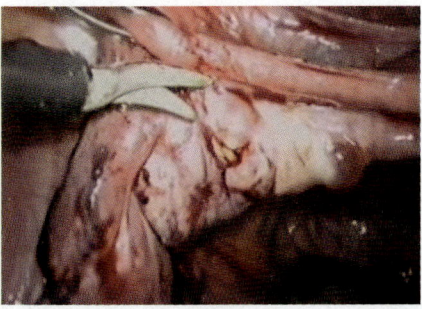

Fig: 9.21: Tube being released from adhesions
to the ovary by sharp dissection

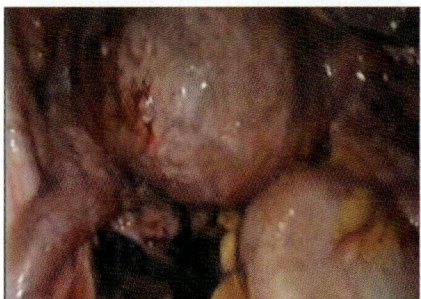

Fig 9.22: Chromotubation shows spill of dye

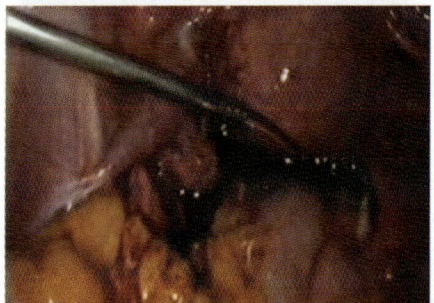

Fig. 9.23: Irrigation and lavage done

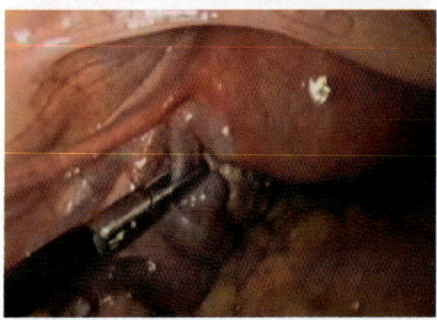

Fig. 9.24: Tubo-ovarian mass with fimbrial phimosis

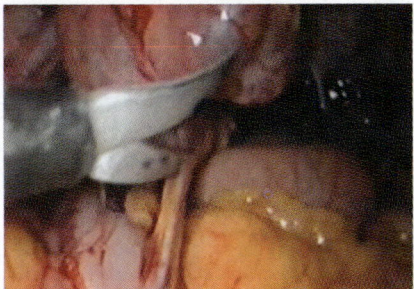

Fig. 9.25: Adhesiolysis to release tube

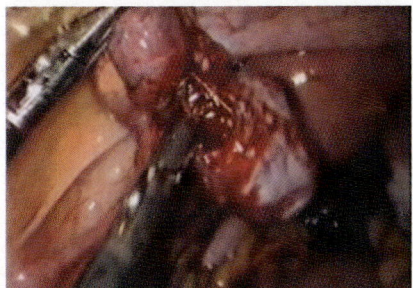

Fig. 9.26: Adhesiolysis being separated from ovary

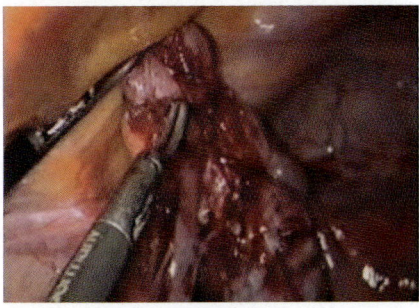

Fig. 9.27: Ostia being accessed by a dissector

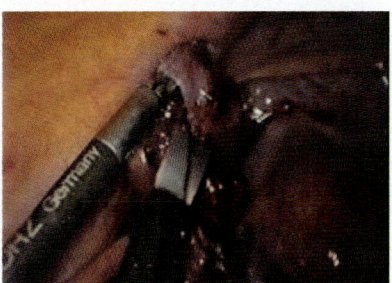

Fig. 9.28: The fibrous band is visualized and released with scissors

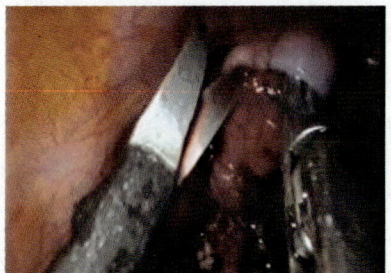

Fig. 9.29: Fibrous band released from other and released with scissors

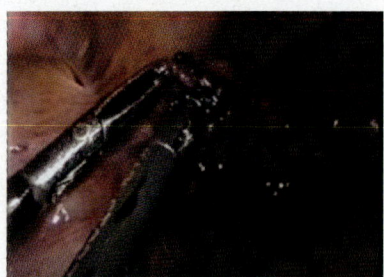

Fig. 9.30: Dissector put in and withdrawn with open prongs

covered by scar tissue, which may need to be incised or excised to gain access to the tubal lumen. The serosa is coagulated to keep fimbria everted (Fig. 9.31). Chromotubation shows tubal patency (Fig. 9.32). Irrigation and lavage, i.e. done before withdrawing the laparoscope.

Frequently, the agglutination can be corrected by just introducing a 3 mm forceps through the small fimbrial aperture and withdrawing it with open jaws gently.[6] The step is repeated a few times in different directions.

Prefimbrial Phimosis

With prefimbrial phimosis, stenosis occurs the level of true abdominal ostia and fimbria that look normal. This stenosis may become apparent only with chromo-pertubation. The treatment requires an incision at the antimesosalpingeal border of the tube extending from the fimbrial end into the distal ampullary part (See Chapter 8).

Salpingostomy (Salpingoneostomy)

It is the creation of new stoma in a tube with complete distal occlusion (hydrosalpinx).

Any associated pelvic and periadnexal adhesions present should be dealt with first. With chromotubation occluded

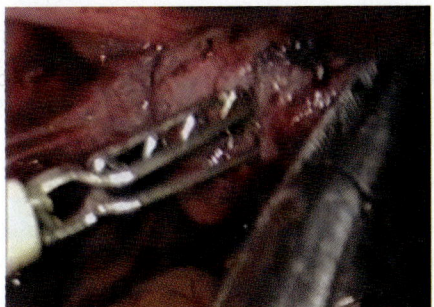

Fig. 9.31: Serosa cauterized to evert mucosa

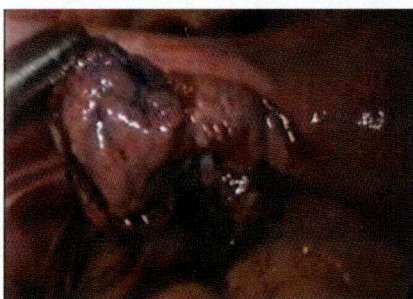

Fig. 9.32: Everted mucosa with dye test positive

terminal end is examined looking for the central punctum. The tube is entered at the central point and the incision extended along an avascular line towards the ovary. This creates a new fimbria ovarica. Now one can view the tube from within and place incisions along avascular areas between endothelial folds.

All bleeding points are identified under irrigating fluid and dessicated discretely. Once stoma is made flaps are everted by dessication of serosal surface (Electrosurgically or Carbon dioxide laser) or by using fine sutures (See Chapter 8).

Laparoscopic Tubal Anastomosis

It is done for tubal block and usually after previous tubal sterilization are giving encouraging results (See Chapter 10).

Salpingectomy

There are number of conditions not amenable to reconstructive surgery or where surgery is contraindicated in view of associated poor prognosis[7] like bipolar disease, presence of extensive intratubal adhesion and severe tubal damage (Grade V category).

In such cases IVF would prove to be a better option.[8,9]

Patients with one or two hydrosalpinges have a lower implantation rate and higher tubal ectopic pregnancy rate when treated with IVF. So, the need of prophylactic salpingectomy arises. The procedure has been described in section of ectopic pregnancy.

This procedure can also be carried out with the use of endoloops or sutures. The proximal end is cauterized – a small window is created in the cauterized mesosalpinx with a dissector and a suture passed through. The suture is carried around the distal end of the fallopian tube and tied. The tube above the suture knot is transected and tube sent for histopathologic examination. Hemostatsis of the pedicle is ensured. Irrigation lavage is done.

Proximal Tubal Cannulation

Proximal tubal Cannulation is the first option for cornual block.[10,11] A 5-7 mm hysteroscope with a 30° scope is used. The occluded tubal ostia is cannulated with a flexible tubal catheter, and methylene blue is injected through the cannula. Spill is observed through the fimbrial end laparoscopically. If no spill is seen, the tube is straightened laparoscopically. The hysterosopic surgeon pushes a guide wire with a soft flexible tip through the initial catheter into the isthmic area of the tube. The wire is withdrawn and dye test repeated (Fig. 9.33).

In spite of tremendous progress being made in ART, there is still a place for reconstructive tubal surgery. Selection of treatment modality should be based on proper investigation,

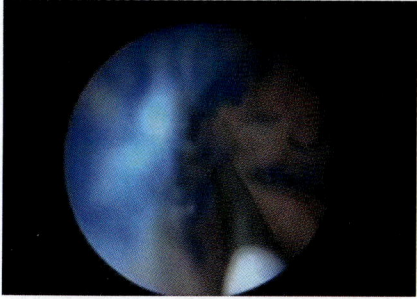

Fig. 9.33: Proximal tubal cannulation

counseling of the couple and honest disclosure with respect to the expertise and the results achieved by the centre in which the couple is to be treated.

REFERENCES

1. Tay JI, Moore J, Walker JJ. 'Ectopic Pregnancy' BMJ 2000; 320:916-9.
2. Natale A, Candiane M, Merlo D, IRRO S, Gruft L, Busacca M. Human chorionic gonadotropin level as a predictor of trophoblastic infiltration into the tubal wall in Ectopic pregnancy a blinded study. Fertil Steril. 2003;79(4):981-6.
3. Hajenius PJ, Mol BW, Borruyt PM, Ankum WM, VanDer Veen F. In comparison Laparoscopic conservative surgery (local Methotrexate) is less successful. Interventions for tubal Ectopic pregnancy. Cochrane Database Syst Rev 2000;(2):CD 000324.
4. Fujishita A, Masuzaki H, Khan KN, Kitajima M, Hiraki K, Ishimaru T. Laparoscopic salpingotomy for tubal pregnancy: Comparison of linear salpingotomy with and without suturing. Hum Reprod 2004;19(5):1195-1200.
5. Gomel V, McComb PF. Microsurgery for tubal infertility. J Reprod Med 2006;51(3):177-84.
6. Kasia JM, Raiga J, Dohas, Bioucle JM, Pouly JL, Kwiatkowshi F, Edgoa T, Bruhat MA. Laparoscopic fimbrioplasty and neosalpingostomy. Experience of Yaounde General Hospital, Cameroon (report of 194 cases). Eur J Obstet Gynecol Reprod Biol 1997;73(1):71-7.
7. Patrick Puttemans, Rudi Campo, Stephen Gordts, IVO Brosens. Hydrosalpinx and ART hydrosalpinx-functional surgery or salpingectomy? Human Reproduction 2000;15:1427-30.
8. Jhonson NP, Malc W, Sowter MC. Surgical treatment for tubal disease in women due to undergo in vitro fertilisation. Cochrane Database Syst Rev 2001;(3):CD 002125.
9. Sabatini L, Daves C. Tubal surgery should be preferred to salpingectomy in mild to moderate tubal dis. The management of hydrosalpinges : tubal surgery or salpingectomy? Curr Opin Obstet Gynecol 2005;17(4):323-8.
10. Musich J, Behrman S. Surgical management of tubal obstruction at the uterotubal junction. Fertil Steril 1983;40:423-40.
11. Sulak PJ, Letterie GS, Coddington CC, Hayslip CC, Woodward JE, Klein TA. Histology of proximal tubal occlusion. Fertil Steril 1987;48:437-40.

CHAPTER 10

Laparoscopic Tubal Anastomosis

Neena Singh Kumar
Surveen Ghumman

Fallopian tube interruption is a common form of contraception worldwide. For a variety of reasons (e.g. change in marital status, wish for additional children, psychological factors), many of these women seek restoration of fertility. Laparoscopic tubal anastomosis is one of the newer approaches by which this can be achieved. It has the advantage of providing a magnified tissue view with minimal tissue handling. Laparoscopic tubal reanastomosis was first done in 1989 using biological glue.[1] This simplified stitchless laparoscopic procedure for reversal of tubal sterilization with the use of a tubal splint, clip fixation of the muscularis and fibrin glue resulted in a promising pregnancy rate, which was similar to the pregnancy rate obtained with the microsurgical re-anastomosis with laparotomy.[2] Laparoscopic tubal anastomosis is now performed in a similar manner to microscopic tubal anastomosis with the advantages of minimally invasive surgery.

Indications

1. Reversal of sterilization
2. Salpingitis isthimica nodosa
3. Tubal occlusion secondary to ectopic pregnancy
4. Failed tubal cannulation for proximal blocks
5. Blocked tubes because of pelvic inflammatory disease

Types of Anastomosis

4 types of anastomosis are possible (See Chapter 8)
• Isthmoisthmic
• Isthmoampullary
• Ampulloampullary
• Tubocornual

Preoperative Preparation

Other factors of infertility are evaluated. Ultrasonography, hysterosalpingography and semen analysis are mandatory investigations (See Chapter 8). The patient should be counseled on the success rate and possibility of conversion to laparotomy if laparoscopy is not feasible. If tubes are unhealthy the option of IVF should be discussed.

Operative Procedure

Diagnostic laparoscopy: The aim of a diagnostic laparoscopy before starting the surgery is to evaluate the extent of fibrosis and length of tubal segment available. This helps to plan the anastomosis accordingly (Fig. 10.1).

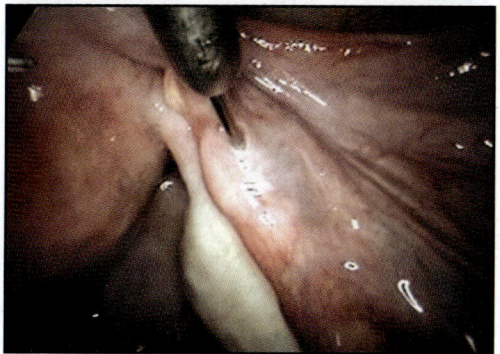

Fig. 10.1: Diagnostic laparoscopy to assess the extent of fibrosis

Transection of tubal stump and removal of fibrous tissue: The uterus is distended with dilute methylene blue. The proximal segment dilates making identification of lumen easier. The tube is held gently at the scarred tissue (Fig. 10.2). A fine forceps grasps the proximal stump and the microscissor is used to transect the proximal end of the tube till patent lumen is reached (Figs 10.3 and 10.4). Excess scar tissue is removed. The lateral end is similarly held and transected (Figs 10.5 and 10.6). Retrograde perturbation through the fimbria may be done to check patency of the transected lumen.

Caution: Mesosalpinx vessels should be avoided while transecting the tubal stump

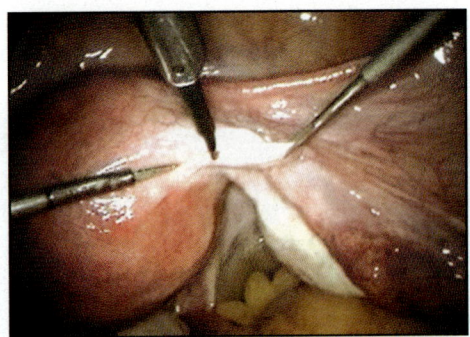

Fig. 10.2: The tube is held at the scar tissue

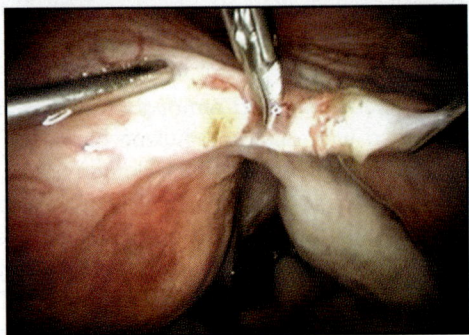

Fig. 10.3: The tube is transected at the medial stump

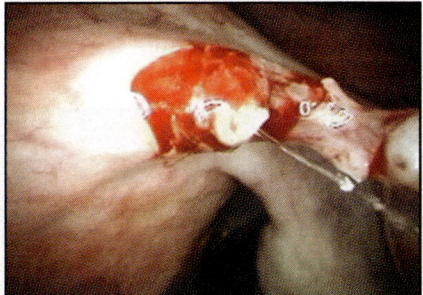

Fig. 10.4: Transection complete at the medial stump

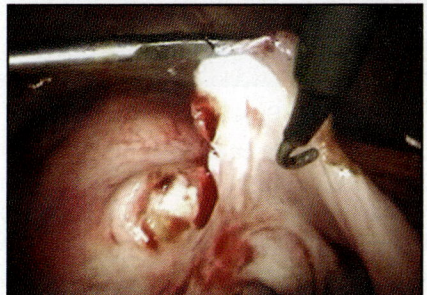

Fig. 10.5: Lateral stump is held

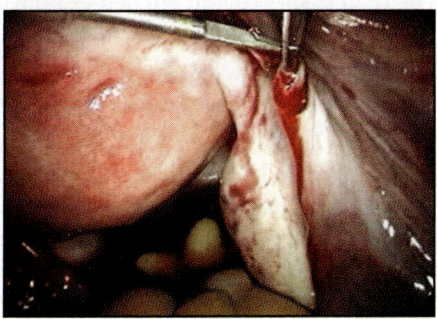

Fig. 10.6: Lateral stump is transected

Approximation of mesosalpinx: 6-0 polyglycon is used for suturing the mesosalpinx. Each suture is tied intra-corporeally (Fig. 10.7).

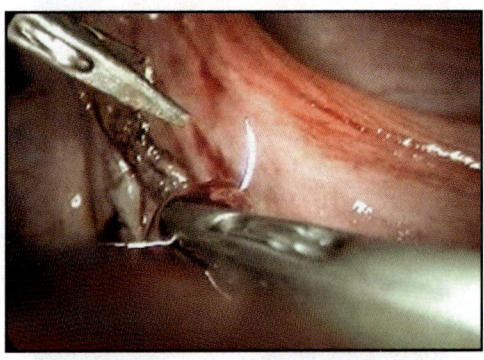

Fig. 10.7: Suturing of mesosalpinx

Anastomosis of the muscle layer: The muscle layer of the tube is sutured with 7-0 polyglactin. The 6 O'clock suture is taken in the proximal and distal segment (Figs 10.8 and 10.9). The suture is taken from outside inside on one side and inside outside on the other so that the knot is outside the lumen (Fig. 10.10). Subsequently sutures are taken at 12 O'clock, 3 O'clock and 9 O'clock position in the muscular layer (Figs 10.11 and 10.12). The sutures at 12 O'clock position are tied last (Figs 10.13 and 10.14). All sutures are tied by intracorporeal technique.

Note: There may be difficulty in applying 3 O'clock and 9 O'clock sutures as movement of laparoscopic instruments occur in a two dimensional plane with limitation of movement in third axis.

The patency of the suturing is checked by chromo-pertubation. Leakage at anastomosis site is acceptable as long as there is a spill at the fimbrial end.[3] Operating field is constantly irrigated with warm ringer lactate to keep it clear. Some surgeons use only 3 sutures. Recently reanastomosis has been described with use of a single stitch at 12 O'clock position with a success rate for tubal patency of 87% and a pregnancy rate of 53%.[4]

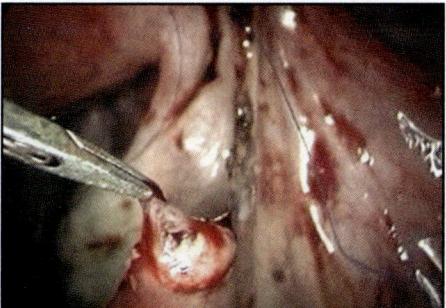

Fig. 10.8: 6 O'clock suture in the muscle layer

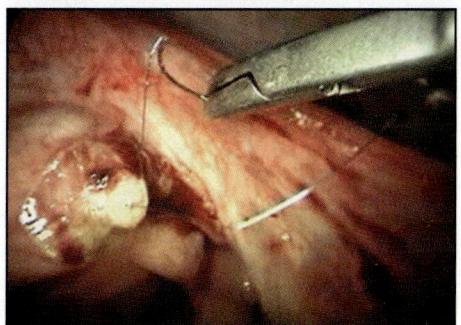

Fig. 10.9: 6 O'clock suture taken in proximal and distal end

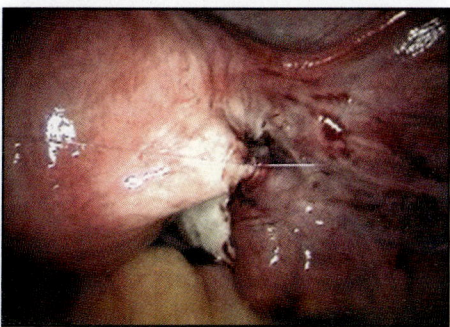

Fig. 10.10: Sutures tied with knot outside the lumen

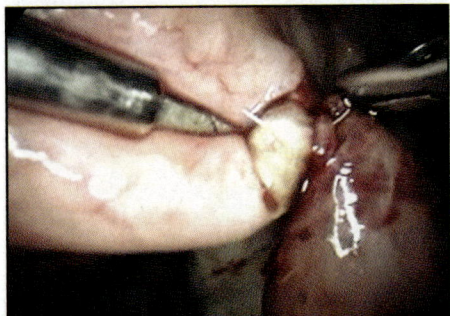

Fig. 10.11: Sutures taken in muscle at 3 O'clock position

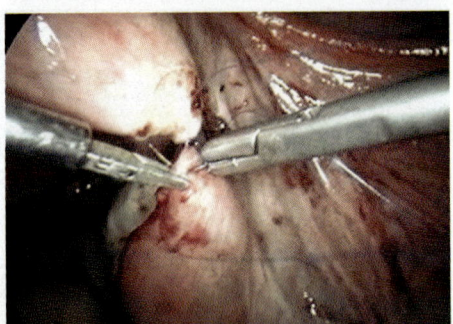

Fig. 10.12: Sutures taken in muscle at 6 O'clock position

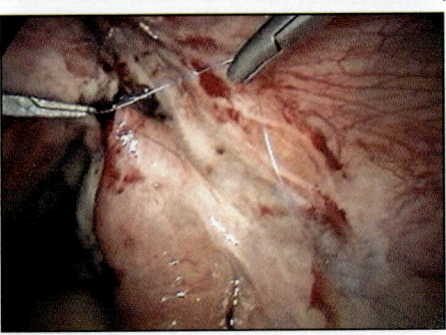

Fig. 10.13: 12 O'clock sutures tied at the end

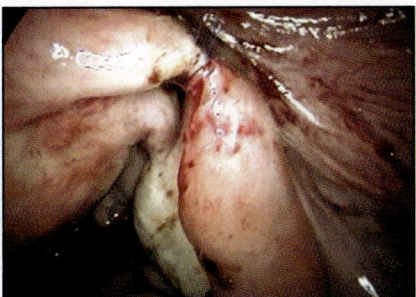

Fig. 10.14: Complete suturing of muscular layer

Suturing of serosal layer: The serosal layer is approximated with 6-0 polyglactin interrupted sutures. It may also be sutured in a continuous manner (Figs 10.15 and 10.16).

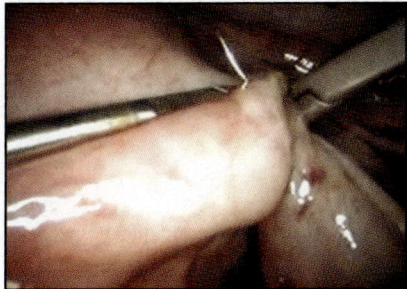

Fig. 10.15: Serosal layer suturing

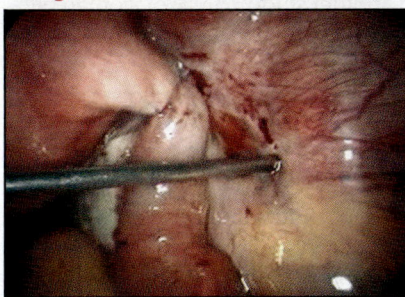

Fig. 10.16: Suturing of both layers completed

Chromopertubation: Chromopertubation is done again to check patency (Fig. 10.17).

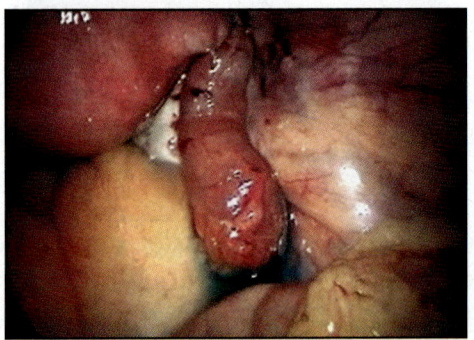

Fig. 10.17: Chromopertubation done to check patency

Postoperative Care

It is as for any minimally invasive surgery. Patient may be discharged after 24 hours.

Results

A 82% success rate has been seen. However, in recent studies pregnancy rate was 56.5% without any ectopic pregnancies. The average time from tubal reversal and pregnancy was 6 months.[5, 6] In another study 78.9% of women became pregnant, and 68.4% carried pregnancies to viability.[7] On comparison with laparoscopy both had similar results with a 80% success rate, laparoscopy taking a longer intraoperative time and shorter hospital stay.[8]

Results depended on:[9]

1. Patient's age
2. Method of tube interruption
3. *Type of anastomosis:* Isthmo- isthmic anastomosis gives a better result than the isthmo-ampullary anastomosis
4. Time lapse between tubal sterilization and reanastomosis

5. Length of fallopian tube segments being anastomosed. A length of more than 5 cm gives a good result
6. Other factors of infertility.

Laparoscopic tubal surgery gives comparable results to classical microsurgical techniques. Further improvement of surgical outcome will be achieved not only through better laparoscopic techniques but also through careful screening for surgical indications. The advent of Robotic surgery would allow movement in the third axis improving surgical techniques.

REFERENCES

1. Sedbon E, Elajolinieres JB, Boudouris O. Tubal desterilization through exclusive laparoscopy. Hum Reprod 1989;4:158.
2. Wiegerinck MA, Roukema M, van Kessel PH, Mol BW. Sutureless re-anastomosis by laparoscopy versus micro-surgical re-anastomosis by laparotomy for sterilization reversal: A matched cohort study. Hum Reprod 2005;20(8):2355-8.
3. Yoon TK, Sung HR, Cha SH Fertility outcome after laparoscopic microsurgical tubal anastomosis. Fertil Steril 1997;67:18-20.
4. Dubuisson JB, Chapron C. Single suture laparoscopic tubal reanastomosis. Curr Opin Obstet Gynecol 1998;10(4):307-13.
5. Ribeiro SC, Tormena RA, Giribela CG, Izzo CR, Santos NC, Pinotti JA. Laparoscopic tubal anastomosis. Int J Gynaecol Obstet. 2004;84(2):142-6.
6. Cetin MT, Demir SC, Toksoz L, Kadayifci O Laparoscopic microsurgical tubal reanastomosis: A preliminary study. Eur J Contracep Reprod Health Care 2002;7(3):162-6.
7. Kaloo P, Cooper M. Fertility outcomes following laparoscopic tubal re-anastomosis post tubal sterilisation. Aust N Z J Obstet Gynaecol 2002;42(3):256-8.
8. Cha SH, Lee MH, Kim JH, Lee CN, Yoon TK, Cha KY Fertility outcome after tubal anastomosis by laparoscopy and laparotomy. J Am Assoc Gynecol Laparosc 2001;8(3):348-52.
9. Barjot PJ, Marie G, Von Theobald P. Laparoscopic tubal anastomosis and reversal of sterilization. Hum Reprod 1999; 14(5):1222-5.

CHAPTER 11

Pelvic Inflammatory Disease

Surveen Ghumman

Pelvic inflammatory disease (PID) refers to infection of the uterus, fallopian tubes, and adjacent pelvic structures that is not associated with surgery or pregnancy. Long-term sequelae such as infertility occur in about 25%.[1] PID comprises a spectrum of inflammatory disorders of the female genital tract including any combination of endometritis, salpingitis, tubo-ovarian abscess and pelvic peritonitis The importance of PID lies in the fact that it is a silent preventable disease taking its toll on the reproductive potential of the woman

ETIOLOGY AND PATHOGENESIS

Pelvic inflammatory disease is almost always an ascending infection in which pathogenic microorganisms spread from the cervix and vagina to the upper portions of the genital tract The most important causative organisms are *Chlamydia trachomatis* and *Neisseria gonorrhoeae;* well over half of the cases being caused by one or both of these sexually transmitted microorganisms. The seroprevalence of chlamydia was found to be 82.7% in patients with infertility who had PID.[2] Women who have an endocervical infection with gonococci or chlamydiae may have a substantially increased risk of 10 to 30% of pelvic inflammatory disease. Perihepatitis may be associated with 10 to 20% of cases. *C. trachomatis* is an obligate intracellular gram- negative bacterium. Infection with this agent can be asymptomatic in up to 80% of women, which can make diagnosis and detection difficult.[3] Chlamydia has its highest prevalence amongst young men and women. More than 13.5% of women under 25 years of age have lower genital tract infection, reducing to 4.9% in women over 25.[4] There are many other organisms responsible for PID (Table 11.1).

The pathogenesis of PID is incompletely understood but involves disruption of standard host immunity, which under normal circumstances protects the upper genital tract from the anaerobes and gram-negative bacteria of the vagina. How this happens remains largely speculative. Damage to cervical

Table 11.1: Bacteriology for PID

Sexually transmitted organisms
- Neisseria gonorrhoea
- Chlamydia trachomatis
- Genital mycoplasma

Aerobic genital bacteria
- Group B streptococcus
- Other streptococci
- Coagulase negative staphylococci
- Escherichia coli
- Gardenella vaginalis
- Haemophilus influenza
- Other facultative gram-negative organisms

Anaerobic genital bacteria
- Peptostreptococci
- Peptococci
- Bacteroides species

mucous and tubal ciliated epithelium by both *Neisseria gonorrhoeae* and *Chlamydia trachomatis* has been well-documented. *N. gonorrhoeae* attaches to and penetrates mucosal epithelial cells, directly causing cell destruction and irreversible damage to ciliary motility. In contrast, it is the host immune response to *C. trachomatis* that causes tubal scarring.

Upper genital tract infection with gonococci, chlamydiae or other microorganisms does not always result in clinically recognizable disease. Infections that are asymptomatic or have atypical presentations also occur.

Risk Factors

1. Young age
2. Multiple sexual partners
3. Intrauterine devices
4. Surgical procedures of female genital tract
5. Previous episode of PID

6. Vaginal douching
7. Cigarette smoking

CLINICAL CHARACTERISTICS

The clinical spectrum of PID ranges from asymptomatic or subclinical endometritis to symptomatic salpingitis, pyosalpinx, tubo-ovarian abscess, pelvic peritonitis and perihepatitis.

1. Lower abdominal pain, usually bilateral, is the most common presenting symptom
2. Abnormal vaginal discharge
3. Abnormal uterine bleeding
4. Dysuria
5. Dyspareunia
6. Constitutional symptoms: nausea, vomiting, fever.
7. Abdominal mass
8. Right upper quadrant abdominal pain is seen in perihepatitis.

Gonococcal pelvic inflammatory disease tends to have a more abrupt onset with more dramatic symptoms of fever and peritoneal irritation than nongonococcal disease. Both gonococcal and chlamydial disease are more likely to begin during the first half of the menstrual cycle than later in the cycle.

Long-term Complications

1. Tubal damage and scarring
2. Recurrent disease
3. Chronic pelvic pain occurred in18% of women even after pelvic inflammatory disease had resolved[5]
4. Ectopic pregnancy occurred about six times more often.
5. Infertility due to tubal occlusion developed in 8% of women after a single episode of pelvic inflammatory disease, in 19.5% after two episodes, and in 40% after three or more episodes.[5] Up to 70% of women who are infertile because of obstructed fallopian tubes have serum antibodies to chlamydiae. Studies have found that 30 to 80% of women were asymptomatic or had mild symptoms.[6]

Screening for Chlamydia

Screening women for lower genital tract infection with *Chlamydia trachomatis* is important in the prevention of pelvic inflammatory disease, ectopic pregnancy and infertility. Currently there is little or no consensus on which diagnostic tool to use as a screening device or which sampling method to be used.

The diagnostic tests are:

1. Nucleic acid amplification including PCR and LCR
2. Gene probe
3. Enzyme immunoassay (EIA)
4. Direct immunofluorescence (DFA)
5. Culture

DIAGNOSIS

The diagnosis of pelvic inflammatory disease should be considered in any woman of reproductive age who has pelvic pain. Because of the potential for serious long-term sequelae, even from mild disease, clinicians should have a high index of suspicion and a low threshold for making the diagnosis and initiating treatment.

Clinical diagnosis: The diagnosis is usually made clinically. The only physical findings that are routinely present are lower abdominal tenderness, adnexal tenderness, and pain on manipulation of the cervix. Other clinical manifestations are fever, leukocytosis, an elevated erythrocyte sedimentation rate, elevated levels of C-reactive protein, and an abnormal vaginal discharge.

Accuracy: The sensitivity and specificity of a clinical diagnosis hovers around 50%.[7] There is a criterion defined by CDC for diagnosis (Table 11.2). However even in women with milder disease, adnexal tenderness was found to be a sensitive marker (96%) of endometritis.[8] The specificity is as low as 4%. Although treating all women with adnexal tenderness is unlikely to miss many cases, a lot of women without PID will receive unnecessary antibiotics. Combining lower abdominal tenderness, adnexal tenderness, and cervical motion tenderness reduced the sensitivity to 83% with a specificity of 22% (Table 11.2).

Table 11.2: Center for disease control and prevention criteria for diagnosis of PID

Minimal criteria
• Lower abdominal tenderness
• Adnexal tenderness
• Cervical motion tenderness

Additional criteria
• Oral temperature more than 38.3° C (101° F)
• Abnormal cervical or vaginal discharge
• Elevated erythrocyte sedimentation rate
• Elevated c-reactive protein
• Laboratory documentation of cervical infection with *Neisseria gonorrhoeae* or *Chlamydia trachomatis*

Definitive criteria
• Histopathological evidence of endometritis on endometrial biopsy
• Tubo-ovarian abscess on sonography or radiological tests
• Laparoscopic abnormalities consistent with PID

Laparoscopy: The "gold standard" of diagnosis is laparoscopy. The appearance of pelvic organs can vary from erythematous, indurated, edematous oviducts to pockets of purulent materials, to a large pyosalpinx or tubo-ovarian abscess.

Advantages
1. Enables microbiological sampling of upper genital tract.
2. Categorizes and grades the PID
3. Surgical interventions like lavage of an abscess may be done
4. Other causes of acute abdomen are ruled out.

Disadvantages
1. Expensive
2. Invasive
3. It cannot detect endosalpingitis

4. Subject to interoperator and intraoperator variability, so not 100% sensitive[9]
5. Requires admission.

Transvaginal ultrasound: Transvaginal ultrasound is useful in detecting fluid collections within the pelvis, such as a tubo-ovarian abscess or pyosalpinx, but cannot visualize the fallopian tube wall which limits its use in diagnosing less severe disease.

Doppler ultrasound: Doppler ultrasound measures blood flow, and power Doppler makes the technique sensitive enough to detect the hyperemia associated with fallopian tube inflammation. A recent study using power Doppler transvaginal ultrasound reports a positive predictive value of 91% and negative predictive value of 100% in a small group of patients, and was of particular value in those with milder salpingitis without pelvic abscess formation which was not detected with "ordinary" transvaginal ultrasound.[10]

Limitation
1. Potential limitations include difficulties in differentiating between endometriosis associated masses and PID
2. The high level of expertise required to interpret the scans.

MRI: In a small study of patients with severe PID, magnetic resonance imaging was found to be superior to transvaginal ultrasound (95% sensitivity, 89% specificity) but cost, lack of access, and limited data preclude its widespread use.[10] MR imaging may reduce the need for diagnostic laparoscopy.[11]

Endometrial biopsy: Endometrial biopsy can be done as an outpatient procedure to diagnose plasma cell endometritis.

Laboratory Diagnosis

Endocervical smear: Endocervical specimens should be examined for *N. Gonorrhoeae* and *C. trachomatis*. Typical gram-negative intracellular diplococci are seen.

Cell culture: The 'gold standard' for detection of chlamydiae is still cell culture. Culture is 100% specific, but estimates of sensitivity are as low as 50%. The majority of laboratories have moved away from culture, as it is expensive, time-consuming and technically difficult.

Nucleic acid amplification and gene probe: Nucleic acid amplification including Polymerase chain reaction (PCR) and ligase chain reaction (LCR). Within the last decade, tests that are based on nucleic acid amplification have become available. Nucleic acid amplification techniques are superior to other methods for detecting asymptomatic chlamydial infection in a young, sexually active population.

Advantages
1. High sensitivity
2. High specificity
3. They can use non-invasive specimen like urine or vulval swabs.

Enzyme immunoassay: The test most often used to detect this sexually transmitted infection, the EIA, has sensitivities in the range 70–80% even when used by experts. If this were to be used in a national screening program, 30% of infections could be missed.[12]

Other laboratory tests: These include erythrocyte sedimentation rate, quantitative C – reactive protein and total white blood cell count.

GRADING

Grading of PID has been done into mild, moderate and severe on the basis of clinical examination and laparoscopic findings.[13] (Table 11.3).

Grade	Clinical Examination	Laparoscopy
	Table 11.3: Grading of acute PID	
Mild	Uncomplicated, limited to tubes/ovaries with or without pelvic peritonitis	Erythema edema, no purulent exudate, tubes freely mobile
Mod	Complicated, inflammtory mass or abscess of tubes and ovaries with or without pelvic peritonitis	Gross purulent material, more marked erythema and edema, tubes freely mobile and fumbrial stoma not patent.
Severe	Spread to structures beyond the pelvis, i.e. ruptured To mass	Pyosalpinx, Inflammed complex abscess

MANAGEMENT

Most women with pelvic inflammatory disease are treated as outpatients.

Indication for Hospitalization

According to guidelines prepared by the Center for Disease Control and Prevention (CDC), hospitalization is particularly recommended when[14]

1. Diagnosis is uncertain
2. Possibility of surgical emergencies such as appendicitis and ectopic pregnancy cannot be excluded
3. Pelvic abscess is suspected
4. Patient is pregnant
5. Patient is an adolescent
6. Severe illness precludes outpatient management
7. Patient is unable to follow or tolerate an outpatient regimen
8. Response to outpatient therapy has not occurred

9. Clinical follow-up cannot be arranged within 72 hours of the initiation of antibiotic treatment
10. HIV infected patients

A pregnancy test should be performed routinely to minimize the possibility of overlooking a tubal pregnancy.

Because a wide variety of microorganisms can be involved in pelvic inflammatory disease and a specific microbial diagnosis cannot be made before the initiation of antimicrobial therapy, treatment must be directed against all potential pathogens. Treatment with single agents such as penicillin or tetracycline does not provide adequate coverage and has been associated with unacceptable failure rates.[15] Monotherapy with cephalosporins has been associated with a clinical response but a failure to eliminate *C. trachomatis.*[16] The antimicrobial regimen should include agents known to be active against *C. trachomatis, N. gonorrhoeae* and broad spectrum of aerobic and anaerobic bacteria commonly detected in upper genital tract of women (Table 11.4). The recommended treatment of Chlamydia during pregnancy is erythromycin or amoxicillin.

Although these regimens have been shown to eliminate gonococci and chlamydiae and to be associated with a clinical response in most treated patients, their efficacy in the prevention of long-term sequelae such as infertility is unproven.

Follow-up: Close follow-up of patients, especially those treated as outpatients, is an integral part of management. Patients should be reassessed 24 to 48 hours after treatment is begun. Clinical improvement should be apparent. If there is no change in condition of patient the diagnosis of pelvic inflammatory disease should be reassessed before addition or substitution of antibiotics. Laparoscopy or ultrasonography should be considered, as should the hospitalization of patients being treated as outpatients.

Medical management is usually sufficient. Intrauterine devices, if present, should be removed once antimicrobial treatment has begun.

Table 11.4: The guidelines of the center for disease control for treatment of pelvic inflammatory disease

Parenteral Regimen

Parenteral regimen A
- Cefotetan, 2 g IV every 12 h
- Cefoxitin, 2 g IV every 6 h

plus

doxycycline,100 mg or IV every 12 h.

Parenteral regimen B
- Clindamycin, 900 mg IV every 8 h,

plus gentamicin loading dose IV or IM (2 mg/kg), followed by a maintenance dose (1.5 mg/kg) every 8 h; single daily dose may be given.

Alternative parenteral
- Ofloxacin 400 mg IV every 12 h, *plus* metronidazole, 500 mg IV every 8 h, *or*
- Ampicillin/sulbactam, 3 g IV every 6 h, doxycycline, 100 mg po or IV every 12 h, *or*
- Ciprofloxacin, 200 mg IV every 12 h, *plus* doxycycline, 100 mg po or IV every 12 h, *plus* metronidazole, 500 mg IV every 8 h.

Oral

Oral regimen A
- Ofloxacin, 400 mg twice a day for 14 d,

plus

Metronidazole, 500 mg twice a day for 14 d.

Oral regimen B
- Ceftriaxone, 250 mg im once, *or*
- Cefoxitin, 2 g im, plus probenecid, 1 g single concurrent dose, *or*
- Other parenteral third-generation cephalosporin (e.g., ceftizoxime or cefotaxime),

plus

Doxycycline, 100 mg twice a day for 14 d.

Surgical Intervention

To drain pelvic abscesses or to resect chronically infected pelvic organs is required occasionally.

Colpotomy: It is done for vaginal drainage of pelvic abscess. There are three requirements for drainage of pelvic abscess.

1. The abscess must be midline
2. The abscess should be adherent to the cul-de-sac peritoneum and should dissect the rectovaginal septum
3. The abscess should be cystic or fluctuant to ensure drainage.

Steps
- The patient is placed in lithotomy position.
- After cleaning and draping, the posterior lip of the cervix is held with the volsellum and a transverse incision is given on the vaginal mucosa of the posterior fornix.
- The cul-de-sac peritoneum and abscess wall are punctured with a long Kelly's clamp
- Fibrous adhesions in the cavity are gently broken by the finger and pus is drained.
- Drain may be inserted in the cavity.

Ruptured tubo-ovarian abscess: This would require a laparotomy for drainage of pus and removal of infected organs if required.

Evaluation of the male sexual partners: Evaluation of the male sexual partners of patients with pelvic inflammatory disease is an integral part of management. Chlamydial and gonococcal infections in these men are often asymptomatic. The men should also be examined for other sexually transmitted infections.

Pelvic inflammatory disease is the most important consequence of sexually transmitted bacterial infections. The current epidemics of infertility and ectopic pregnancy are the result of this important medical, social, and economic problem. It is imperative to develop better diagnostic techniques and treatments that can prevent the long-term sequelae of this disease.

GENITAL TUBERCULOSIS

Genital tuberculosis is an important cause of tubal factor infertility in developing countries. In India the incidence of genital tuberculosis in the infertile population varies from 2 to 10% and accounts for 5% of pelvic infections.[17] In developed countries incidence has dropped down to 1%. With increasing HIV infection and drug resistance the incidence of tuberculosis is increasing worldwide. Since this disease often has a symptomless presentation and a insidious course it reniains a diagnostic dilemma. A recent study quoted a 7.2% incidence of gemtal tuberculosis in infertile patients.[18]

Etiopathogenesis

Genital tuberculosis is almost always secondary to a focus elsewhere in the body. The primary focus is usually healed by the time the genital lesion becomes evident and a long latent period may intervene between primary disease and genital tuberculosis. Genital tuberculosis is concomitantly present in 5 to 10% of cases of pulmonary tuberculosis.

The blood stream is the commonest method of spread and infection as it is mainly caused by *M. tuberculosis*. Bovine organisms may spread directly from peritoneum, bowel lesions or infected mesenteric lymph nodes in 7% of cases. In 1-2% cases the primary infection may be sexually transmitted and ascends to upper genital tract.[19] Usually both tubes are involved in 85 to 100% cases. The uterus is involved in 50-60% cases, ovaries in 20 to 30%, cervix in 5% and vulva in 1% cases.[20] It may start as endosalpingitis and progress to generalized peritonitis with small grayish white tubercles covering the peritoneal surfaces. There could be dense adhesions leading to pyosalpinx, bowel obstruction, tubal block and infertility. Tubercular endometritis may cause intrauterine adhesions.

Clinical Presentation

1. Infertility: Infertility is a common symptom and often may be the only presenting symptom. Latent tuberculosis should be considered in patients presenting with unexplained infertility with apparently normal pelvic and non-endometrial tubal factors and repeated IVF failure.[21]

2. Pelvic pain: It does not respond to antibiotics.
3. Menstrual irregularity: Menorrahagia, oligomenorrhoea, amenorrhoea may be present
4. Vaginal discharge
5. Generalized malaise
6. Low grade fever
7. Adnexal mass
8. Bilateral adnexal tenderness

Diagnosis

Tuberculosis presents a diagnostic dilemma as there may be non-availability of affected tissue for sampling and inaccuracy of tests to detect tuberculosis. Its long latent period prevents early diagnosis.

Erythrocyte sedimentation rate (ESR): ESR may be raised as in any infection

Mantoux test: Mantoux is a non-specific test. It showed a specificity of 80% and a sensitivity of 55% in women with tuberculosis.[22]

Endometrial biopsy: Endometrial biopsy is still one of the most commonly used methods. The biopsy is best done premenstrually when the tubercles reach their maximum growth. The cornu is the best site to take the biopsy as spread from the tubes first reaches there. The biopsy is then sent for smear, culture and histopathology.

- Histopathological diagnosis was possible in 50% cases which show a typical tubercle.
- Smear preparation should contain 10,000 AFB/ml for detection.
- Culture: The biopsy culture is positive in 10 to 60% of cases and requires a bacterial load of 10 AFB/ml for positivity
  1. *Conventional culture:* It takes 6 to 8 weeks which is a constraint. Sensitivity would take another 6 to 8 weeks.

2. *Newer culture Techniques*
   i. Radiometric methods (BACTEC): It is a rapid culture method where radioactive carbon labelled substrates for bacterial growth like formic acid and palmitic acid are detected. The radioactive labeled carbon dioxide released by the growing bacteria is measured as a marker of bacterial growth. The results take 5 to 7 days.
   ii. Mycobacterial growth indicator tubes (MGIT): It is a rapid culture technique which does not rely on radiometric detection
   iii. Septi check AFB: Since it is a biphasic culture technique it has a better mycobacterial recovery than conventional methods.

Laparoscopy: Tubercles may be seen on the serosal surface of uterus and tubes. There may be inflamed stiff tubes, peritoneal fluid and caeseation. Chromotubation is not encouraged if tuberculosis is suspected, but if done, the dye may drip slowly. Biopsy can be taken.

Polymerase chain reaction (PCR): PCR involves amplification of a given sequence of DNA using an enzyme Taq polymerase so that even minute amounts can be detected. Limitation of PCR.
- Sensitivity is 85 to 99%
- Specificity is poor
- Cannot differentiate between MTB and MOTT.
- Cannot differentiate between live and dead bacteria.

Results are available in 3 days.

PCR for RNA: rRNA is an integral part of bacterial ribosome and its presence indicates bacterial multiplication and active infection. Genus and species specific probes are being developed for detection of active bacteria.

Nucleic acid sequence based amplification (NASBA): Detection of binding of specific gene sequencing with denatured complimentary single strand DNA/RNA. This is done by chemiluminescence.

Ligase chain reaction (LCR): DNA ligase links two DNA strands. The fragmented primers are added excess in amount and the enzyme ligase binds them to complimentary strands on bacterial DNA.

Immunodiagnosis: **Antibody/Antigen Detection (ELISA):** These tests have a poor specificity due to cross reactivity between various bacterial constituents.

ESTAT: ESTAT test is based on the production of the cytokine Interferon Gamma by the patient's whole blood when injected with the specific antigen.

Treatment

It is important to treat these patients at the initial stage of the disease in order to prevent irreparable damage to the tubes and preserve fertility. Treatment is usually medical. The drug treatment consists of INH, Rifampicin, Ethambutol and Pyrizinamide given for a period of 6 to 9 months.

Surgical treatment is indicated if there is
- Hydrosalpinx and pyosalpinx not responding to medical treatment
- Tuboovarian mass
- Pelvic adhesions and peritonitis
- Asherman's syndrome

Future fertility: Microsurgical reconstructive tubal surgery is not recommended because of the reactivation of silent infection if patient is not adequately treated. Prognosis for conception is poor with pregnancy occurring in 5% and live birth in 2.2% cases. Results after IVF have been quoted as 5 to 16.5%. Surrogacy may be the only option in destroyed endometrium.

Tuberculosis is a disease with a diagnostic dilemma. Early diagnosis and treatment is important to preserve fertility. Newer diagnostic techniques are improving accuracy of diagnosis. With increase in multidrug resistant tuberculosis and HIV infection, tuberculosis is becoming a major cause of infertility.

REFERENCES

1. Rolfs RT, Galaid EI, Zaidi AA. Pelvic inflammatory disease: trends in hospitalizations and office visits, 1979 through 1988. Am J Obstet Gynecol 1992; 166:983-90.
2. Vidhani S, Mehta S, Bhalla P, Bhalla R, Sharma VK, Batra S. Seroprevalence of Chlamydia trachomatis infection amongst patients with pelvic inflammatory diseases and infertility. J Commun Dis 2005; 37(3):233-8.
3. Gaydos CA, Howell MR, Pare B, et al. Chlamydia trachomatis infections in female military recruits. N Engl J Med 1998; 339: 739-44.
4. Svensson LO, Mares I, Olsson SE, Nordstrom ML. Screening for Chlamydia trachomatis infection in women and aspects of the laboratory diagnostics. Acta Obstet Gynecol Scand 1991; 70: 587-90.
5. Westrom L. Effect of acute pelvic inflammatory diseases on fertility. Am J Obstet Gynecol 1975;121:707-13.
6. Wolner-Hanssen P, Kiviat NB, Holmes KK. Atypical pelvic inflammatory disease: subacute, chronic, or subclinical upper genital tract infection in women. In: Holmes KK, Mardh P-A, Sparling PF, Wiesner PJ, (Eds). Sexually Transmitted Diseases. 2nd ed. New York: McGraw-Hill, 1990; 615-20.
7. CDC. CDC guidelines on sexually transmitted diseases. MMWR 1998; 47:RR02.
8. Peipert JF, Ness RB, Blume J, et al. Clinical predictors of endometritis in women with symptoms and signs of pelvic inflammatory disease. Am J Obstet Gynecol 2001; 184:856-63.
9. Sellors J, Mahony J, Goldsmith C, et al. The accuracy of clinical findings and laparoscopy in pelvic inflammatory disease. Am J Obstet Gynecol 1991; 164:113-20.
10. Molander P, Sjoberg J, Paavonen J, et al. Transvaginal power Doppler findings in laparoscopically proven acute pelvic inflammatory disease. Ultrasound Obstet Gynecol 2001;17: 233-8.
11. Timo A. Tukeva, Hannu J. Aronen, Pertti T. Karjalainen, Pontus Molander, MD, Timo Paavonen, and Jorma Paavonen, MR

Imaging in Pelvic Inflammatory Disease: Comparison with Laparoscopy and US Radiology. 1999;210:209-16.

12. Watson EJ, Templeton A, Russel I, Pavonen J, Mardh PA, Stary A, Pederson BS The accuracy and efficacy of screening tests for Chlamydia trachomatis: a systematic review J. Med. Microbiol 2002; 51:1021-31.

13. Hegan WD, et al. Criterion for diagnosis and grading of salpingtis Obstet Gynecol 1983;61:113-7.

14. Pelvic inflammatory disease: guidelines for prevention and management. MMWR Morb Mortal Wkly Rep 1991;40:1-25.

15. Thompson SE, Brooks C, Eschenbach DA, et al. High failure rates in outpatient treatment of salpingitis with either tetracycline alone or penicillin/ ampicillin combination. Am J Obstet Gynecol 1985; 152:635-41.

16. Sweet RL, Schachter J, Robbie MO. Failure of beta-lactam antiobiotics to eradicate Chlamydia trachomatis in the endometrium despite apparent clinical cure of acute salpingitis. JAMA 1983;250:2641-5.

17. Malkani PK Pelvic Tuberculosis Obstet Gynecol 1959;14:600-4.

18. Jindal UN. An algorithmic approach to female genital tuberculosis causing infertility. Int J Tuberc Lung Dis. 2006; 10(9):1045-50.

19. Noglas: Pathophysiology of female genital tuberculosis. A 31-year study of 1436 cases. Obstet Gynecol 1979; 53: 422-8.

20. Arora VK, Johri A, Arora, R Rajarat P. Tuberculosis of the vagina in an HIV seropositive case. Tubercle Lung Dis 1994;75:239-43.

21. Dam P, Shirazee HH, Goswami SK, Ghosh S, Ganesh A, Chaudhury K, Chakravarty B. Role of latent genital tuberculosis in repeated IVF failure in the Indian clinical setting. Gynecol Obstet Invest 2006; 61(4):223-7.

22. Raut VS, Mahashur AA, Sheth SS. The Mantoux test in diagnosis of tuberculosis in women. Int J Gynecol Obstet 2001;72:165-9.

CHAPTER 12

Endometriosis

Surveen Ghumman

Endometriosis is defined as the presence of endometrium at places other than the normal uterine cavity. It is found in 3 to 10% of all women in the reproductive age group. In the infertile women the incidence is 20 to 40%.[1]

Theories for Histogenesis of Endometriosis

1. *The coelomic metaplasia theory*: It is thought that there is stimulation of the multipotential cells of the coelomic epithelium to transform into endometrial cells.
2. *Reflux and direct implantation theory*: Endometriosis is thought to occur because of implantation of viable endometrial cell on the surrounding tissues after they are refluxed through the fallopian tube (Sampson's theory).
3. *Vascular dissemination theory*: The endometrial cells are transported to distant sites through the vascular and lymphatic systems.
4. *Autoimmune theory*: Ectopic endometrial implants grow because of an autoimmune disorder.

Anatomic Locations of Endometrial Implants

It is usually limited to pelvis and lower abdominal organs namely ovaries, uterosacral ligaments, broad ligaments, cardinal ligament, round ligament, peritoneum of the lower anterior abdominal wall, urinary bladder, rectovaginal pouch, rectum, sigmoid colon, ureters, vermiform appendix, ileum, cecum, ascending colon, umbilicus, abdominal scars. Occasionally diaphragm, portiovaginalis of the cervix, posterior vaginal fornix, vagina and perineum at the site of episiotomy may also be involved.

About 0.7 to 1 % of patients may have malignant transformation. Rapidly enlarging endometriomas or those more than 10 cm have a greater chance of malignancy.

CLINICAL FEATURES

There is the classic triad of dysmenorrheal, dyspareunia and infertility. Intervention is usually indicated for pain, infertility or impaired function of bladder, ureter or intestines.

Women with minimal endometriosis may have extensive symptoms and those with marked endometriosis may be symptom free.

Pain

1. *Dysmenorrhea*:
   - Progressive.
   - Usually presents after 20 years of age but can be seen in adolescents.
   - Does not respond to oral anti-inflammatory agent or oral contraceptives.
   - Pain could be referred to rectum, lower sacral or coccygeal region because of premenstrual or menstrual swelling of ectopic implants.
2. *Dyspareunia*: It may be due to:
   - Fixed retroversion of the uterus
   - Ovarian fixation by adhesions
   - Uterosacral or vaginal infiltration
3. *Chronic pelvic pain*: It is a common symptom
4. *Sciatica*
5. *Acute pelvic pain*: Nearly 10% of patients present with acute symptoms. It is usually due to a leaking endometrial cyst or rupture of the cyst.

Infertility

Nearly 40 % of the women are infertile. The causes of infertility could be tubal, ovulatory or defects in implantation.

Tubal factor:
- Anatomic distortion due to extensive scarring.
- Inflammatory response in the tube due to endometriotic implants can alter tubal function.
- Cornual block due to endometriosis of the tube.

Ovulatory dysfunction:
- There is an altered rate of follicular growth.
- Asynchronization of oocyte maturation, uterine receptivity and ovulation.

- Luteinized unruptured follicle
- Shortened luteal phase.

Fertilization and preimplantation development: Due to increased production of prostaglandins, cytokines and activated macrophages there may be a deleterious effect on fertilization and implantation. Several mechanisms have been postulated.

- Decline in sperm motility.
- Adverse effect on sperm binding.
- Decreased rate of cleavage and development of blastocyst.
- Enhanced phagocytosis of sperms.
- Endometriosis may also cause subfertility by causing more sperm binding to the ampullary epithelium thereby affecting sperm-endosalpingeal interactions.[2]

Implantation:

- Poor uterine receptivity due to loss of integrin expression.

Abnormal immune system response:

- Increase cell mediated gamete injury.
- Increased prevalence of autoantibodies.
- Anti-endometrial antibody production.
- Recurrent pregnancy loss: Based on results from controlled prospective studies, there is no evidence indicating that endometriosis is associated with recurrent pregnancy loss. Furthermore no evidence indicates that medical or surgical treatment of endometriosis reduces the spontaneous abortion rate.[3]

Urinary symptoms

- Hematuria
- Ureteral obstruction
- Urgency
- Frequency.

Gastrointestinal symptoms

- Dyschezia
- Constipation
- Hemochezia.

Others
- Catamenial pneumothorax
- Hemoptysis
- Swollen and painful scars.

Symptoms depend on:
- Location of the implant
- Presence of adhesions
- Distortion of ovarian anatomy by endometriosis
- Involvement of other organs like ureter or rectum.

Association between stage of endometriosis and severity of symptoms is poor. [4] Presence of pelvic pain did not correlate with the total area of endometriosis, type of lesion or volume of disease. The important parameter was the depth of infiltration. Endometriotic lesions more than 1 cm in depth were associated with severe discomfort. [5]

PHYSICAL FINDINGS

- Tender uterosacral ligaments: There is a painful swelling of the implant before and at menstruation
- Cul-de-sac nodularity: It may reach 1 cm or more in size
- Induration of the rectovaginal septum
- Fixed retroversion of the uterus
- Adnexal mass: This may be a tender irregular mass
- Generalized or localized pelvic tenderness.

INVESTIGATIONS

This is a disease which may be difficult to diagnose. Diagnosis may be missed in upto 7% of patient and under staged in 50% during laparoscopy.

Lab Studies

- *Serum cancer antigen 125 test:* It has a low sensitivity in detecting endometriosis, but the results are useful as prognosticators of treatment outcome.[6] A normal value does not mean that endometriosis is absent.

- *Placental protein 14 (PP14):* This could be raised in endometriosis.

Imaging Studies

- *Ultrasonography:* Cannot provide definitive diagnosis. It is useful to perform before a laparoscopy as it identifies presence of small endometriotic cysts. The typical appearance is that of a cyst containing low-level homogenous internal echoes consistent with old blood.
- *MRI:* MRI is helpful in detecting rectal involvement and has been shown to accurately detect rectovaginal endometriosis and cul-de-sac obliteration in more than 90% of cases.[7] MRI can detect lesions upto 4 mm.
- *Sigmoidoscopy and intravenous pyelography:* Patients with symptoms suggestive of deep invasive endometriosis of the cul-de-sac should have a sigmoidoscopy and intravenous pyelography.

Procedures

Laparoscopy:
Laparoscopy is considered the primary diagnostic modality for endometriosis. It can provide definitive diagnosis and quantify the severity of disease. A methodical thorough inspection of the lateral pelvic wall, ovarian surface, both sides of the broad ligament, the bladder and bowel serosa and the cul-de-sac is made.

Sequence of diagnostic laparoscopy movements for scoring
The pelvic cavity is explored in the customary alpha sequence i.e. examination of the anterior abdominal wall, round ligament, urinary bladder, anterior uterus, fundus, posterior uterus, uterosacral ligaments, and rectovaginal pouch (Fig. 12.1). The assessment proceeds to the left anterior broad ligament, left fallopian tube from cornual angle laterally, left ovary on all surfaces, left ureter from pelvic brim to the ureteric tunnel, and posterior broad ligament. Finally the right anterior broad

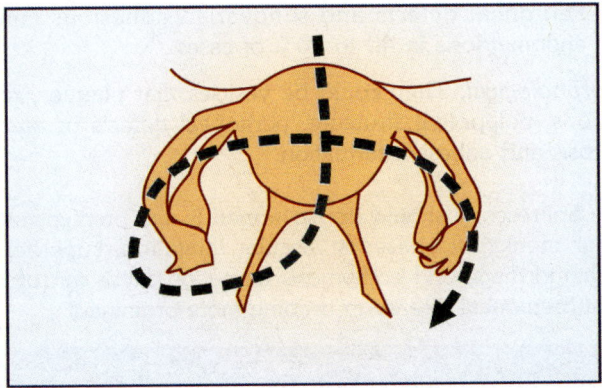

Fig. 12.1: Alpha sequence for diagnostic laparoscopy in endometriosis

ligament, right fallopian tube, right ovary, ureter and posterior broad ligaments are seen. Furthermore the extent of the disease is assessed, anomalies or distortions of the pelvic organs are identified, and upper abdominal organs, abdominal walls, liver, diaphragm, omentum, small bowels and appendix are evaluated. Per-rectal examination is important to evaluate rectovaginal endometriosis. An implant which has penetrated several cm retroperitoneally is known as an iceberg lesion and can be detected by palpation with a palpation probe/spatula. 2% of patients with endometriosis have peritoneal defects as against 7% in normal population.

Range of Appearance (Table 12.1)

1. Darkly pigmented : Yellow, brown ,blue or black discoloration Depends on how much hemosiderin there is in the lesion
2. Red raspberry colored: Red polypoidal lesions are active and closest to endometrial histology
3. White lesions are predominantly fibromuscular scarring with scattered glandular elements
4. Blebs: They are non-pigmented implants which are active endometriotic stroma

5. Peritoneal defects and subovarian adhesions contain endometriosis in 40 to 70% of cases.

Morphological: They could be vesicles, flat plaques, raised lesions, polypoidal structure, peritoneal defects or areas of fibrosis and adhesion formation.

> Laparoscopy should be performed in the premenstrual or menstrual phase as vascular dilatation, superficial hemorrhage and ecchymosis formation cause microfoci in peritoneal disease to become more prominent.

Table 12.1: Terminology used to describe peritoneal endometriosis

- Powder burn puckered black lesion
- Vascular glandular papule
- Vesicular lesions
- Red flame like
- Petechial lesions
- Hypervascular area
- Discolored area
    - Yellow brown
    - Blue
    - White
- White scarring
- Peritoneal defects
- Cribriform peritoneum
- Subovarian adhesions

Visual characteristics for diagnosis of endometrioma
- Size smaller than 12 cm
- Adhesions to the lateral pelvic wall, posterior broad ligament or both
- The presence of powder burn lesion
- Superficial endometriosis with adjacent puckering on the surface of the ovary
- Chocolate colored fluid content.

Deep Endometriosis

It can best be evaluated by palpation. Three types have been described. [8]

- *Type I:* Large pelvic area of typical or subtle lesions surrounded by white sclerotic tissue. During excision their section is in the shape of a cone
- *Type II:* Small lesion associated with retraction of the bowel. Excision reveals a nodule
- *Type III:* It is a nodular endometriosis of the rectovaginal septum and may spread laterally to involve the ureter.

CLASSIFICATION

Endometriosis has been classified into minimal, mild, moderate and severe according to The American Fertility Society (Table 12.2). Point scores are assigned based on the number of lesions

Endometriosis	<1cm	1 to 3 cm	> 3 cm
Table 12.2: The American Fertility Society revised classification of endometriosis			
Peritoneum			
Superficial	1	2	4
Deep	2	4	6
Ovary			
Right superficial	1	2	4
Right deep	4	16	20
Left superficial	1	2	4
Left deep	4	16	20
Posterior cul-de-sac obliteration	Partial 4		Complete 40
Adhesions	<1/3 enclosure	<1/3 to 2/3 enclosure	>2/3 enclosure
Ovary			
Right filmy	1	2	4
Right dense	4	8	16
Left filmy	1	2	4
Left dense	4	8	16
Tube			
Right filmy	1	2	4
Right dense	4	8	16
Left filmy	1	2	4
Left dense	4	8	16

and their bilaterality. Lesion size is also a scoring factor. This classification is a fairly accurate method of recording laparoscopic findings. However, high intraobserver and interobserver variability precludes its use in comparing the outcomes of therapeutic studies.[9] There is poor correlation with pain and dyspareunia and fecundity rates. [10]

Stage I	(Minimal disease)	-	1 to 5 points
Stage II	(Mild disease)	-	6 to 15 points
Stage III	(Moderate disease)	-	15 to 40 points
Stage IV	(Severe disease)	-	> 40 points.

If fimbriated end of fallopian tube is completely enclosed, it changes the points to 16. Endometriotic cyst must be confirmed by histology or presence of the following features:

- Cyst diameter less than 12 cm
- Adhesions to pelvic side wall and/or broad ligament
- Endometriosis on the surface of the ovary
- Tarry thick chocolate colored fluid content.

Complete obliteration of cul-de-sac is when no peritoneum is visible below uterosacrals.

TREATMENT

Treatment is initiated in the symptomatic patient presenting with pain, infertility or adnexal mass.

Expectant

Expectant line of treatment evolved when it was realized that in mild to moderate endometriosis hormonal therapy did not give better results than expectant management in patients of infertility.[11] Laparoscopic laser ablation of minor disease of endometriosis appears to lessen the interval to conception although the cumulative pregnancy rate remains nearly the same as that of women managed conservatively. In advanced disease the surgical therapy is more successful in comparison to expectant or medical treatment as it removes mechanical factors causing infertility. The potential benefit of cytoreductive therapy must be weighed against the risk of adhesion formation through surgical devitalization of peritoneal surfaces.

Medical Therapy

Medical therapy is given as treatment of choice to relieve pain in endometriosis but it is not the first line of treatment if her presenting complaint is infertility. It has the disadvantage of high recurrence after cessation of treatment.

Medical therapy can be given as

- Non-steroidal anti-inflammatory drugs
- Oral contraceptives
- Progestogens
- Danazol
- GnRH agonists

All these therapies have similar clinical efficacy in terms of reduction in dysmenorrhea, dyspareunia, pelvic pain, bulk of endometriotic tissue and in duration of relief, as has been shown in a Cochrane meta-analysis of randomized controlled trials.[12]

Meta-analysis which compared surgical with non-surgical treatment confirms superiority of surgical treatment with a crude pregnancy rate 38% higher than non-surgical treatment.[13] The difference in rates for medical and surgical therapy for stage I and II is primarily due to lost time in providing medical treatment especially in older women.

Progestogens

All progestational agents act by decidualization and atrophy of the endometrium.

1. *Medroxy progesterone acetate:* 30 mg / day of medroxy progesterone acetate is given and it relieves the pain, nodularity and tenderness in 80% of patients.[14]

2. *Parenteral depot medroxy progesterone acetate:* It is given in a dose of 150 mg every 3 months for one year. The time to resumption of ovulation is longer and variable with depot preparations.

3. *Megesterol acetate:* 40 mg/day of megesterol acetate may be given.[15]

4. *Dydrogesterone:* Dydrogesterone is a derivative of progesterone and is very similar to endogenous progesterone in molecular structure and pharmacological effects. It is very useful in the medical treatment of endometriosis especially in patients with infertility as it does not prevent ovulation and can be given in the postoperative period. It has no effect on body weight, blood pressure, blood clotting factors and cholesterol. Furthermore it has no androgenic, corticosteroid or estrogenic side effects. It corrects luteal phase asynchrony and causes complete secretory transformation of endometrium.

   Dose: Dydrogesterones are given as 10 mg. twice a day from day 5 to day 25 of the cycle and continued for 3 cycles or may be given continuously.

Combined oral contraceptive pills (COCP)

COCPs act by ovarian suppression and continuous progestin administration. Oral contraceptives were originally prescribed in high doses. High dose estrogen and progestogens transform endometrial tissue into decidua that ultimately undergoes necrosis and involution. The original high dose regimen is no longer given. Low dose oral contraceptive pills (20 to 35 μg of ethynyl estradiol may be used for mild symptoms in women not attempting pregnancy. It is given in a continuous manner for one year. The dose may be increased to 2 tablets a day to prevent breakthrough bleeding. Initially, a trial of continuous or cyclic COCPs may be administered for 3 months. If pain is relieved, this treatment is continued for 6 to 12 months. Subsequent pregnancy rates upon discontinuation of the pill are 40 to 50%. The long-term efficacy of multiphasic preparations remains unproven.

Danazol

Danazol has been shown to be as effective as any of the newer agents, but with a higher incidence of adverse effects. Danazol acts by inhibiting the midcycle follicle-stimulating hormone and luteinizing hormone surges and preventing steroidogenesis in the corpus luteum. The recommended dose is 600-800 mg/d. However, smaller doses have been used with success.

Adverse effects:

They are related to the anabolic, androgenic and antiestrogenic properties and may be dose related.

The adverse effects are weight gain, muscle cramps, decreased breast size, vasomotor symptoms, acne, oily skin, deepening of voice, increase in low density lipoprotein and decrease in high density lipoprotein and idiopathic drug reactions like gastrointestinal disturbances, weakness, dizziness, skin rashes, headaches, and muscle cramps.

Results

1. *Pain:* 95% of the patients get pain relief. Mild to minimal endometriosis responded well to 400 mg of danazol but severe form of the disease required higher doses. Ovarian endometriomas greater than 1 cm did not show a good response.

2. *Recurrence:* Recurrence of symptoms occurs in 50% of patients within 4 to 12 months of stoppage of drug.[16]

3. *Fertility:* Danazol does not enhance fertility and conception is delayed while patient is on danazol.

Gonadotropin releasing hormone antagonists: GnRH analogs produce a hypogonadotropic-hypogonadic state by down-regulation of the pituitary gland. Goserelin and leuprolide acetate are the commonly used agonists. Treatment is usually restricted to monthly injections for 6 months (Table 12.3). There is an initial flare followed by a down regulation. It results in improvement of all stages of the disease. 80% of patients show visible reduction in implants after 6 months. A better response was seen with subcutaneous route than intranasal route. This may be due to the greater consistency in drug levels with subcutaneous route. However, efficacy is limited to pain suppression and fertility rates may show no improvement.[17]

Disadvantages
1. Recurrence: In 57 % of patients there was a return of pain within 6 months of cessation of therapy.
2. Decreased bone density: A decrease in trabecular bone content occurs in two-thirds of patients during the course of the therapy. Add back therapy is given to avoid this side effect
3. Vaginal dryness
4. Superficial dyspareunia
5. Headaches
6. Depression

There is no place for medical treatment with drugs that are also potent contraceptives in the treatment of patients who are infertile.[17, 18]

Table 12.3: Indications for GnRH analogues in Endometriosis

1. *Preoperative:* In cases of acute inflammation due to endometriosis.
2. *Postoperative:* Followup treatment with GnRH agonists seems to improve pain and pregnancy rate in patients with severe endometriosis.
3. In patients with pain so as to avoid recurrent surgeries.
4. Severe endometriosis such as frozen pelvis and rectovaginal endometriosis where surgery is not possible or incomplete surgery has been done.
5. In stimulation protocols for ART in patients with endometriosis of all grades.
6. In patients with adenomyosis with infertility

Newer Drugs
1. *Mifepristone:* Mifepristone is another antiprogestin with no menopausal side effects.
2. *Aromatase inhibitors:* These include anastrozole, letrozole, exemestane and vorozole. They inhibit an enzyme, aromatase, which is a major source of estrogen.

3. *Leukotrine antagonists*: Leukotrine antagonists block these powerful immune system factors that in excess produce chemicals which cause inflammation and spasms in smooth muscles. Drugs like zafirlukast, montelukast and zileuton are being used, as the levels of luekotrines have been found to be high in some women with dysmenorrhea.

4. *Selective estrogen-receptor modulators (SERMs)*: Selective estrogen-receptor modulators (SERMs) drugs act like estrogens in some tissues and like estrogen blockers in others. Though tamoxifen may worsen endometriosis, the action of other SERM like raloxifene or tibolone may be beneficial.

5. *GnRH antagonist*: Cetrorelix in a 3 mg dosage once weekly over 8 weeks has shown promising results for medical treatment of symptomatic endometriosis.

6. *Gestrinone*: Gestrinone is an antiprogestin which reduces both estrogen and progesterone receptors. It has fewer menopausal symptoms vis-à-vis GnRH agonist. Adverse effects include male hormone symptoms such as acne and unhealthy cholesterol levels

Surgery

Surgery aims for restoration of anatomy by complete excision of all endometriosis and associated adhesive disease. Surgical care can be broadly classified as

1. *Conservative surgery:* When reproductive potential is retained,

2. *Semi-conservative Surgery:* When reproductive ability is eliminated but ovarian function is retained,

3. *Radical surgery:* When the uterus and ovaries are removed.

Therapy depends on

- Age of the patient
- Desire for fertility
- Pain relief
- Duration and intensity of symptoms
- Extent of disease
- Previous treatment undertaken

Indication

1. Correction of pain, infertility or other symptoms in patients with extensive pelvic endometriosis. Surgery has a better prognosis for pregnancy in advanced disease and is more successful in relieving pain.
2. Cases of mild to moderate endometriosis where hormonal treatment has failed to relieve the pain.
3. Asymptomatic or mild endometriosis: Surgical ablation of asymptomatic endometriosis has also been shown to improve fecundity rates on a 3-year follow-up.[19] Hence on doing diagnostic laparoscopy if one finds endometriotic implants they should be dealt with in the same sitting even if patient has no symptoms of pain. This decision has to be weighed against the risk of postoperative adhesion formation and its effect on fertility.

Conservative Surgery

Conservative surgery is indicated in all cases of infertility. Conservative procedures are carried out to remove all implants, resect adhesions, relieve pain, reduce the risk of disease recurrence, reduce post operative adhesion formation and restore involved organs to a normal anatomic and physiologic condition. For the infertile patient, restoration of the normal tuboovarian relationship is necessary to increase fertility. These surgeries are cytoreductive and recurrence is caused by progression of microscopic residual disease.

Many cases of recurrence are actually due to residual disease and not a true recurrence.

The objective in infertile patient endometriosis is to have all endometriotic disease removed and functionality of the pelvic organs enhanced

The laparoscopic approach is the method of choice for treating endometriosis conservatively.[20] It provides magnification to identify subtle implants and superior visualization of the cul-de-sac.

Laparotomy is preferred to laparoscopy if
1. There is difficulty in establishing tissue planes of dissection.
2. Improved access is necessary for atraumatic manipulation.
3. Extensive dense pelvic adhesions.
4. Large endometriomas.
5. Deep involvement of the rectovaginal septum with fibrotic extension into the peri rectal fossa.
6. Invasion of bowel muscularis.
7. Endometriotic infiltration in the region of the uterine vessel and ureter.

Laparoscopic procedures which can be performed are
- Ablation of endometriotic implants
- Adhesiolysis
- Ovarian cystectomy
- Oophorectomy

Anesthesia: Carried out under general anaesthesia with intubation in Trendelenburg's position with cushioned leg rests making it convenient for the surgeon.

Endoscopic Ablation

The basic techniques available for surgical treatment of endometrial implants are
1. Excision
2. Coagulation
3. Vaporization

Coagulation can be done by
- Monopolar or bipolar cautery
- Thermocoagulation
- Laser

Extent of tissue penetration is related to
- Power and type of current
- Duration of application
- Size of electrode

    Bipolar cautery has the advantage of less tissue damage than monopolar cautery.

Principles of Conservative Surgery

1. The involved peritoneum is separated with hydrodissection. This retroperitoneal placement of fluid dissipates CO_2 energy, leading to safer dissection.
2. Laser beam is applied till bubbling of retroperitoneal areolar tissue is noted.
3. A 2 to 4 mm of clear margin is desired around each lesion. The zone of thermal necrosis is minimal with Co_2 laser.
4. Excision of involved peritoneum is better than vapourization of the implants when the extent of the tissue penetration cannot be recognized.
5. Deep cul-de-sac nodules may require a combined vaginal – laparoscopic approach or a laparotomy to palpate and recognize all nodules.
6. With extensive dissection, electrosurgery should be avoided as it leads to widespread tissue damage and difficulty in identifying planes.

Co_2 laser may not be ideal for ablation of cyst wall as it is absorbed by fluid and incomplete ablation may occur in the presence of blood and hemosiderin though it has the advantage of being more fine than other lasers.

Surgical Technique

Lysis of Bowel Adhesions

Adhesions are excised by scissors, electrosurgery or ultra pulse CO_2 laser. The structures are separated by forceps and a cleavage plane formed. Hydrodissection helps in identifying and developing dissection planes especially during CO_2 laser use on the ureter, bladder, etc.

Peritoneal Implants

Implants should be destroyed in the most effective and least traumatic manner so as to minimize postoperative adhesion formation.

1. *Small lesion less than 5 mm:* Small lesion less than 5 mm in diameter on the peritoneum are treated with laser or bipolar coagulation or excised.
2. *Deep lesions or lesions more than 5 mm:* Deep lesions or lesions more than 5 mm in diameter must be excised with a tissue margin of 2 to 4 mm as microscopic lesions are commonly found close to the visible implant. Ablation leads to greater tissue destruction and subsequent adhesion formation. There may be inadequate tissue destruction. It may further create difficulty due to proximity of vital structures like ureter, bladder or vessels. The deep lesions need to be assessed by rectovaginal palpation preoperatively and laparoscopic blunt probe palpation.

Excision is preferable to ablation in an infertile patient as it leaves less chance of deep residual disease and there is lesser tissue destruction and subsequent adhesion formation

Direct excision technique: Lesions are grasped with a fenestrated forceps, elevated and excised with scissors, laser, harmonic scalpel or electric needle.

All peritoneal defects should be ablated as they often have microscopic disease

Genitourinary Involvement

Genitourinary involvement is seen in 1-11% of patients having endometriosis. Bladder lesions are removed as the peritoneal lesions followed by cystoscopy to rule out any mucosal involvement.

Rectovaginal Involvement

Rectovaginal involvement occurs in 10% of cases. They present with symptoms of deep rectal pain often worsening with bowel movements or at the time of menstruation. There may be alternating diarrhea and constipation. In cases with more advanced disease there may tenesmus or feeling of incomplete rectal emptying. Diagnosis is made by per rectal examination and laparoscopy. The extent of muscularis involvement in serosal sigmoid deposits is assessed by the movement of the muscularis of the bowel wall independent of the deposits limited to the serosal layer. Sufficient radical surgery is the preferred treatment and it is necessary to remove all nodules completely. Preoperative medical treatment with GnRH agonists seems to reduce recurrence rates. But medical treatment by itself is insufficient and leads to high rate of recurrence.

Surgical treatment: This is possible to achieve laparoscopically based on the following principles:
- Dissection is always from normal tissue towards the diseased tissue.
- Constant tissue traction.
- Best modality of treatment here is CO_2 laser though some prefer scissors to any energy modality since it gives an indirect palpation and tissue feel while dissecting and cutting.

Steps: A bogie probe is placed in the rectum with a sponge forceps in the vagina before dissection of the rectovaginal space. The peritoneum is opened above the ureter and retracted medially, dissection carried out till a 0.5 cm margin. Further the pararectal spaces are opened and rectum mobilized laterally and from the posterior cervix till the areolar tissue of the normal rectovaginal septum is reached. The anterior rectum is dissected first, followed by lateral dissection and finally posterior dissection. Superficial invasion of the muscularis of the bowel or bladder should be treated with electrocoagulation or laser vaporization because of precision and lack of deeper penetration of the energy sources. The uterosacral disease is excised to whatever depth necessary to achieve eradication while the residual rectal disease is shaved from the anterior rectal wall. If there is rectal stricture formation either due to disease or fibrosis then anterior segmental resection is to be considered along with transanal staple anastomosis. The cavity is copiously irrigated.

Postoperative Therapy: Postoperative suppression with GnRH agonist depot preparations is given for three months followed by active fertility treatment in infertile patients.

Ovary

Endometriomas are a common problem occurring in an infertile patient with endometriosis. Small lesions can be ablated by laser or electrocautery taking care not to destroy surrounding tissues by thermal injury. With larger lesions, a cystectomy is done either with removal of cyst wall or the cyst wall is fulgurated. Usually complete removal is preferred as it has better results.

Steps
1. Flimsy adhesions should be resected.
2. Ovary should be carefully inspected for extent of involvement.
3. Shallow longitudinal incision is made on the endometrioma.

> *Caution*:
> 1. Shallow longitudinal incision on the ovary should be made in such a way so as to not disturb the normal anatomical relationship of the ovary with utero ovarian ligament and fimbria ovarica.
> 2. Care should be taken while dissecting hilar region to maintain hemostasis.

4. A cleavage plane is created between the cyst and the ovarian tissue with the help of a scissor or knife handle. As much of the normal ovarian tissue should be preserved as possible.
5. After placing purse string sutures to eliminate the dead space, running 5-0 sub cortical sutures are placed. Sutures on the surface are avoided because they cause adhesions.

Endoscopic Management (See Chapter 13 and DVD ROM)
Endometriomas greater than 5 cm in diameter may be difficult to remove endoscopically because of dense adhesions and difficulty in removing the entire wall.

With larger cysts contents are drained and wall is inspected after irrigation. The lining is destroyed by electrocoagulation in small endometriomas. With larger endometriomas the cyst wall is stripped off from the bed of the normal ovarian tissue. This may be facilitate by hydrodissection .The remaining fragments are vaporized with laser or fulgurated by electrocautery.

Ovarian defect is left to heal spontaneously as suture placement may cause adhesion formation. The incised capsule can be inverted by application of low power CO_2 laser or bipolar cautery.

Other Conservative Surgery for Pain Relief

Conservative surgery for pain relief could be done in cases where there is persistent pain. Two methods are used.
1. Presacral neurectomy
2. Laparoscopic uterine nerve ablation (LUNA)

Presacral Neurectomy

Division of the superior hypogastric plexus is a useful adjunctive procedure to reduce pain. This plexus consists of fine strands of nerves embedded in the delicate areolar tissue and is formed as a continuation of the aortic and inferior mesenteric plexuses over the bifurcation of the Aorta. After placing the patient in a reverse Trendelenburg's position, the intestines are displaced cephalad and the bifurcation of the aorta and sacral promontory is exposed. The nerve segments of superior hypogastric plexus are transected at the level of the third sacral vertebra, and the distal ends are ligated. Bleeding is controlled by bipolar cautery.
Complications
1. Hemorrhage: Hemorrhage can occur from middle sacral vessels located in the midline between the presacral nerve and the periosteum of the sacral promontory. This is controlled by ligation or coagulation. Injury to the left common iliac vein or vena cava may require an immediate laparotomy.
2. Ureteric injury.
3. Urinary urgency
4. Persistent postoperative constipation was seen in 32% of cases.

Laser Uterine Nerve Ablation (LUNA)

Sympathetic fibres T-10 to L-1 are present within the inferior hypogastric plexus and course along the inferior vena cava and sacrum to enter the uterus through the nerves of the uterosacral ligaments and accompanying uterine arteries. The parasympathetic components of the paracervical nerves originate from S-1 to S-3 or S-4 traveling through the nerve erigentes to emerge in the lateral pelvis forming the Frankenhäuser on ganglion lateral to the cervix. Division of the uterosacral ligaments at the point of their attachments to the cervix should interrupt many sensory nerve fibres of the cervix and uterine corpus.

Technique

The uterosacral ligaments are stretched by anteverting the uterus with the uterine manipulator. The CO_2 laser transects the ligaments at their insertion into the cervix, using a vertical motion from medial to lateral. The depth of the incision should be adequate so as to completely transect the ligament. If the ureter is close to the uterosacral ligament, relaxing incision is made along the outer side of the uterosacral ligament.

Complication

1. Bleeding
2. Ureteric injury.
3. Pelvic denervation
4. Loss of uterine support leading to uterine prolapse.
5. Adhesion formation
6. Ureteral transaction.

Postoperative Therapy

Postoperative adjunctive hormonal treatment has been shown effective in reducing pain but has no impact on fertility. GnRH analogs, danazol, and medroxy-progesterone have all been found to be useful for this indication[21] LNG IUD is effective in controlling pain episodes postoperatively. [22]

Results of Conservative Surgery

Endometriosis was found to resolve spontaneously in one third of women who were not actively treated.[23] Overall, the recurrence rate is 19% and is similar for all techniques.[24] Laparoscopic ablative surgery with bipolar diathermy or laser for endometriomas were shown to be effective for relieving pelvic pain in 87% of patients.[25] Laparoscopic cystectomy was found to yield better pain relief and pregnancy rates than drainage.[26] In patients with subfertility, tissue ablation significantly increased the cumulative pregnancy rate.[19] In women who wish to preserve their reproductive potential, the rates of recurrent pain symptoms are 44% with surgical management and 53% with medical management.[27]

Semi Conservative Surgery

The indication for this type of surgery is mainly in women who have completed their childbearing and are too young to undergo surgical menopause, having severe symptoms where medical therapy has failed. Hysterectomy and cytoreduction of pelvic endometriosis is done with ovarian conservation. Ovarian endometriosis should be removed surgically as they may cause persistence of symptoms. There is a risk of premature menopause but since only one tenth of functioning ovarian tissue is all that is needed for hormone production it is a theoretical risk in a carefully performed surgery. A 6-fold higher rate of recurrence is seen with ovarian conservation compared to women who undergo oophorectomy.[28]

Radical Surgery

This involves total hysterectomy with bilateral oophorectomy and cytoreduction of visible endometriosis. Ureteric obstruction may warrant surgical release. Resection anastomosis may be needed in bowel obstruction. Endometriosis may recur in 15% of women after extirpative surgery.[29]

RECURRENT ENDOMETRIOSIS

The rate of repeat surgical intervention is directly related to the extent of disease and ability to conceive postoperatively. Only 10% of those who achieve pregnancy after initial surgery require further intervention. Pelvic pain and deep dyspareunia due to incomplete excision may recur within weeks or months after conservative surgical treatment. This is preventable in many instances with adequate surgical technique and adequate suppression with GnRH agonists in cases of severe endometriosis. The principles of recurrent surgery are:

1. Preferable to under treat rather than over treat in cases of infertility.
2. Dissection is to be meticulous because of increased adhesion formation especially in cases who had initial laparotomy.
3. Good preoperative bowel preparation is required as there are high chances of bowel injuries due to adhesions.

Laparotomy vs laparoscopic resection for recurrent endometriosis

Laparoscopy was as efficacious as laparotomy in conservative surgical management of recurrent endometriosis There was no significant difference in recurrence of dymenorrhea 34% vs 42% (laparoscopy vs laparotomy), pelvic pain and clinical findings. The clinical pregnancy rate was 45% vs 54%.[30] Laparoscopy should be performed when cleavage planes are not identified at laparoscopy or optimal conservative surgery is not feasible. Laparoscopy offers the additional advantage of magnification. Patients also respond better to repeat courses of medical therapy given for pain.

MANAGEMENT OF ENDOMETRIOTIC CYSTS ASSOCIATED WITH INFERTILITY

The ovary is one of the more frequent sites of pelvic endometriotic lesions. Management of ovarian endometriosis, though a frequent clinical issue in routine practice, has various aspects that are still uncertain or debated. The pathophysiology, correlation with attributed symptoms (pain and subfertility) and the optimal therapeutic strategy to apply are still controversial.

Incidence

Ovarian endometriomas are identified in around 22 % of patients with endometriosis, associated with subfertility or pelvic pain. In unilateral lesions the left side is more frequently affected than the right side.

Impact on Fertility

For unilateral endometrioma, the causal relationship with infertility is uncertain. According to the revised AFS classification (1995), the presence of an ovarian endometrioma, of 3 centimeters size, leads to such a score, that the resulting stage is inevitably III, or moderate endometriosis. Moderate endometriosis is associated with an impairment of fecundity, with a spontaneous conception rate of 22.3 %. Predictive value of this classification is still very controversial. After surgical treatment of ovarian endometriomas the reported conceptions rate are in the range of 50 %. These findings suggest that an ovarian endometrioma might impair fertility. However, this negative effect is not always demonstrated. The impact of endometrioma on the results of IVF is also controversial.

Treatment

Removal of lesions is usually considered as the gold standard, for endometrioma of at least 3 centimeter size, especially more when pain is associated. In case of infertility, the main objective of the treatment is to improve the fecundity. An accessory objective is to have a histological proof of the type of the cyst and its benign nature which would require surgical removal of the whole cyst. However, other therapeutic options have been proposed.

1. **Expectant:** The impact of endometriomas, less than 3 cm size, on fertility is probably minimal. (Fig. 12.2) For young women, the probability of a malignant lesion is very low. These patients can be treated expectantly along with a regular imaging control of the cyst.

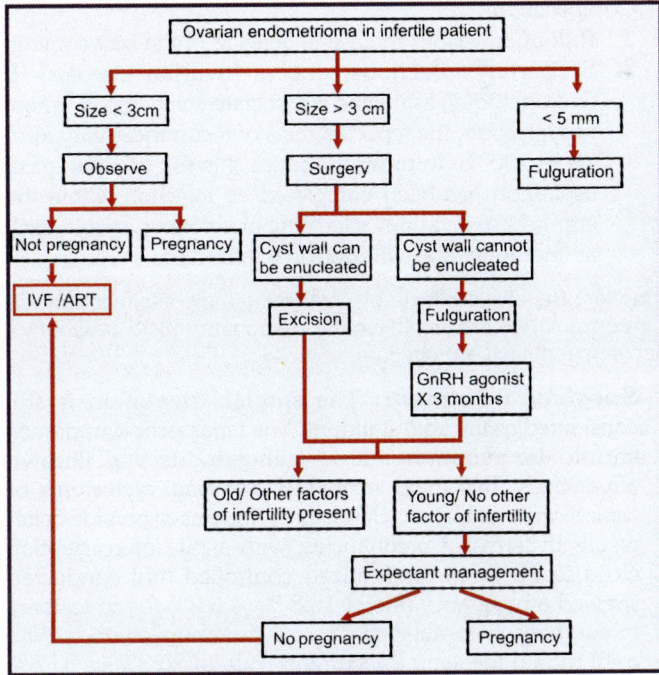

Fig. 12.2: Treatment of ovarian endometrioma in infertility

2. ***Hormonal suppression:*** As medical treatment has little impact on ovarian endometriomas larger than 3 centimeters size it should not be recommended in such situations. A decrease of size of the cyst after medical treatment has been observed reaching in some cases to 50%. Medical treatment combined with surgery has been done, but no beneficial effect on fertility has been demonstrated.

3. ***Ultrasound guided cyst aspiration:*** Transvaginal ultrasonic aspiration of an ovarian endometrioma is usually a simple procedure, performed without general anesthesia.

Complication
1. Risk of adhesions in case of spillage of the cyst content.
2. Secondary infectious process (ovarian abscess). If endometrioma aspiration is associated with improvement of symptoms, the reported rates of recurrences vary from 28 to 100 %. In order to reduce this risk of recurrence, aspiration has been completed by injection within the empty cyst of various sclerosing or cytotoxic agents, such as methotrexate, ethanol or tetracycline.

Caution: Beneficial effects of ultrasonographic aspiration prior to perform IVF are insufficiently demonstrated to presently recommend such a procedure.

4. ***Surgical treatment:*** The surgical treatment is still considered as the gold standard. The laparoscopic approach should be recommended, owing to its well known advantages. Two main techniques are used: cystectomy or aspiration and ablation. Cystectomy appears to provide better results in terms of pregnancies, with a rate of conception close to 50 %. A randomized controlled trial conducted showed a pregnancy rate of 18.8 % vs 6.2% for cystectomy in comparison to ablation in a 24 month followup.[31] With a 42 month followup a recurrence rate of 26.3% vs 57.8% was seen with cystectomy and ablation respectively.[32] Three major issues have to be assessed, in addition to technical aspects and results:
   a. *Post operative adhesions:* Post operative adhesions are frequently encountered after surgery.
   b. *Recurrence:* Recurrence after surgery varies from 0 to 30% depending on the surgical procedure, the definition and the length of follow-up. Cummulative reoperation rate of 8.2 % after 48 months in a recent study.[33] Cystectomy seems to lead to fewer recurrences, as demonstrated by randomized controlled studies.
   c. *Impact of surgery on ovarian function and ovarian reserve:* Raised FSH levels have been found in patients after surgery as there may be removal of healthy tissue leading to a

decreased ovarian reserve. On histopathological analysis 54% of patients had ovarian tissue on the cyst wall.[34] However, none of the tissue had follicles.

5. **IVF:** IVF is the option for the 50 % of patients who have not conceived after surgery. The impact of an ovarian endometrioma on the results of IVF does appear very limited, and the presence of an ovarian endometrioma is not a contra-indication to perform an IVF. Pregnancy and delivery rates are not altered but cancellation rate is increased. A decreased responsiveness to ovarian stimulation by gonadotropins has been reported for repeat surgery and in cases of severe endometrioses with large sized bilateral ovarian endometriomas, but without effect on pregnancy rates. Aspiration of an ovarian endometrioma, incidentally identified during ovarian hyperstimulation or ovum pick up for IVF, does not appear to be required, except in cases of large size cyst or associated pain. One should be aware of the risk of infection and abscess formation in these patients. Unexpected puncture of an ovarian endometrioma during ovum pick up has no impact on the results of IVF, but bears a risk of infection. It is not necessary to operate and definitely not reoperate on endometriomas before IVF. If found accidentally during IVF cycle stimulation it should be ignored and cycle continued.

Note: Recurring ovarian endometriomas should not be systematically removed before performing an IVF. Iterative surgery may impair ovarian reserve and the presence of the ovarian endometrioma does not impair the expected results of IVF.

MANAGEMENT OF INFERTILE PATIENT FOLLOWING SURGERY

Following surgery further decision must be made regarding management of previously infertile patient who wishes to conceive. Management decisions are difficult because of

variability of endometriosis presentation, concomitant disease, outcome of surgery , other infertility factors, multiple treatment options and until recently a paucity of good studies. However, current concepts have an evidence based approach.

Evaluation of endometrial surgery: The first step is evaluation of the surgery done for these patients with regard to operative finding approach, energy source used, technique and skill of the surgeon.

In light of evidence supporting the equivalent if not better outcome of laparoscopy compared to laparotomy the laparoscopic approach is preferable in most cases of endometriosis associated infertility

Factors Affecting Management of Infertility Following Surgery

Recently endometriosis fertility index has been presented to evaluate postsurgical probability of pregnancy.[35] This includes surgical findings, pelvic status, age, duration of infertility, number of prior surgeries, prior gravidity, and other associated causes of infertility. The clinician must evaluate all these in addition to outcome of surgery before recommending a treatment plan.

Early Stage Endometriosis: In early stage disease surgical treatment gave a pregnancy rate of 58% compared to 45% for expectant management.[36] The Cochrane review concluded that the use of laparoscopic surgery in the treatment of minimal and mild endometriosis may improve success rates.[37] For any 12 patients with Stage I or II endometriosis found on laparoscopy there would be one additional pregnancy if the lesions are excised or ablated compared to giving no treatment at all.

Invasive adhesive endometriosis: For invasive adhesive endometriotic disease the available evidence supports surgical approach compared to non surgical approach.[13] In extensive endometriosis GnRH suppression is given followed by surgery This has better pregnancy rates than surgery alone.

Rectovaginal nodules: Rectovaginal nodules have the same prognosis for pregnancy rates as superficial endometriosis. If there are severe tubal adhesions consider IVF.

Culde sac obliteration: Laparoscopy and laparotomy both give a 25% life table pregnancy rate.[38]

Post Surgical Medical Treatment

A recent Cochrane review showed that medical therapy does not have a role in treatment of endometriosis related infertility either after surgery or alone.[39]

Presurgery Ovarian Suppression

It has been suggested that presurgical ovarian suppression is a useful adjunct. Improved pregnancy rates have been reported with presurgical medical treatment using Danazol or GnRH. However, these data are sufficiently inconclusive to recommend preoperative ovarian suppression.[39]

Controlled Ovarian Stimulation and Intrauterine Insemination (COS and IUI)

Control population fecundity in endometriosis is 2 to 4% per cycle and treated population with COS and IUI is 5 to 18%.[40] The addition of IUI increases fecundity only slightly in clomiphene group but doubles it when gonadotropins are used. Pregnancy rates are 6-8% with clomiphene IUI and 12-20% with gonadotropin and IUI. COS with IUI is helpful in stage I and II disease. 3-4 cycles being appropriate. Maximum 6 cycles of clomiphene with IUI and 6 cycles of gonadotropins with IUI can be done in selected young patients. Randomized controlled trials in moderate to severe endometriosis are lacking. However, results of COS with IUI would be poor because of anatomical distortion.

Repeat Surgery vs IVF

IVF-ET usage in an infertile patient of endometriosis removes the critical step of fertilization and early embryo development

from an invivo environment which is perceived to be hostile to these steps.

There is no randomized controlled trial that support repeat surgery for infertility patients especially for patients who have stage III and IV endometriosis, IVF is a better option (Table 12.4).[41] In one study the pregnancy rate after 2 IVF cycles was 70% whereas it was 24% after repeat surgery.[42] Hence, IVF is an preferable alternative to repeat surgery for most patients. IVF was also superior to COS and IUI.[43] It is self evident that IVF will be of value in advanced disease due to its low background pregnancy rate of the disease and tangible rate of success with IVF. The value of IVF in early stage disease is unproven.

Table 12.4: Treatment strategies based on specific situations

- Younger patients with minimal endometriosis ⟶ expectant management.
- Patients more than 35 years age ⟶ COH/IUI or IVF
- Patients with severe endometriosis, tubal disease, male factor or combination of etiologies ⟶ IVF at an earlier stage.

IUI COS should be second line of therapy after expectant management unless there is an absolute indication for IVF like older women, male factor infertility, long standing infertility or tubal adhesions in which case it is justifiable to refer patients for ART where estimated prognosis after surgery is poor. They should be referred immediately after surgery (Fig. 12.3).

Impact of Endometriosis on IVF

Deleterious effect on outcome have been reported because of difficulty in monitoring, reduced response to gonadotropins, decreased oocyte retrieval, decreased fertilization and implantation rates and impaired oocyte and embryo quality. There are studies which show no difference Hence, evidence is inconclusive

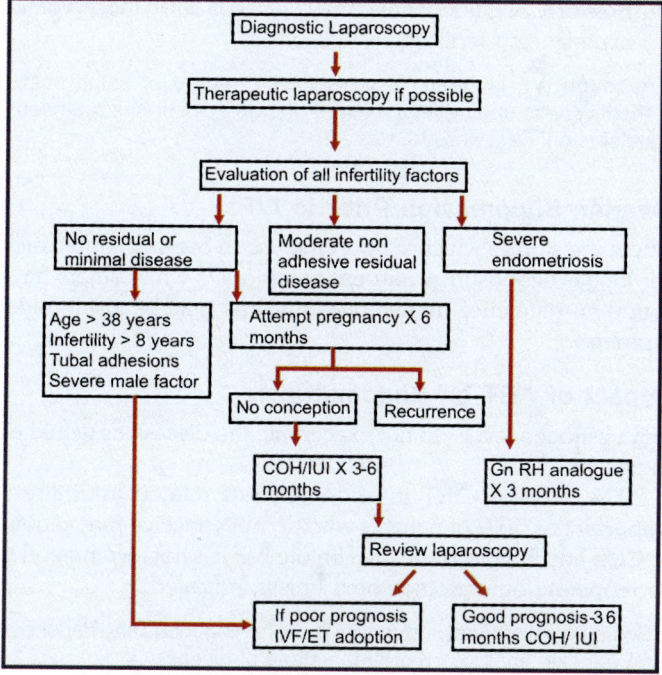

Fig. 12.3: Postsurgical management of an infertility patient

Limitations of IVF in Endometriosis:

i.   Reduced oocyte yield in such patients leads to impaired folliculogenesis and difficulties for oocyte retrieval

ii. Fertilization rates are significantly reduced

iii. There is a lower cleavage rate and fewer embryos reach the 4 cell and blastomere stage hampering the ART process.

iv. Impairment of implantation

v.   Incidence of aberrant nuclear and cytoplasmic morphology is higher in these embryos.

vi. Long protocol GnRH agonist usage leads to suppression of endometriosis thus improving IVF outcome.

vii. Role of ICSI is unclear and may be beneficial in those women experiencing fertilization difficulties.

Although IVF is clearly worthwhile its degree of value cost, effectiveness and optimal method of employment has not been satisfactorily answered.

Ovarian Suppression Prior to IVF

There are studies which support the use of ovarian suppression for longer periods in severe endometriosis[44] while others have found no difference. In fact precious time may be lost in older women.

Impact of ART on Endometriosis

High estrogen levels do not exacerbate the disease as would be expected.

The place of ART in endometriosis related infertility is important as 50% of patients who do not conceive may require it. COS and IUI should be tried before IVF It is not recommended to reoperate on endometrioma unless indicated.

Postsurgical prognosis of fertility is not homogenous and depends on adnexal adhesion more than stage of disease.

Medical or Surgical Treatment?

Endometriosis remains a difficult clinical problem. Once the diagnosis is made before deciding the treatment of the disease it is important to determine what underlying problem should be treated infertility or alleviating painful symptoms. First line treatment for painful symptoms should be medical and surgery should be reserved for cases in which medical treatment has failed or for patients with more severe disease. In infertility, surgery and assisted conception have a role in moderate and severe disease, but the appropriate management of less severe cases is still uncertain. The benefit of surgery in these patients may be entirely due to the mechanical clearance of adhesions and obstructive lesions. Evidence based guidelines also support the role of surgery.[17] Medical treatment of minimal or mild endometriosis has not shown to increase pregnancy rates.[45] In milder cases it would be appropriate to use assisted conception techniques and treat the patient as if she had unexplained infertility before going in for surgery. Furthermore other analyses have shown improvement in vitro fertilization pregnancy rates with pretreatment with gonadotropin-releasing hormone (GnRH) agonists in stage 3 and 4 endometriosis. In a case-controlled study, pregnancy rates with intracytoplasmic sperm injection were not affected by the presence or extent of

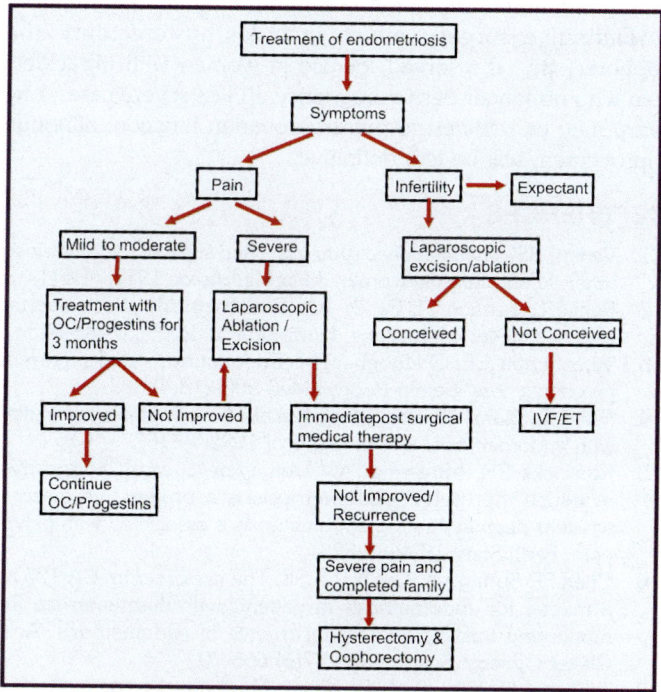

Fig. 12.4: Treatment of Endometriosis

endometriosis.[46] ICSI appears to be an efficient treatment option after fertilization failure with IVF in unexplained and stage I endometriosis-associated infertility.[47] Figure 12.4 shows the approach to management of endometriosis based on whether pain or infertility is the presenting complaint.

> The treatment of endometriosis focuses upon amelioration of two symptoms: pain and infertility. The treatment of endometriosis-associated pain can be well treated medically and all medical treatments are equally effective. In treatment of endometriosis-associated infertility surgical treatment improves fertility, probably for all stages of disease. Assisted reproduction are efficacious.

Definitive surgery, which includes hysterectomy and oophorectomy, is reserved for use in women with intractable pain who no longer desire pregnancy. In less severe cases, one ovary may be retained to preserve ovarian function, although improvement will be less definitive.

REFERENCES

1. Verlauf BS. The incidence symptoms and signs of endometriosis in fertile and infertile women J Fla Med Assoc 1987;74:671.
2. Reeve L, Lashen H, Pacey AA: Endometriosis affects sperm-endosalpingeal interactions. Hum Reprod. 2005;20:448-51
3. Vercammen EE, D'Hooghe TM: Endometriosis and recurrent pregnancy loss. Semin Reprod Med 2000;18(4):363-8
4. Fedele L, Bianchi S, Bocciolone L et al. Pain symptoms associated with endometriosis. Obstet Gynecol 1992;79:767
5. Konincks PR, Mueleman C, Demeyere S et al. Suggestive evidence that pelvic endometriosis is a progressive disease whereas deep infiltrating endometriosis is associated with pelvic pain. Fertil Steril 1992;57:523.
6. Chen FP, Soong YK, Lee N, Lo SK: The use of serum CA-125 as a marker for endometriosis in patients with dysmenorrhea for monitoring therapy and for recurrence of endometriosis. Acta Obstet Gynecol Scand 1998;77(6):665-70.
7. Takeuchi H, Kuwatsuru R, Kitade M: A novel technique using magnetic resonance imaging jelly for evaluation of rectovaginal endometriosis. Fertil Steril 2005;83:442-7

8. Kroninckx PR, Martin DC. Deep endometriosis: a consequence of infiltration or retraction or possible adenomyosis externa? Fertil Steril 1992;58:924.

9. Hornstein MD, Gleason RE, Orav J, et al: The reproducibility of the revised American Fertility Society classification of endometriosis. Fertil Steril 1993;59(5):1015-21.

10. Koninckx PR, Meuleman C, Demeyere S, et al: Suggestive evidence that pelvic endometriosis is a progressive disease, whereas deeply infiltrating endometriosis is associated with pelvic pain. Fertil Steril 1991;55(4):759-65

11. Hull ME, Moghissi KS, Magyar DF, et al Comparison of different treatment modalities of endometriosis in infertile women. Fertil Steril 1987;47:40.

12. Prentice A, Deary AJ, Goldbeck-Wood S, et al. Gonadotrophin-releasing hormone analogues for pain associated with endometriosis (Cochrane Review). In: The Cochrane Library, Issue 1, 2002. Oxford: Update Software.

13. Adamson GD, Pasta DJ Surgical treatment of endometriosis associated infertility – metanalysis compared with survival analysis Am J Obstet Gynecol 1994;171:1488-1505.

14. Kauppila A: Changing concepts of medical treatment of endometriosis. Acta Obstet Gynecol Scand 1993;72(5):324-36.

15. Schlaff WD, Dugoff L, Damewood MD, Rock JA: Megestrol acetate for treatment of endometriosis. Obstet Gynecol 1990; 75(4):646-8.

16. Puleo JG, Hammond CB Conservative treatment of endometriosis externa: the effect of danazol therapy. Fertil Steril 1983;40:164.

17. Hughes E, Fedorkow D, Collins J, Vandekerckhove P: Ovulation suppression for endometriosis. Cochrane Database Syst Rev 2000;(2):CD000155

18. Royal College of Obstetricians and Gynaecologists. The investigation and management of endometriosis. London: RCOG, 2000. (Guideline No 24.)

19. Marcoux S, Maheux R, Berube S, et al: Laparoscopic surgery in infertile women with minimal or mild endometriosis. Canadian Collaborative Group on Endometriosis. N Engl J Med 1997 Jul 24;337(4):217-22.

20. Saidi MH, Vancaillie TG, White AJ, et al: Complications of major operative laparoscopy. A review of 452 cases. J Reprod Med 1996 Jul; 41(7):471-6.

21. Selak V, Farquhar C, Prentice A, Singla A: Danazol for pelvic pain associated with endometriosis. Cochrane Database Syst Rev 2001;(4):CD000068 .

22. Abou-Setta AM, Al-Inany HG, Farquhar CMLevonorgestrel-releasing intrauterine device (LNG-IUD) for symptomatic endometriosis following surgery. Cochrane Database Syst Rev. 2006 Oct 18;(4):CD005072

23. Harrison RF, Barry-Kinsella C: Efficacy of medroxyprogesterone treatment in infertile women with endometriosis: a prospective, randomized, placebo-controlled study. Fertil Steril 2000;74(1): 24-30

24. Revelli A, Modotti M, Ansaldi C, Massobrio M: Recurrent endometriosis: a review of biological and clinical aspects. Obstet Gynecol Surv 1995;50(10):747-54.

25. Jones KD, Sutton C: Patient satisfaction and changes in pain scores after ablative laparoscopic surgery for stage III-IV endometriosis and endometriotic cysts. Fertil Steril 2003;79(5): 1086-90.

26. Alborzi S, Momtahan M, Parsanezhad ME: A prospective, randomized study comparing laparoscopic ovarian cystectomy versus fenestration and coagulation in patients with endometriomas. Fertil Steril 2004 Dec;82(6):1633-7.

28. Sutton CJ, Pooley AS, Ewen SP, Haines P: Follow-up report on a randomized controlled trial of laser laparoscopy in the treatment of pelvic pain associated with minimal to moderate endometriosis. Fertil Steril 1997;68(6):1070-4

29. Namnoum AB, Hickman TN, Goodman SB, et al: Incidence of symptom recurrence after hysterectomy for endometriosis. Fertil Steril 1995;64(5):898-902

30. Redwine DB: Endometriosis persisting after castration: clinical characteristics and results of surgical management. Obstet Gynecol 1994; 83(3):405-13.

31. Bucassa M Fedele L , Biarchi S et al Surgical treatment of recurrent endometriosis laparotomy vs laparoscopy Hum Reprod 1998;13: 2271-4.

32. Berreta P, Franchi M , Ghazzi F et al Randomized controlled trials of two laparoscopic treatment of endometrioma Cystectomy vs drainage and coagulation Fertil Steril 1998;70:1176-80.

33. Sutton CSG, Ewen SP, Jacob SA et al Laser laparoscopic surgery in treatment of ovarian endometriomas J Am Assoc Gynecol Laparoscop 1997;4:319-23.
34. Bucassa M, Marana M, Caruana P et al Recurrence of endometrioma after laparoscopic excision. Am J Obstet Gynecol 1999;180:519-23.
35. Muzii L, Biandu A, Croce C et al Laparoscopic examination of ovarian cyst: Is stripping technique a tissue sparing procedure. Fertil Steril 2002;77:609-14.
36. Adamson GD, Pasta DJ Pregnancy rates can be predicted by validated endometriosis fertility index (EFI) Fertil Steril 2002;77: S48.
37. Olive DL, Schwartz LB, Endometriosis N Eng J Med 1993;328: 1759-69.
38. Jacobson TZ Barlow DH, Koninckv PR et al. Laparoscopic surgery for subfertility associated with endometriosis Cochrane database Syst Rev 2002;4:CD 001398.
39. Donnez J, Nisolle M, Casanas Roux F. Rectovaginal septum endometriosis or adenomyosis.: Laparoscopic management I a series of 231 patients Hum Reprod 1995;10:630-5.
40. Yap C, Furness S, Farquhar C. Pre and postoperative medical therapy for endometriosis surgery Cochrane database Syst Review 2004; (3):CD 003678.
41. The Practice Committeee Of American Society of Reproductive Medicine Use of Clomiphene citrate in women Fertil Steril 2004; 82:90-96.
42. The Practice Committeee Of American Society of Reproductive Medicine Endometriosis and infertility. Fertil Steril 2004;81:1441-6.
43. Pagidas K, Falcone T, Hemmings R, et al. C of reoperation for moderate (Stage III) and severe (Stage IV) endometriosis related infertility withIVF- ET Fertil Steril 1996;65:791-5.
44. Drowski WP, Pry M, Ding J, et al. Cycle specific and cumulative fecundity in patients with endometriosis who are undergoing COH IUI or IVF- ET Fertil Steril 2002;78:750-6.
45. Zikopanulos K, Kolibianakis EM, Derroey P. Ovarian stimulation for IVF in patients with endometriosis Acta Obstet Gynecol Scand 2004;83:651-5.
46. Badawy SZ, ElBakry MM, Samuel F, Dizer M. Cumulative pregnancy rates in infertile women with endometriosis. J Reprod Med 1988; 33(9):757-60.

47. Bukulmez O, Yarali H, Gurgan T. The presence and extent of endometriosis do not affect clinical pregnancy and implantation rates in patients undergoing intracytoplasmic sperm injection. Eur J Obstet Gynecol Reprod Biol 2001; 96(1):102-7

48. Omland AK, Bjercke S, Ertzeid, Fedorcsak P, Oldereid NB, Storeng R, Abyholm T, Tanbo T. Intracytoplasmic sperm injection (ICSI) in unexplained and stage I endometriosis-associated infertility after fertilization failure with in vitro fertilization (IVF). J Assist Reprod Genet 2006;23(7-8):351-7.

CHAPTER 13

Ovarian Endometriosis— Laparoscopic Management

Neena Singh Kumar
Surveen Ghumman

Endometriosis has remained an enigma with its etiology still not clearly defined. It affects 10 to 15% of women during reproductive years. The ovary is a common site leading to formation of endometriotic cyst. The classic triad of dysmenorrhea, dyspareunia and infertility is characteristic of the disease. Endometriosis can be classified as mild , moderate or severe according to the American Fertility Society (See Chapter 12). There may be a tender mass in adnexa if an endometriotic cyst is present. Laparoscopy is the gold standard of diagnosis (Fig. 13.1). Ultrasound may diagnose chocolate cyst of ovary as an enlarged cyst with uniform granular hypoechoic fluid collection or a tubo-ovarian mass (for details see Chapter 12).

Typically these cysts generate fibrosis turning the cortex outwards and invaginating it. These are actually pseudocysts and the lining is the ovarian cortex becomes difficult to peel off. Upto 7% of endometriomas will be intraovarian and will have a true lining which can be easily peeled off.

Caution: One may often mistake a hemorrhagic corpus luteum for a chocolate cyst. It can be differentiated by the colour of the base which is yellow in corpus luteum.

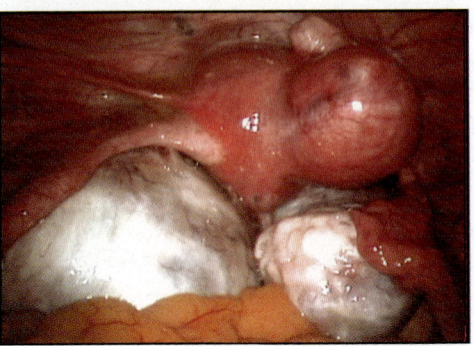

Fig. 13.1: Bilateral endometriomas with fibroid uterus

Superficial Small Ovarian Endometrioma

Superficial endometriosis of the ovary usually presents as small dark, punctuate lesions immediately beneath the cortical surface. Tiny surface lesions can be vaporized or coagulated by bipolar cautery. Layer by layer vaporization can be done by short bursts of laser. Occasionally the visible lesion may be a tip of a larger deeper lesion.

If a deeper lesion is suspected with a superficial endometrioma the implant should always be excised and the ovary explored.

Moderate Endometriomas

There may be difficulty in stripping the pseudocapsule and it may often have to be excised. The endometrioma is incised with a monopolar hook or scissors after stabilizing the ovary by grasping the ovarian ligament. A small claw forceps pulls the inner surface of the cyst wall and the cyst lining is gently excised. Laser coagulation helps in achieving hemostasis. Ovarian wound is left open.

Large Endometriomas

Large endometriomas may be adherent to the adjoining tissues. (Fig. 13.2). They are difficult to remove endoscopically because of extensive adhesions and care must be taken in identifying the ureter.

Technique

The steps of surgery are–

Adhesiolysis

Adhesiolysis is done and ovaries and tubes are released. The ureter is identified. (See accompanying DVD ROM)

Decompression of the Cyst

The cyst is decompressed and irrigated till clear to minimize spill. If spill occurs copious irrigation and suction is done to prevent an inflammatory reaction (Fig. 13.3).

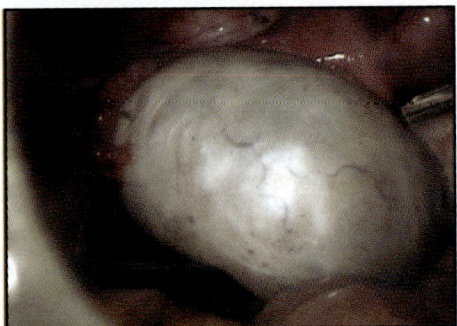

Fig. 13.2: Big endometrioma
(11/10 cm) of left ovary

Opening the cyst wall : The endometrioma is opened and cyst wall identified (Fig. 13.4). The cavity is inspected for papillary structures or any other suspicious structures (Fig. 13.5).

Stripping the Cyst Wall

The cyst wall is stripped from the ovary by a teasing and twisting motion combined by countertraction within the ovary (Fig. 13.6).

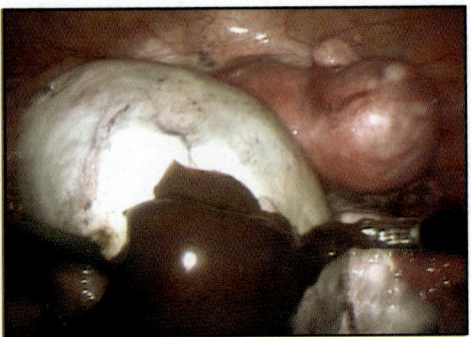

Fig. 13.3: Chocolate material drained and irrigated to prevent inflammation

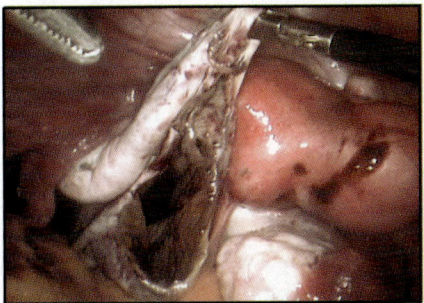

Fig. 13.4: Cyst opened and wall identified

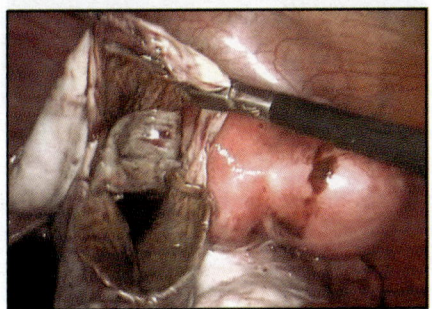

Fig. 13.5: Inspecting cavity of cyst

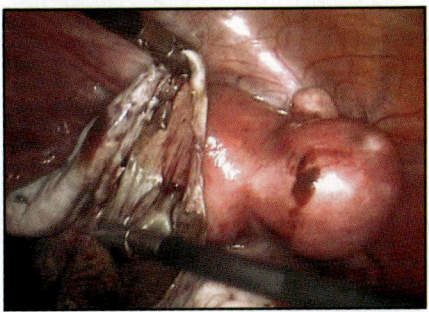

Fig. 13.6: Peeling the cyst wall

Control of Bleeding

Bleeding is controlled by coagulation with laser or bipolar forceps and hemostasis is ensured. (Fig. 13.7). The remaining fragments are vaporized with laser or fulgurated by electrocautery.

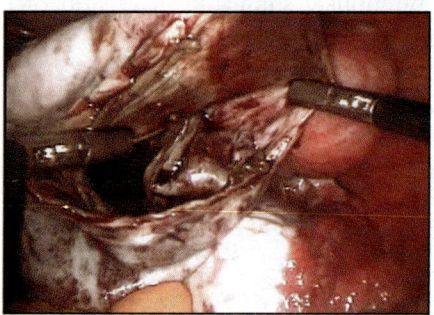

Fig. 13.7: Completion of removal of cyst wall and ensuring hemostasis

After excision the edges are left open to heal. Ischemia associated with suture placement can provoke adhesion formation after laparoscopic reconstruction.

Most endometriotic cysts are not true cysts. They are formed by invagination of the ovarian cortex. Oocytes may be lost by removal of the ovarian cortex that forms the pseudocyst. CO_2 laser vaporizes the cyst wall layer by layer with superficial depth and prevents excessive destruction of the cortex. With cautery, damage may be more widespread as there is scattering. Scissor excision may have a role as it gives a tissue feel. However, it can be argued that since the ovarian cortex invaginates, it is unavailable for external ovulation and removal causes no harm. Excision also provides histopathological specimen for diagnosis.

Note: It is important to avoid excessive destruction of ovarian tissue in the infertile patient justifying undertreatment of these patients.

In a recent cochrane review it was stated that there is some evidence that excisional surgery for endometrioma provides for a more favorable outcome than drainage and ablation, with regards to the recurrence of the endometrioma, recurrence of symptoms and subsequent spontaneous pregnancy in women who were previously subfertile.[1] Excision of cyst wall in endometrioma was strongly recommended especially in infertile patients.[2]

Recurrent Ovarian Endometrioma

Recurrent endometriomas, as detected by TVS, can remain asymptomatic and do not necessarily progress in size without medical treatment. The decision to reoperate depends on symptoms, like severe pain, and failure of medical treatment rather than on its size. However, such patients are more likely to have signs of deep nodules and adnexal/bowel adhesions along with larger endometriomas on TVS scan, thus predisposing them to require a second procedure.[3] Laparoscopic excision of recurrent ovarian endometriomas may be done and the recurrence of pain and the reproductive outcome is comparable with those found after primary surgery.[4] Caution must be used in all recurrent procedures for ovarian endometriomas in infertile patients, to ensure preservation of ovarian tissues, as these patients may have ovarian failure. The success rates of IVF are not affected by recurrence.

Removal of Endometrioma before IVF (See Chapter 12)

Laparoscopic cystectomy for small endometriomas before commencing an IVF cycle does not improve fertility outcomes. Proceeding directly to controlled ovarian hyperstimulation in women with asymptomatic ovarian endometriomas might reduce the time to pregnancy, the costs of treatment, and the hypothetical complications of laparoscopic surgery. Conversely, conservative surgical treatment of ovarian endometriomas in symptomatic women does not impair IVF or intracytoplasmic sperm injection success rates.[5] The number of oocytes and embryos obtained was not significantly decreased by laparoscopic cystectomy, suggesting that in experienced hands this procedure may be a valuable surgical tool for the treatment of large ovarian endometriomas. However, great care must be taken to avoid ovarian damage.[6,7]

Ovarian endometriomas can be managed laparoscopically. However, large endometriomas with extensive adhesions may be a problem and laparotomy may be needed. In treating the infertile patient maximum amount of ovarian tissue should be conserved so that ovarian reserve is not disturbed.

REFERENCES

1. Alborzi S, Zarei A, Alborzi S, Alborzi M. Management of ovarian endometrioma. Clin Obstet Gynecol 2006;49(3):480-91.
2. Hart RJ, Hickey M, Maouris P, Buckett W, Garry R. Excisional surgery versus ablative surgery for ovarian endometriomata. Cochrane Database Syst Rev 2005; 20(3):CD004992.
3. Exacoustos C, Zupi E, Amadio A, Amoroso C, Szabolcs B, Romanini ME, Arduini D. Recurrence of endometriomas after laparoscopic removal: sonographic and clinical follow-up and indication for second surgery. J Minim Invasive Gynecol 2006; 13(4):281-8.
4. Fedele L, Bianchi S, Zanconato G, Berlanda N, Raffaelli R, Fontana E. Laparoscopic excision of recurrent endometriomas: long-term outcome and comparison with primary surgery. Fertil Steril 2006;85(3):694-9.
5. Garcia-Velasco JA, Mahutte NG, Corona J, Zuniga V, Giles J, Arici A, Pellicer A. Removal of endometriomas before in vitro fertilization does not improve fertility outcomes: a matched, case-control study. Fertil Steril 2004; 81(5):1194-7.
6. Canis M, Pouly JL, Tamburro S, Mage G, Wattiez A, Bruhat MA. Ovarian response during IVF-embryo transfer cycles after laparoscopic ovarian cystectomy for endometriotic cysts of >3 cm in diameter. Hum Reprod 2001; 16(12):2583-6.
7. Marconi G, Vilela M, Quintana R, Sueldo C Laparoscopic ovarian cystectomy of endometriomas does not affect the ovarian response to gonadotropin stimulation. Fertil Steril 2002; 78(4):876-8.

CHAPTER 14

Ectopic Pregnancy

Sudha Salhan
Surveen Ghumman

Pregnancy occurring anywhere other than the uterine cavity is termed as an ectopic pregnancy. It is a life-threatening condition and one of the leading causes of maternal mortality in the developed countries. Patient could present either with acute symptoms where she may be hemodynamically unstable or as a chronic presentation.

Incidence

Ectopic pregnancy may be the only life-threatening disease in which prevalence has increased as mortality has declined. The incidence of ectopic pregnancy has increased from 4.5 per 1000 to 19.7 per1000 over the last 20 years. There are various reasons for it.

1. Increased incidence of sexually transmitted disease.
2. Increased ability to detect the disease early.
3. More tubal surgeries being performed on patients.
4. Popularity of contraception that prevents intrauterine but not extrauterine pregnancies.
5. Unsuccessful tubal sterilization.
6. Induced abortion followed by infection.
7. Assisted reproductive technology.

Etiology

1. Tubal damage secondary to inflammation[1,2]
2. Intrauterine contraceptive devices (IUD)
3. Oral contraceptive pill
4. Prior tubal surgery
5. Endometriosis
6. Assisted reproductive technologies[3]
7. Developmental or acquired tubal anomalies: Intramural polyps and tubal diverticula can
8. Other causal factors: Cigarette smoking increases the risk of ectopic pregnancy.

Sites of Ectopic Pregnancy
1. Tubal – 95 to 97%
   - Ampullary – 55%
   - Isthmic – 20 to 25%
   - Infundibulum or fimbrial – 17%
   - Interstitial or cornual – 2 to 4%
2. Ovarian – 0.5%
3. Cervical – 0.1%
4. Abdominal - 0.03%

Clinical Presentation

Abdominal pain, bleeding per vaginum and adnexal mass are the classical triade of findings of ectopic pregnancy.
1. Abdominal pain could be
   - Generalized
   - Localized in pelvis
   - Referred to shoulder
2. Abnormal uterine bleeding is present in 75% cases
3. Adnexal mass is present in only 50% of cases and its accurate detection is dependant on the diagnostic skills of examiner, degree of peritonitis, presence or absence of tubal rupture and cooperation of the patient.

There could be mild to severe tenderness on palpation, guarding or rigidity in the lower abdomen. Cervical excitation pain may be present on bimanual examination. Uterus may be slightly enlarged. A tender boggy mass in the pouch of Douglas is due to collection of blood.

Diagnostic Aids

β hCG

Single β hCG: It is of little use if positive. When negative it rules out an ectopic pregnancy.

Serial measurement: The quantification of β hCG is useful in determining the viability of pregnancy. Doubling time for β hCG is 1.9 days. In normal intrauterine pregnancy there is an increase of more than 66% in 48 hours. In ectopic pregnancy this increase is less than 66%. β hCG levels increase between 30 to 50% for an interval of 24 hours in normal intrauterine pregnancy.

Fallacy

1. In early ectopic pregnancy the increase may be similar to a normal pregnancy.
2. In 15% of normal pregnancies there may be a less than 66% increase.[4] Negative results from a qualitative serum β hCG test indicate that ectopic pregnancy is not present, except in rare cases of chronic ectopic pregnancy. Therefore, in high-risk asymptomatic patients, use of endovaginal sonography is indicated only if the qualitative serum β hCG test is positive.

Human chorionic gonadotrophin (β HCG) ratio (β hCG 48 hours/β hCG 0 hour) of <0.87 predicted failing pregnancy of unknown location (PUL), with a sensitivity of 93.1% and a specificity of 90.8%. Using this cutoff a non-interventional approach in women with pregnancy of unknown location can be adopted.[5]

Urinary pregnancy tests can detect β hCG at a level of 25 to 50 IU/L and hence are useful in initially triaging a patient who in reproductive age group presents with abdominal pain or abnormal vaginal bleeding.

Serum Progesterone Assay: During the first 8 – 10 weeks of gestation serum progesterone levels change little and are usually more than 20 ng/ml. Patients with ectopic pregnancy have levels of less than 15 ng/ml. All pregnancies which are non-viable have a level of less than 5 ng/ml. However, this test is not done routinely for diagnosis. It can exclude ectopic pregnancy with 97.5% sensitivity (levels of ≥25 ng/milliliter exclude the diagnosis), obviating the need for further testing serum progesterone levels of less than 5 ng/ml can identify nonviable pregnancies with 100% sensitivity.

Transvaginal Sonography: Features which point towards an ectopic pregnancy are:

a. *Adnexal findings:*

Mass in adnexa – TVS can identify a mass in the adnexa of 10 mm diameter. Extraovarian mass with mixed echogenicity is the most common ultrasonographic finding seen in 86 to 100% of patients.[6]

Extrauterine cardiac motion: May be seen in 8 to 26% of cases.

Tubal ring: This is present in 42 to 68% of patients and is the second most common ultrasound finding.[7] This sign is highly specific for ectopic pregnancy (98.9%).

b. *Endometrial findings*

Empty uterine cavity – Usually gestational sac is seen at 34 days pregnancy on transvaginal sonography, with a serum β hCG level of 1500 IU. Fetal heart rate is seen at 4.5 weeks of gestational age when the crown rump length was 3 mm.

Pseudogestational sac: A decidual cast can be mistaken for a gestational sac. A double line image is present in the true sac where there is a hypoechoic decidual lining of the uterus and hyperechogenic rim of the trophoblast surrounding the gestational sac. A double-sac sign is the earliest reliable indication of an intrauterine pregnancy (IUP) on endovaginal sonograms. The parietal decidua creates the outer ring, and the capsular decidua makes up the inner ring of the double sac. A true sac of IUP and a pseudo sac of ectopic pregnancy can be confidently distinguished on the basis of a typical double-sac sign. The pseudosac of ectopic pregnancy is caused by either the presence of intrauterine fluid surrounded by a thick decidual reaction or a detached decidual cast containing fluid centrally

c. *Fluid in pouch of Douglas*

Intraperitoneal fluid in ectopic pregnancy is usually echogenic and may be the only abnormal endovaginal sonographic finding of ectopic pregnancy. Fluid may be present in patients with ectopic pregnancy, regardless of its nature (intact, ruptured, or aborting). However, pelvic fluid is a nonspecific finding that may be found in other conditions that can clinically mimic ectopic pregnancy, such as a ruptured ovarian cyst, pelvic inflammatory disease, and ovarian torsion.

Adnexal mass with empty uterine cavity has a sensitivity of 97% and a specificity of 99%. Endovaginal sonography is a readily available, cost-effective, and indispensable tool in the diagnosis and management of ectopic pregnancy.

3D ultrasonography: 3D ultrasonography shows an asymmetry in the endometrial configuration in intrauterine pregnancy which is absent in cases of ectopic pregnancy. It is also accurate in detecting ectopic gestational sac in asymptomatic patients prior to sixth gestational week.

Color Doppler ultrasonography:
  It can detect
  • Peritrophoblastic flow associated with adnexal mass.
  • Increased tubal blood flow on the side of ectopic pregnancy.
  • Decreased impedance to flow and increased peak blood velocity in uterine arteries.
  • Differentiates between viable and non-viable pregnancy.

Culdocentesis: It is positive if blood is aspirated with a syringe from the pouch of Douglas.

Fallacy
  • It does not rule out other intraperitoneal causes of bleeding
  • It is positive only if ectopic pregnancy is ruptured.

Laparoscopy:
  It is indicated if
  • Ectopic pregnancy is strongly suspected and ultrasonography is negative.
  • There are no products of conception on D & C with a positive pregnancy test.

- In unstable patient with an uncertain diagnosis
- Significant intraperitoneal fluid is present.

The disadvantage of laparoscopy is that it is an invasive procedure which carries some risk of complications. It may not be able to detect a small ectopic sac. Diagnostic laparoscopy is still considered the standard reference for the diagnosis of ectopic pregnancy, although this invasive approach has a reported false-negative rate of 3-4% and a false-positive rate of 5%.[8]

When the diagnosis is uncertain and condition of patient is unstable or there is significant intraperitoneal bleed evaluation should start with laparoscopy.

Dilatation and curettage:

It is helpful in only selected situations where—

   i. Level of β hCG is low, to detect the presence of degenerating villi.

   ii. Excessive bleeding per vaginum is present.

> The combined use serum b hCG and high-resolution endovaginal sonography with its high sensitivity and specificity is the current noninvasive approach for diagnosing ectopic pregnancy and is replacing the routine use of invasive procedures such as culdocentesis, dilation and curettage, and diagnostic laparoscopy.

With the increasing interest in the conservative nonsurgical management of ectopic pregnancy, endovaginal sonography can have a role in both the selection and follow-up of these patients.

Treatment

1. Expectant treatment:

If the trophoblast gets separated from blood supply by localized hemorrhage and blood clots, atresia of trophoblast is induced. In such cases the gestational tissue is eventually reabsorbed leading to spontaneous resolution. This is seen in 64% of ectopic pregnancies with an average resolution time of 20 ± 13 days. Success rate was higher with lower β hCG levels.[9]

Criterion for expectant management
- β hCG threshold of 1000IU/L
- Hemoperitoneum of less than 50 ml
- Hematosalpinx of less than 2 cm
- Absence of recognizable fetal parts or fetal heart on ultrasound
- Absence of clinical symptoms.

Protocol for expectant management
- i. Establish reliable diagnosis
- ii. Inform patient of other treatment options
- iii. Obtaining consent for acceptability of this method of management.
- iv. Monitoring β hCG levels every 3 to 4 days until they decrease to 10 IU/L.

Disadvantages

Nearly 30% women have tubal occlusion following spontaneous resolution of ectopic pregnancy and this unfavorable outcome may limit its application in women who desire fertility.[10]

Laparoscopy is indicated if
- Abdominal pain is increasing
- Increase in cul-de-sac fluid volume
- Plateauing or increasing β hCG levels

2. Medical treatment:

With introduction of accurate non-surgical diagnostic techniques, primary medical treatment of ectopic pregnancy has become possible.

Indications

1. Contraindication to surgery like multiple abdominal surgeries or extensive pelvic adhesions.
2. Interstitial pregnancy.
3. Sites where conservative surgical treatment is relatively unsuccessful like cervix, ovary and abdomen.[11]
4. May be preferred as first line of treatment if there is no contraindication.

1. *Methotrexate:* Usually Methotrexate is the drug of choice. Methotrexate is an antifolic acid metabolite. It interferes with synthesis of DNA by inhibiting pyrimidines. This prevents proliferation of trophoblastic cells leading to cell death.

Single Dose Protocol

A single dose of 50 mg/m^2 may be sufficient. Protocol is as given in Table 14.1.

Table 14.1: Single dose methotrexate protocol	
Day 1:	Baseline studies Methotrexate 50 mg/m^2
Day 4:	β hCG titer
Day 7:	β hCG titer Complete blood and platelet count Liver and renal function tests
Weekly:	β hCG titer till it is negative.

Follow-up:
- β hCG levels are measured on day 1, 4 and 7. Initially there may be a rise in the levels.
- If there is a less than 15% decline in levels between day 4 and 7 another dose of methotrexate is given
- Serum β hCG levels were measured weekly till it reaches 15 IU/L if there was a decrease of more than 15%.
- Declined of less than 15 % of β hCG levels in any subsequent week required methotrexate protocol to be repeated.

Inclusion criterion
1. Unruptured ectopic
2. Patient hemodynamically stable
3. Mass of less than 3.5 cm in diameter.

4. Absent fetal heart
5. β hCG levels of less than 10,000 mU/ml
6. Patient should be able to return for follow-up.

Contraindication

1. Hepatic, renal or peptic disease
2. Elevated baseline liver enzymes
3. Thrombocytopenia or neutropenia

Prerequisites to methotrexate treatment

1. Administration of Anti D if patient is Rh negative and greater than 8 weeks gestation.
2. Obtain baseline liver and renal function tests, complete blood and platelet count.
3. Counsel patients of failure rate of 5 to 10% and need for subsequent surgery.

Precautions

1. Avoid exposure to sun as photosensitivity is a complication.
2. Refrain from sexual intercourse during therapy.
3. Avoid folate containing vitamins and alcohol till β hCG is negative.
4. To report immediately if there is worsening of symptoms such as vaginal bleeding, abdominal and pleuritic pain, dizziness or syncope.

Monitoring

1. Clinical signs like pain and adnexal mass
2. USG for size of mass and presence of hemoperitoneum
3. β hCG
4. Hematological indices
5. Liver biochemistry

Side effects of methotrexate

Mylosuppression, stomatitis, gastritis, diarrhea, alopecia, liver toxicity, abdominal pain, photo-sensitivity, pneumonitis, renal toxicity and anaphylaxis.

Usually these effects are seen in 20 to 30% of patients on multi-drug regimen and are not present in single drug regimens They take 72 hours to resolve once the drug is stopped.

Predictors of the Success of Therapy

The most commonly identified predictors of the success of methotrexate therapy for ectopic pregnancy are chorionic gonadotropin levels, progesterone levels, size and volume of the gestational mass, presence or absence of fetal cardiac activity, and presence or absence of free peritoneal blood

Serum beta-human chorionic gonadotropin levels on day 4 following methotrexate treatment of patients with ectopic pregnancy do not predict successful single-dose therapy.[12] However in another study transvaginal ultrasound findings are as important as serum βhCG level on the first day of methotrexate treatment. In unruptured cases, day 3 serum β hCG level is important to reevaluate the decision to continue follow-up or perform early surgery for increased risk of treatment failure.[13]

Advantage: As compared with the multiple-dose protocols, single-dose methotrexate is less expensive, has fewer side effects, requires less intensive monitoring of patients, is more readily accepted by patients, and may not require rescue therapy with Leucovorin. Single-dose treatment with MTX could be as successful as multiple doses with no difference in incidence of complications.[14]

Disadvantage: Single dose protocol may have problems of resolution pain and having a prolonged time to resolution. Also patients with high serum β hCG levels have a poor success rate.

Results: There is a success rate of 94% with an average resolution time of 35 days. Tubal patency on ipsilateral side was present in 82% cases. 80% of those attempting pregnancy got pregnant with a 12.5% repeat ectopic rate.[15] Resolution pain occurs in 20% of cases. There may be a prolonged resolution time occasionally. Repeat ectopic is seen in 7 % cases.

Multiple Dose Protocol

1 mg/kg of methotrexate is administered on day 1, 3, 5 and 7 along with 0.1 mg/kg CF administered intramuscularly on day 2, 4, 6 and 8.

In the variable dose protocol β hCG was measured 2 days after the first methotrexate injection. If the decrease in β hCG was more than 15% no more methotrexate was given and weekly β hCG was done. If plateau of β hCG was observed at two consecutive times methotrexate was administered 4 weeks after the first dose. Maximum of 4 doses are given.

Complications of Medical Therapy

Pain: After methotrexate therapy, abdominal pain commonly increases, presumably as a result of either tubal abortion or stretching of the tube by hematomas. The pain is generally self-limiting and usually controlled with orally administered non-steroidal anti-inflammatory drugs. If such drugs do not relieve the pain, reevaluation is indicated. Although many physicians believe that surgical therapy is necessary in such cases, a recent study indicated that observation alone is appropriate in many cases.[16]

Formation of hematomas: After treatment with methotrexate, up to 56% of ectopic gestational masses that are monitored ultrasonographically increase in size.[17] Although masses of 7 to 8 cm have been noted; most of the women with masses of this size are asymptomatic. These masses may persist even after serum chorionic gonadotropin levels have decreased to less than 15 mIU per milliliter; the time to resolution could be upto 108 days.[17] These masses should not be interpreted as representing treatment failure, since they are probably resolving hematomas rather than persistent trophoblastic tissue.

Methotrexate is also used to treat persistent ectopic pregnancy which results from proliferation of residual trophoblastic tissue remaining after conservative surgical procedure. The trophoblast can be located within the muscular layer of the oviduct or between the muscularis and serosa so that at the time of salpingostomy only portion of the trophoblast within the tubal lumen is removed. These patients are managed expectantly, by methotrexate therapy or by surgery. If the titer of serum β hCG is elevated then a serial β hCG is required. If titer continues to fall, expectant treatment can be done. If the levels remain same or increases, a single dose of methotrexate or repeat surgery is indicated.

Medical Therapy by Local Injections

1. *Methotrexate*: A dose of 1mg/kg may be instilled locally under transvaginal sonography or laparoscopically. Although laparoscopic approach seems to be more accurate, it is difficult to justify using a single injection of medication as the only treatment for a women receiving general anaesthesia and undergoing laparoscopy, when a linear salpingostomy can be easily performed. Placement of transvaginal injection is less precise and one cannot be certain that the medication has actually been deposited in the ectopic site. It is also uncertain whether the solution containing the medication is able to stay in the location where it is deposited or it is extruded out. An 83% success rate was noted.[18] The theoretical advantage of lower systemic levels of the drug with local administration was proved wrong in a recent study.[19]

2. *Prostaglandins:* Prostaglandin F2 was injected locally. It is unacceptable now due to poor efficacy and systemic effect.

3. *Hyperosmolar glucose*: When injected locally a success rate of 82 to 92 % is reported.[20] Success rate of ultrasonographically directed local injection therapy is 72% whereas it is 90% in patients where it is laparoscopically directed.

Surgical Treatment

Surgery could be conservative or radical. It is an important decision to make whether or not the patient is physiologically stable enough to undergo a lengthy conservative microsurgical procedure. When ectopic occurs in a sole remaining tube one must make all possible attempts to repair it.

Conservative Surgical Treatment

This approach is possible if the diagnosis is made considerably early before rupture of the oviduct. It consists of:
  1. Linear salpingostomy
  2. Segmental resection

Linear Salpingostomy

It is the surgical treatment of choice if fertility needs to be preserved. Linear salpingostomy has now become the standard laparoscopic operation when an ectopic mass is unruptured but measures more than 4 cm by ultrasound.

The surgery can be done laparoscopically or by laparotomy.

Steps

1. Expose, elevate and stabilize tube.
2. The incision is made in the antimesenteric wall till lumen is entered (Fig. 14.1A).
3. Products of conception are expressed by gentle pressure from the opposite side of the tube. Gentle traction by forceps or suction may be needed to completely remove the products of conception. (Figs 14.1B and C). Remaining fragments can be removed by irrigation of lumen with ringer lactate.
4. Hemostasis: Hemostasis is obtained along the border of the incision using bipolar electrocoagulation or fine needle unipolar coagulation. Hemostasis is secured at implantation site with bipolar electrocoagulation under constant irrigation. Manual compression of the vessels in the mesosalpinx with periodic release allows the surgeon better visualization of bleeding points. It may be necessary to coagulate a portion of the vascular arcade below the fallopian tube. Collateral circulation to the tube will prevent necrosis and preserve structure and function. Vascular interruption is a preferred alternative to excessive intraluminal coagulation with damage to tubal mucosa and muscularis.
5. The tubal serosa and muscularis is sutured in a single layer with 5-0 non-reactive material (Fig. 14.1D) The incision may be left to heal by secondary intension. (Fig. 14.1E) or margins may be sutured separately for hemostasis (Fig. 14.1F).

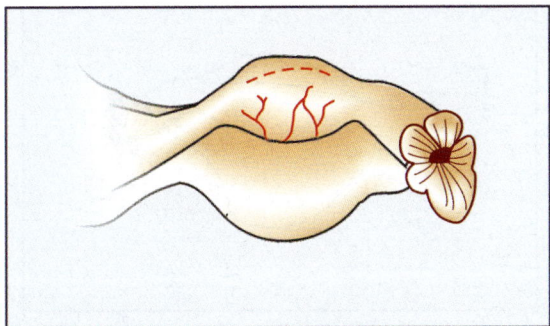

Fig. 14.1A: Incision given on antimesenteric border

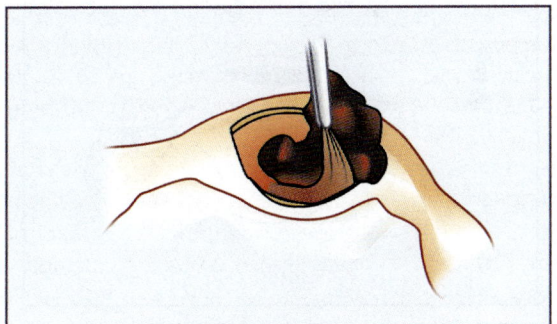

Fig. 14.1B: Removal of products of conception

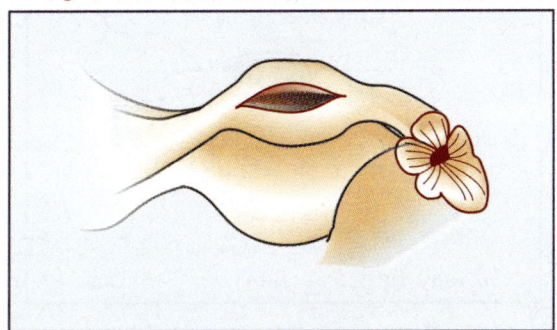

Fig. 14.1C: Products of conception completely removed

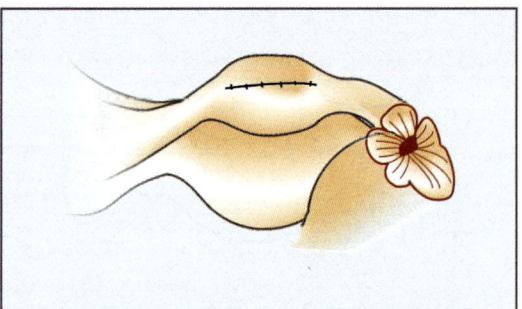

Fig. 14.1D: Muscularis and serosa sutured

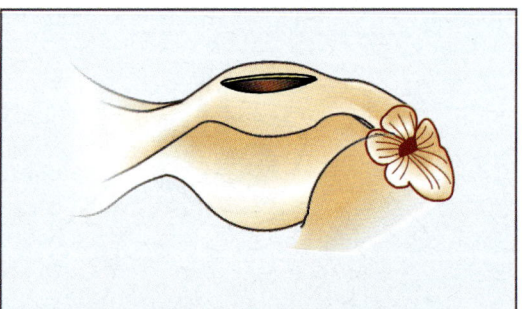

Fig. 14.1E: Edges left unsutured

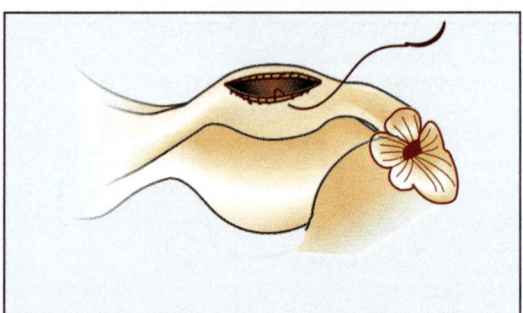

Fig. 14.1F: Margins sutured separately for hemostasis

Precautions

1. Care is taken to provide complete hemostasis in tubal mucosa as postoperative bleeding can lead to intraluminal adhesions.
2. No suture material should be retained on the mucosal surface as it may cause inflammation and lead to adhesion formation.
3. If there is possibility that attempts to remove all trophoblastic tissue will damage the tubal mucosa, the tissue should be left *in situ*.

Results: The intrauterine pregnancy rate was 61% with a repeat ectopic rate of 15%.[21] The best results are seen in unruptured ectopic without serosal invasion, in young patients with no history of infertility and patients with grossly normal oviducts. Tubal patency is seen in 70 to 100% in various studies. Repeat ectopic is seen in 10 to 20% of pregnancies being 7.7% if contralateral tube is normal and 28.5% if the contralateral tube is blocked .80% of the times the repeat ectopic occurs on the same side.[22] The reproductive outcome depends on

1. History of prior infertility – Intrauterine pregnancy rate is 25% if there is history of prior infertility and increases to 68%. When history is absent.[23]
2. Condition of contralateral tube. If intact and healthy pregnancy rate is 87% and decreases to 51% in unhealthy tube.
3. Age of the patient.

Laparoscopic Conservative Management

Laparoscopic management is preferred provided there are no contraindications.

Contraindications

1. Hemodynamically unstable patient
2. Severe pelvic adhesions
3. General contraindications to laparoscopy.

Hemoperitoneum is not a contraindication as suction can be done.

Steps

1. Two auxiliary puncture sites are made suprapubically to allow manipulation of fallopian tube.
2. A dilute solution of vasopressin is injected into the tubal wall.
3. Laser, unipolar needle cautery or scissors can be used to make a salpingotomy incision, on the antimesenteric border of the tube in area of maximal distention. It should be large enough to allow for extrusion of complete products of conception. It is important to keep the tube taut. The tube is opened and hemostasis is obtained simultaneously. The CO_2 laser is excellent for placing the incision and the products of conception protect the tubal mucosa of the opposite side from damage.
4. *Hemostasis is achieved:*
   - Before placement of the incision, by creating a line of coagulation with bipolar forceps.
   - While incision is being made, by using a fine unipolar needle and blended low voltage current.
   - After the incision is made, by using bipolar coagulation along the margin
5. If products do not extrude they are removed by gentle pressure of the probe, hydrodissection or suction irrigation. Suction is used if the product are viable and irrigation if they are non-viable and surrounded by blood clots. Occasionally biopsy forceps are needed to dislodge pregnancy tissue specially those located in the extraluminal site between serosa and muscularis. Care is taken to remove all placental tissue to avoid persistent ectopic pregnancy.
6. The tissue is placed in an endoscopic bag.
7. Tube is irrigated and checked for hemostasis.

8. The tube then heals by secondary intention or is sutured. Healing by secondary intension is preferred as closure may result in stenosis of the lumen increasing chances of a repeat ectopic. The tube repairs itself within a month.

Results: The results are similar to those of open technique.

Laparoscopic Salpingostomy vs. Medical Management:

On comparison of methotrexate and laparoscopic salpingostomy the fertility rate was 82% with a mean interval time to conceive of 9.4 months after the treatment with methotrexate and a 82.6% fertility rate with the mean interval time to conceive of 11.7 months in laparoscopic salpingostomy. Both therapeutic methods constitute reliable solutions for managing ectopic pregnancy.[24]

Persistent Tubal Ectopic Gestation

It is defined as continual growth of viable trophoblastic tissue after initial treatment of the disorder. Persistent trophoblastic tissue can remain after linear salpingostomy in 8.3% treated laparoscopically and 3.9% treated by laparotomy.[21] There may be an initial decline in serum β hCG level followed by a rise. Hence levels should be monitored weekly after linear salpingostomy. Usually levels fall to undetectable levels in 12 days. The tendency is to find persistent trophoblastic tissue in proximal part of the tube. Trophoblastic tissue can be easily flushed out of distal portion of the oviduct and it may be difficult to identify particles of trophoblastic tissue wedged in the proximal portion of the oviduct. Tubal rupture with intrabdominal hemorrhage can occur with persistent ectopic pregnancy.[25]

Hydrodissection to flush out the gestational products is better than piecemeal removal by forceps.

Risk Factors for Persistent Ectopic Gestation

1. Small ectopic pregnancy (<2 cm)[26]
2. Early therapy ($<$ 42 days from last menstrual period)
3. High levels of serum β hCG ($>$ 3000 IU/L)
4. Rapidly rising levels of β hCG or serum progesterone higher than 5 nmol / L: This is because normally growing tissue of ectopic pregnancy may be more fragile and more difficult to remove from the functioning implantation site than aborted tubal tissue that has been partially separated from the oviduct by thrombi and necrosis.
5. Less than 50% decrease in levels of serum β hCG on day 1.[27]

Treatment

1. Medical: A single dose of methotrexate (50 mg/m^2) is effective.
2. Surgical reoperation and removal of oviduct if there are signs of hemodynamic instability, increasing abdominal pain combined with sonographic presence of free intrabdominal fluid.
3. Expectant: Only if patient is asymptomatic and hCG levels are not rapidly increasing.

Persistent ectopic has no effect on the patient's reproductive function.

As persistent ectopic can present at a later stage following initial appropriate decrease in β hCG concentration weekly β hCG concentration measurement is recommended until they return to normal range.

Segmental Resection

1. *Segmental resection of the involved portion of oviduct with primary microsurgical anastomosis:* Tissue edema may cause difficulty in reanastomosis.
2. *Segmental resection with reanastomosis at a later date:* Patients need to be subjected to a second surgery.

Indications

1. Isthmic ectopic pregnancy
2. Ruptured tube
3. Continued bleeding after salpingostomy

Prerequisite: Patients with minimal bleeding should be taken up for this surgery.

Advantage

Since implantation site is removed it cannot be involved in a subsequent ectopic pregnancy and a more normal architecture of oviduct is restored.

Steps: Bipolar forceps are introduced and the tube is desiccated on either side of damaged site and divided (Fig. 14.2A). The underlying mesosalpinx is desiccated and tubal segment excised and removed (Figs 14.2B and C). Alternatively an endoloop suture is placed proximally and distally around the tubal segment. The sutures are placed deep enough to include the vessel arcade just below the tube. The tube is divided between the sutures. If on examining the lumen, the site implantation is not clear then more tube should be excised until normal mucosa is reached, Reanastomosis may be done in the same sitting or at later time, depending on patient's condition and state of the tubes. It is best done under a microscope with microsurgical techniques discussed in Chapter 8. The seromuscular sutures are placed under magnification using 6-0 or 7-0 absorbable material. Serosa is sutured with interrupted sutures. Adjacent mesosalpinx should be excised and removed with care to avoid formation of hematoma in the broad ligament.

Segmental resection is preferred to salpingostomy in isthmic pregnancy as

1. The narrow tubal lumen and thick muscularis of the isthmus is more prone to postoperative damage and obstruction with linear salpingostomy.
2. Narrow lumen limits exposure needed to remove the pregnancy successfully and achieve hemostasis.
3. Isthmic area is usually in a state of advanced rupture and is better treated by excision than repair

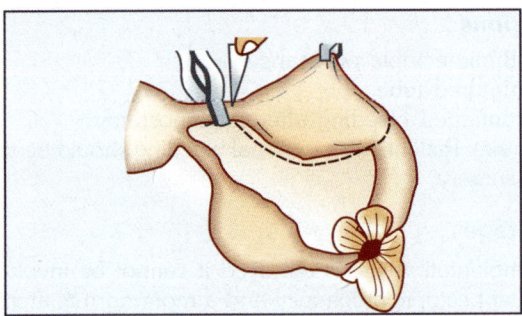

Fig. 14.2A: Tube is desiccated proximal and distal to the ectopic gestation sac

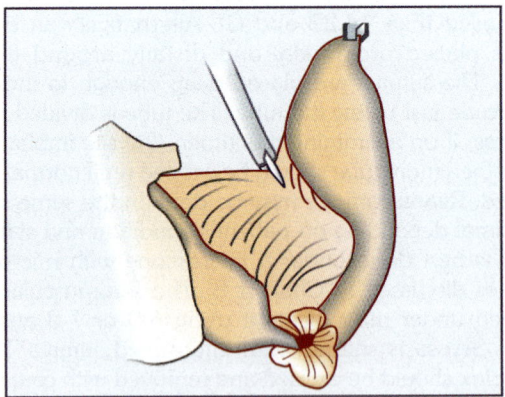

Fig. 14.2B: Mesosalpinx is desiccated and cut below the sac

Comparison of partial resection and linear salpingostomy shows that each has advantages and disadvantages (Table 14.2).

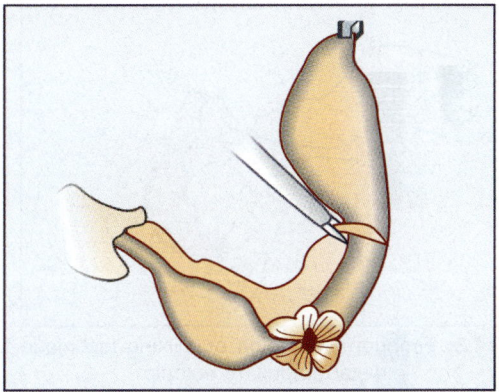

Fig. 14.2C: Tube is cut just distal to the sac and segment removed

Table 14.2: Partial ressection vs. linear salpingostomy

Advantage of linear salpingostomy
1. Create minimum tubal damage
2. Preserve tubal length
3. Eliminate need for another procedure.

Disadvantage of linear salpingostomy
1. Damaged part of tube left in situ.
2. Higher chance of persistent ectopic pregnancy.
3. Increased chance of repeat tubal ectopic.

Advantage of segmental resection
1. The tube with the localized tubal pathology responsible for occurrence of ectopic pregnancy is removed
2. Less chance of persistent ectopic pregnancy

Disadvantage of segmental resection
1. Increased surgery time if anastomosis is done
2. Need for subsequent surgery if anastomosis not performed along with primary surgery.

Fimbrial Evacuation

It is done when pregnancy is in the fimbrial segment of fallopian tube by pushing out the sac with pressure from the fingers (Fig. 14.3).

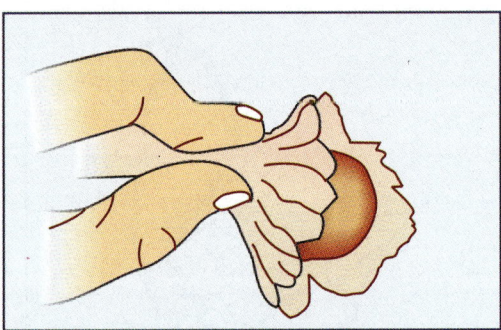

Fig. 14.3: Fimbrial evacuation or milking technique for distal ampullary ectopic

Disadvantage:

1. It is not recommended in ampullary tubal pregnancy as may cause damage to the tubal mucosa.
2. It is associated with a two-fold increase in recurrent ectopic pregnancy.
3. There is a high rate of surgical reexploration for recurrent bleeding from persistent trophoblastic site.

Laparoscopically it can be removed by irrigation, suction or grasping forceps.

Aquaexpression of Tubal Pregnancy

This consists of inserting the distal tip of the aquadissector into the tubal lumen through the fimbrial end to extract a non-viable ampullary pregnancy with surrounding blood clot. The pregnancy is dislodged and irrigated out of the tube with pressurized fluid from the aquadissector (Fig. 14.4).

Radical Surgical Treatment

This includes removal of the fallopian tube. Salpingectomy can be done by both laparoscopy as well as laparotomy.

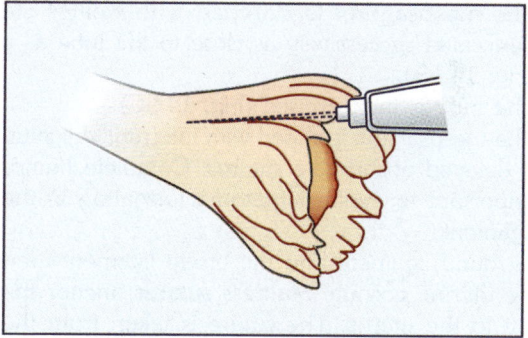

Fig. 14.4: Irrigation technique

Indications

1. Ruptured tubal pregnancy with severely damaged tube.
2. Recurrent ectopic pregnancy in same fallopian tube
3. Previous tubal surgery for infertility.
4. Ectopic pregnancy in a woman who has completed her family.
5. Cornual pregnancy.

Removal of a healthy ovary is now considered unjustified. With partial cornual resection a residual tract may develop leading to an interstitial pregnancy. Complete peritonization of the cornual incision and advancement of the round and broad ligament over the uterine cornua should prevent an interstitial pregnancy. An attempt to resect the cornua completely can lead to a residual myometrial defect which can cause uterine rupture, interstitial recanalization or placental encroachment during a subsequent intrauterine pregnancy. Excessive resection is avoided by resecting only one-third thickness of cornual portion of the myometrium.

Steps:

1. The tube proximal to the gestational sac is desiccated and cut (Fig. 14.5A).

2. The mesosalpinx is clamped with Kelly's clamp or desiccated successively as close to the tube as possible (Fig. 14.5B).
3. The tube is then excised (Fig. 14.5C).
4. The mesosalpinx is closed with interrupted ligatures of 2-0 delayed absorbable sutures. Complete hemostasis is important to avoid hematoma formation in the broad ligament.

The round ligament and the broad ligament are sutured over the uterine cornua. Mattress sutures anchor the broad ligament to the uterus. The suture is taken from the broad ligament anteriorly 2 to 3 cm below the round ligament. A second bite is taken from the fundus of the uterus posterior and superior to the uterine incision. A third bite is taken through the posterior surface of the broad ligament. When tied it completely covers the cornua.

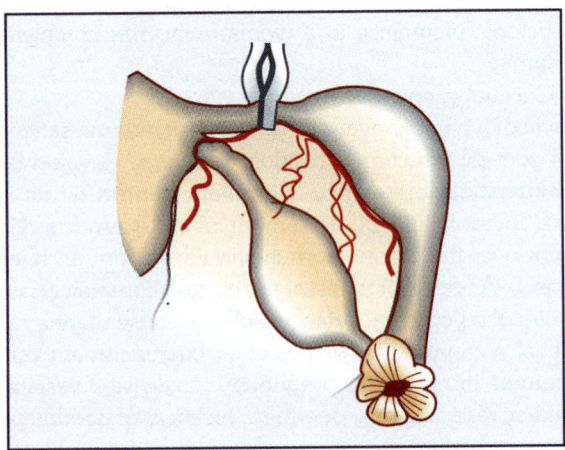

Fig. 14.5A: The proximal end of the tube is desiccated and cut

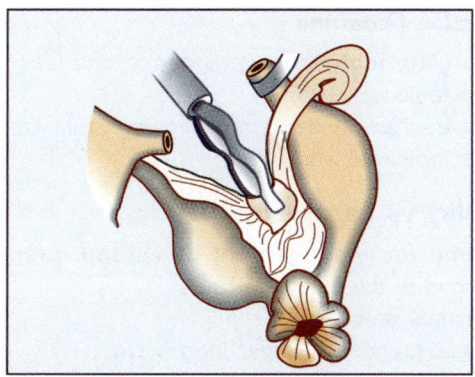

Fig. 14.5B: The mesosalpinx is cut close to the tube

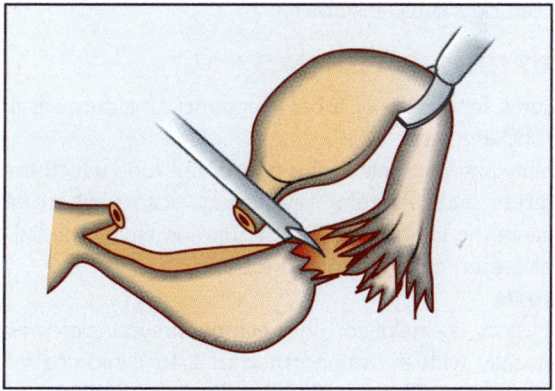

Fig. 14.5C: The tube is removed

Laparoscopic Salpingectomy

Immediate treatment success rate was similar for methotrexate (94.7%) and laparoscopic salpingostomy (91.4%). The mean time for hCG to decrease to less than 15IU/L was significantly less in laparoscopic salpingostomy group[28] (see Chapter 9 and accompanying DVD ROM).

Reproductive Outcome

Radical surgery: Intrauterine pregnancy rate was 50% and recurrent ectopic was 10%.

Conservative surgery: Intrauterine pregnancy rate was 53% and recurrent ectopic rate was 14%.

Laparotomy vs Laparoscopy

Laparotomy for management of ectopic pregnancy is recommended in the following cases.

1. Interstitial pregnancy
2. Ectopic pregnancy larger than 6 cm
3. hCG value greater than 15,000 mIU/ml
4. Hemoperitoneum greater than 2000 ml
5. Hemodynamic instability.

INTERSTITIAL PREGNANCY

It accounts for 2- 4% of tubal pregnancy. Incidence is 1:2500 to 1: 5000 live birth.

The zygote implants in the part of the tube which traverses the uterine wall. Angular pregnancy occurs when embryo implants in the lateral angle of the uterine cavity medial to the internal ostium of the fallopian tube.

Diagnosis

- History is similar to other ectopic pregnancies presenting usually with an amenorrhea of 2 to 3 months followed by spotting. The gestational sac in the interstitial pregnancy is better protected in the interstitium than other parts of the tube.
- May present with symptoms of severe hemorrhage when the developing chorionic villi erode into blood vessels of uterine cornua as this is the area where uterine and ovarian vessels anastomose.
- The uterus is asymmetrically enlarged.

Timor-Trisch's transvaginal criterion: It is used for diagnosis and includes

1. Empty uterine cavity
2. Chorionic sac seen separately and less than 1 cm from the most lateral edge of the uterine cavity
3. Thick myometrial layer surrounding the chorionic sac.

It has a good specificity (88 to 93%) but a poor sensitivity (40%).

'Interstitial line sign' refers to visualization of an echogenic line extending from the endometrial cavity into the cornual region and abutting the interstitial mass or gestational sac. It is 80% sensitive and 98% specific for diagnosis of interstitial pregnancy.[29] Often laparoscopy is needed to confirm diagnosis.

Treatment

Medical: Methotrexate in a single dose is successful in 83% of cases. Success rate was 91% with multiple dose.[30]

Surgical: Cornostomy or corneal resection and reconstruction of uterine wall. The excision of the cornual section of the uterus is done in a stepwise fashion until normal tubal lumen is visualized. The tube is then excised by cutting a wedge in the myometrium at the uterine cornua. Deep suture should not be taken in the myometrium.

A figure of eight mattress suture is taken at the site of wedge resection to close the myometrium (Figs. 14.6A to E). The damage caused will require a tubal implantation to be performed at a later stage to restore tubal patency if needed. Immediate laparotomy is needed in massive intra-abdominal bleed. Maternal mortality could be upto 2 to 2.5%.

It is time to fine tune our surgical approaches to ectopic pregnancies. During the previous years we defined what procedures should be performed. In the coming years we need to determine how best to perform them. Attempts to maximize fertility rates with conservative procedures have resulted in a term delivery rate of upto 50%. With the advent of operative laparoscopy there is decreased hospital stay and morbidity in patients with unruptured ectopic pregnancy. The choice of

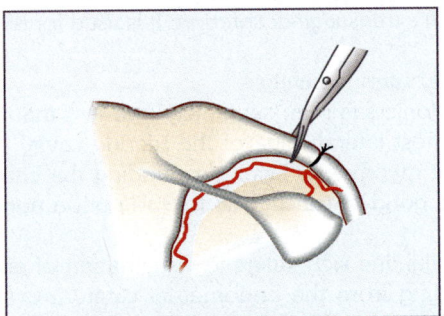

Fig. 14.6A: Distal end of tube is cut

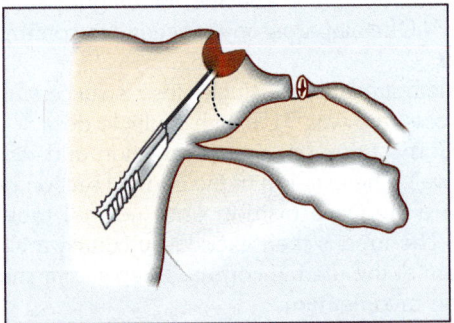

Fig. 14.6B: A wedge is cut in the myometrium proximally

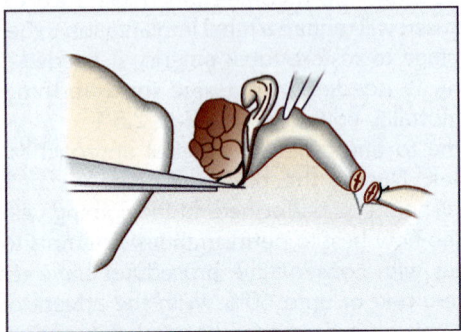

Fig. 14.6C: Products are removed

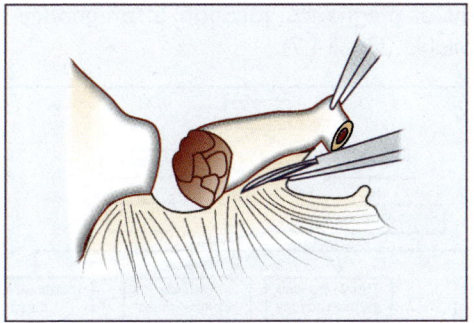

Fig. 14.6D: Diseased segment of tube removed

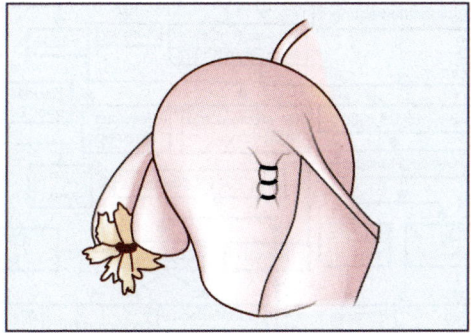

Fig. 14.6E: Mattress sutures taken in myometrium

therapeutic management of unruptured tubal pregnancy has become a controversial issue in recent years. Primary medical treatment appears to be as effective as conservative surgery and the latter has similar subsequent reproductive outcome as do radical procedure. For more advanced pregnancies or in the presence of hemoperitoneum, surgical treatment remains the treatment of choice. Multiple treatment options allow the physician to individualize ectopic pregnancy management according to the history, reproductive plans, size and stage of development of pregnancy, location of pregnancy and the facilities available (Fig. 14.7).

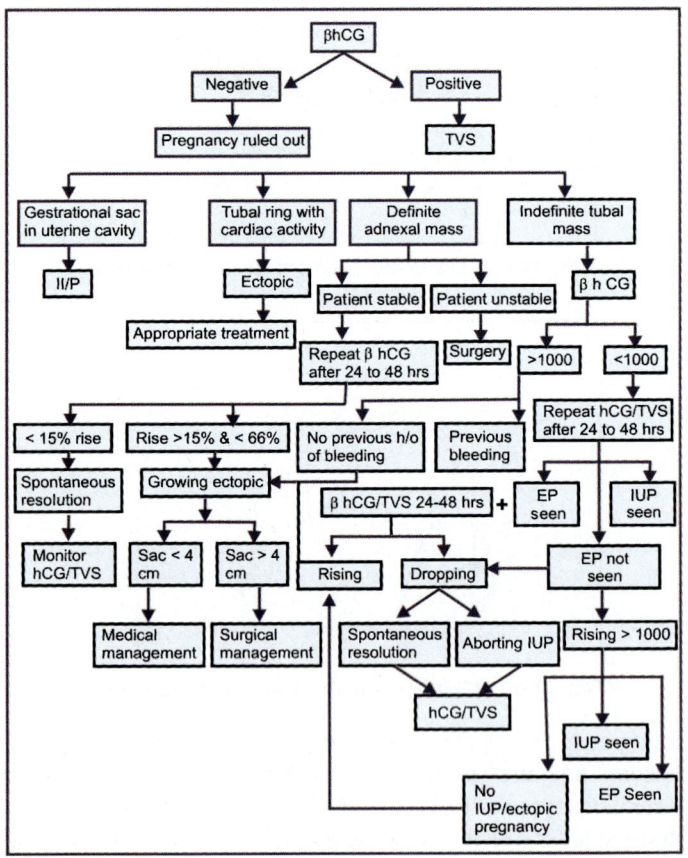

Fig. 14.7: Approach to pregnancy of unknown location on the basis of hCG and TVS (EP-Ectopic pregnancy, IUP-Intrauterine pregnancy)

REFERENCES

1. Westrom L Effect of acute pelvic inflammatory disease on fertility. Am J Obstet Gynecol 1975;121:707-13.

2. Karaer A, Avsar FA, Batioglu S. Risk factors for ectopic pregnancy: A case-control study. Aust N Z J Obstet Gynaecol 2006; 46(6):521-7.

3. Society for assisted Reproductive Technology and American Society of Reproductive Medicine. Assisted Reproductive Technology in the United States: 1997 results generated from the American Society for Reproductive Medicine /Society for Assisted Reproductive Technology Registry. Fertil Steril 2000;74:641-53.

4. Kadar N, CaldwellBV, Romero R. A method of screening for ectopic pregnancy and its indications. Obstet Gynecol 1981; 58: 162-6.

5. Condous G, Kirk E, Van Calster B, Van Huffel S, Timmerman D, Bourne T. Failing pregnancies of unknown location: a prospective evaluation of the human chorionic gonadotrophin ratio. BJOG. 2006 May; 113(5):521-7.

6. Cacciatore B, Stenman UH, Ylostalo P. Early screening for ectopic pregnancy in high-risk symptom-free women. Lancet 1994; 343:517-8.

7. Atri M, deStempelJ, Bret P. Accuracy of transvaginal ultrasonography for detection of hematosalpinx in ectopic pregnancy. JCU 1992;20:255-61.

8. Taylor RN, Padula C, Goldsmith PC. Pitfall in the diagnosis of ectopic pregnancy: immunocytochemical evaluation in a patient with false-negative serum f3- hCG levels. Obstet Gynecol 1988; 71:1035-8.

9. Korhonen J, Stenman UH, Ylostalo P. Serum human chorionic gonadotropin dynamics during spontaneous resolution of ectopic pregnancy. Fertil Steril 1994;61:632-6.

10. Trio D, Strobelt N, Picciolo C,et al. Prognostic factors for successful expectant management of ectopic pregnancy . Fertil Steril 1995; 63:469-72.

11. Kirk E, Bourne T. The nonsurgical management of ectopic pregnancy. Curr Opin Obstet Gynecol. 2006;18(6):587-93

12. Gabbur N, Sherer DM, Hellmann M, Abdelmalek E, Phillip P, Abulafia O. Do serum beta-human chorionic gonadotropin levels on day 4 following methotrexate treatment of patients with ectopic pregnancy predict successful single-dose therapy? Am J Perinatol. 2006;23(3):193-6.

13. Dilbaz S, Caliskan E, Dilbaz B, Degirmenci O, Haberal A Predictors of methotrexate treatment failure in ectopic pregnancy. J Reprod Med 2006;51(2):87-93.

14. Alleyassin A, Khademi A, Aghahosseini M, Safdarian L, Badenoosh B, Hamed EA. Comparison of success rates in the medical management of ectopic pregnancy with single-dose and multiple-dose administration of methotrexate: a prospective, randomized clinical trial. Fertil Steril 2006 Jun; 85(6):1661-6.

15. Stoval TG, Ling FW. Single dose methotrexate: an expanded clinical trial. Am J Obstet Gynecol 1993;168:1759-62.

16. Lipscomb GH, Puckett KJ, Bran D, Ling FW. Management of separation pain after single-dose methotrexate therapy for ectopic pregnancy. Obstet Gynecol 1999;93:590-3.

17. Brown DL, Felker RE, Stovall TG, Emerson DS, Ling FW. Serial endovaginal sonography of ectopic pregnancies treated with methotrexate. Obstet Gynecol 1991;77:406-9.

18. Carson SA, Buster JE. Ectopic pregnancy. N Engl J Med 1993; 329:1174-81.

19. SchiffE, Shalev E, Bustan M, et al. Pharmacokinetics of methotrexate after local tubal injection for conservative treatment of ectopic pregnancy. Fertil Steril 1992;57:688-90.

20. Gjelland K, Hordnes K, Tjugum J, et al. Treatment of ectopic pregnancy by local injection of hyperosmolar glucose: A randomized trial comparing administration guided by transvaginal ultrasound or laparoscopy. Acta Obstet Gynecol Scand 1995; 74:629-34.

21. Yao M, Tulandi T. Current status of surgical and nonsurgical management of ectopic pregnancy. Fertil Steril 1997;67:421-33.

22. Langer R, Golan A,Razier A,et al. Reproductive outcome after conservative surgery for unruptured tubal pregnancy – a 15 year experience. Fertil Steril1990;53:227-31.

23. Fernandes H, Pauthier S,Doumerc S, et al Ultrasound guided injection of methotrexate verus laparoscopic salpingotomy in ectopic pregnancy. Fertil Steril 1995;63:25-9.

24. Dalkalitsis N, Stefos T, Kaponis A, Tsanadis G, Paschopoulos M, Dousias V: Reproductive outcome in patients treated by oral methotrexate or laparoscopic salpingotomy for the management of tubal ectopic pregnancy. Clin Exp Obstet Gynecol 2006;33(2):90-2

25. Kelly RW, Martin SA, Strickler RC. Delayed hemorrhage in conservative surgery for ectopic pregnancy. Am J Obstet Gynecol 1979;133:225-6.

26. Seifer DB, Diamond MP, DeCherney AH. Persistent ectopic pregnancy. Obstet Gynecol Clin North Am 1991;18:153-9.

27. Graczykowski JW. Misell DR. Methotrexate prophylaxis for persistent ectopic pregnancy after conservative treatment for by salpingostomy. Obstet Gynecol 1997;89:118-22.

28. Saraj AJ, Wilcox JG, Najmabadi S, et al. Resolution of hormonal markers of ectopic gestation: A randomized trial comparing single dose intramuscular methotraxate with salpingostomy. Obstet Gynecol 1998;92:989-94.

29. Ackerman TE, Levi CS, Dashefsky SM, et al. Interstitial line sonographic finding in interstitial (cornual) ectopic pregnancy. Radiology 1993;189:83-7.

30. Tang A, Baartz D, Khoo SK. A medical management of interstitial ectopic pregnancy: A 5-year clinical study. Aust N Z J Obstet Gynaecol 2006;46(2):107-11.

CHAPTER 15

Prevention of Postoperative Adhesions

Surveen Ghumman

In all infertility surgeries there lies the risk of postoperative adhesions. Acquired adhesions are subdivided into inflammatory or postsurgical. The problem of offering elective surgery with apparent risk and difficult to quantify benefit to an otherwise healthy women needs to be individually evaluated in each case. All couples must be informed of the potential risks and benefit and the likelihood of each. Also any alternative approach to their problem should be discussed. These considerations put a constraint on the surgeon. A 97% incidence after open gynecologic pelvic procedures has been reported.[1] In clinical and autopsy studies of patients who had prior laparotomies, the incidence of intra-abdominal adhesions was 70-90%.[2] It was found that all patients who had undergone at least one prior abdominal surgery developed one to more than ten adhesions.[3]

Adjunctive procedures which are helpful in preventing the formation of postoperative adhesions favorably tip the balance of risk and benefits and broaden the therapeutic window. The development of postoperative reformation after lysis is a major cause of failure of reconstructive surgery. To meet these challenging problems the surgeon must understand how peritoneal injury normally heal adhesion free, and be familiar with modalities that may impede the process or reduce adhesion formation.

Etiology

1. Infection: Adhesions are seen in pelvic inflammatory disease subsequent to first episode in 23%, second episode 35% and third episode 75%.
2. Endometriosis.
3. Pelvic surgery.

Mechanism of Infertility

1. Adhesions may encapsulate or seclude the ovary sufficiently to cause a mechanical barrier preventing either ovum escape or ovum pick-up.

2. Alter the anatomy, motility and function of the tubes.
3. Tubal occlusion secondary to intraluminal occlusion
4. Intrauterine adhesions preventing implantation.

Pathophysiology of Adhesion Formation

The peritoneum is composed of two layers, a superficial layer of polygonal mesothelial cells and a submesothelial stromal layer composed of connective tissue, collagen, reticular or elastic fibers with abundant vasculature and lymphatics. Adhesions represent abnormal attachment between two structures.

Adhesions may be caused when peritoneal surfaces are subjected to:
• Ischemia
• Mechanical trauma
• Inflammation
• Presence of foreign material.

A serosal injury causes release of vasopermeability factors and chemotactic mediators that initiate the inflammatory reaction. Disruption of stromal mast cells result in release of histamine and vasoactive kinins. There is an increase in capillary permeability. Chemotactic factors cause movement of leucocytes to the site of injury, causing production of peroxide and superoxide radicles and initiate enzyme release causing further tissue damage. Thromboplastin is released and activates the clotting cascade leading to formation of serosanguinous discharge. This coagulates within a period of 3 hours causing fibrinous agglutination of peritoneal surfaces. Normally fibrinous attachments are lysed within 72 to 96 hours of formation. Plasminogen activators in the mesothelium and submesothelial blood vessels convert plasminogen in blood and fibrinous exudates to plasmin, a fibrin splitting enzyme. Only fibrinous attachments that persist for 3 days longer are susceptible to fibroblast migration and proliferation, producing permanent adhesions (Fig. 15.1). Factors that impair fibrinolysis or those which produce heavy fibrin deposits are therefore causative of adhesion formation.

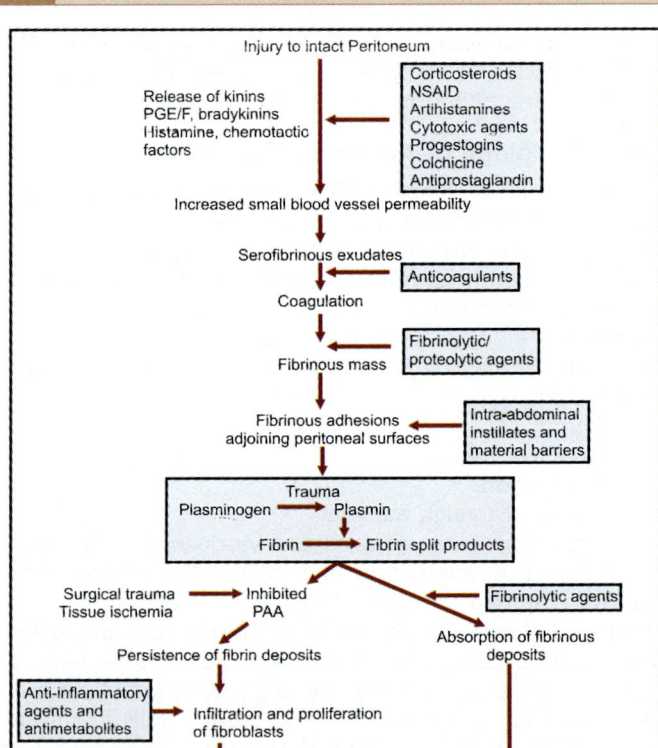

Fig. 15.1: Stages of normal peritoneal healing and adhesion formation and drugs used for prevention

Hence factors which suppress plasminogen activator ultimately suppress fibrinolysis and allow adhesion development. Foremost among these is tissue ischemia which impairs the intrinsic ability of the peritoneum to lyse fibrin by reducing plasminogen activator activity. Intraoperatively, crush injury, interrupted vascular supply, undue tension on peritoneal surfaces and peritoneal and vascular grafts without adequate vascular supply are the most common causes (Table 15.1).

Table 15.1: Factors predisposing to adhesion formation

Injury to peritoneal surfaces
- Crushing instruments
- Harsh handling of tissues
- Intra-abdominal packs
- Drying of serosal surface

Tissue ischemia
- Interruption of vascular supply
- Undue tension or oversuturing
- Over vigourous reperitonization
- Pertoneal or omental grafts
- Overadequate pedicles

Foreign material
- Talc or cornstarch
- Lint
- Reactive suture material

Infection

Overwhelming of normal fibrinolytic mechanism
- Endometriosis

When packs are placed in the abdominal cavity they may abrade the serosa. Drying of serosal surface is another common insult which cause production of fibrinous attachment.

Blood: Blood provides
- An additional source of fibrin
- Cellular elements that make lysis more difficult.
- Platelets which stimulate the serosal inflammatory reaction and fibroblastic proliferation.

Infection: Infection causes adhesions as the:
- Bacteria release enzymes that induce inflammatory exudates and impair fibrinolytic activity. The duration of the infectious process is significant in determining whether these attachments are lysed before fibroblast migration into them. Infections persisting for more than 3 days permit this to occur.

- There is alteration in tissue oxidation - reduction potential secondary to infection or inflammation and this may potentiate the role of ischemia in surpressing normal fibrinolytic mechanism.

Extensive soft adhesions will form within 72 hrs after laparotomy. These seem most extensive at about 10 days to 2 weeks, by which time they become dense and vascular. Over 20% of adhesive obstructions occur within 1 month of surgery, and up to 40% occur within 1 year. The problem of postsurgical adhesions increases with the patient's age, the number of laparotomies, and the complexity of surgical procedures.[4] The number of prior episodes a patient has experienced is the strongest predictor of recurrence.

Types of Adhesions

There are various types of adhesions encountered according to degree of insult faced There may be flimsy adhesions between vicera and abdominal wall (Figs 15.2 and 15.3) or they may be curtain like (Fig. 15.4). Gut may be seen suspended from the adhesions in the abdomen (Fig. 15.5).

Medical Approach to Prevention of Postoperative Adhesions

1. *Dexamethasone and promethazine*: Dexamethasone inhibits all phases of inflammation including capillary dilatation and fibrin deposition during early stages and capillary and fibroblast proliferation and deposition of collagen in later stages. All these events are critical to formation of adhesions. Promethazine is a H_1 receptor antagonist which blocks release of histamine from mast cells and thus prevents increase in vascular permeability induced by histamines. This effect diminishes the extravasation of serosanguinous exudates into interstitium of the damaged tissue, thereby decreasing inflammation and edema. Both promethazine and dexamethazone stabilize the lysosomal membranes thus minimizing the effect of autolytic enzymes in the lyosomes

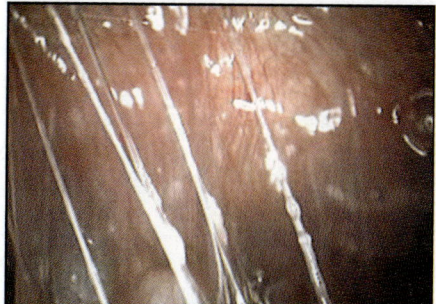

Fig. 15.2: Filmy adhesions between viscera and abdominal wall

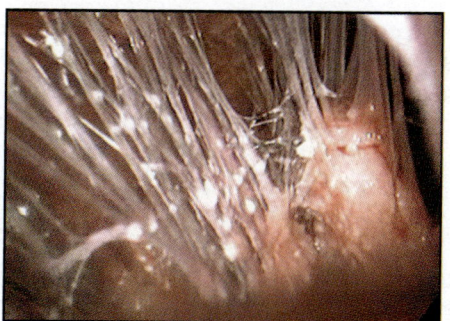

Fig. 15.3: String type of adhesions

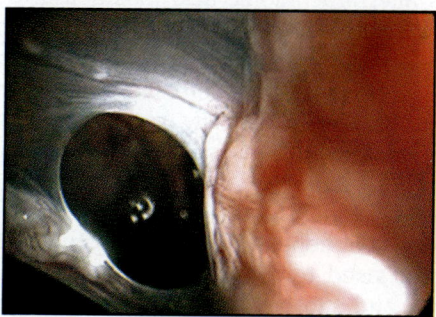

Fig. 15.4: Curtain like adhesions

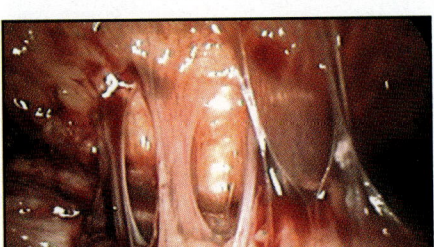

Fig. 15.5: Gut suspended in mid abdomen from adhesions

and consequently reducing the risk of tissue damage. Each of these effects may reduce the likelihood of adhesion formation by reducing the fibroblastic response to injury. With these effects in mind the regime of Dexamethasone 20 mg and promethazine 25 mg given 4 hourly after surgery for 48 hours was thought to block the adhesion cascade. However, subsequent studies did not consistently prove the same.[5]

2. *Non-steroidal anti-inflammatory agents:* It is thought that nonsteroidal anti-inflammatory drugs (NSAIDs) may act through the antiprostaglandin and anti-platelet effect. NSAIDs alter arachidonic acid metabolism by changing cyclooxygenase activities, inhibiting the formation of end products, including prostaglandins and thromboxane. By inhibiting prostaglandin and thromboxane synthesis, NSAIDs decrease vascular permeability, plasmin inhibition, platelet aggregation, coagulation and also enhance macro-phage function.

3. *Antibiotics:* Cephalosporin, doxycycline or penicillins are used to prevent adhesions. Broad-spectrum antibiotics are commonly used for prophylaxis against postoperative infections and subsequent adhesion formation.

Surgical Approach to Prevention of Postoperative Adhesions

1. General principles (Table 15.2)
- Talc or cornstarch should be wiped from surgical gloves with a moistened sponge.
- Surgical packs and sponges are minimally used as they abrade the tissue and create raw surfaces.
- Pedicles should be cut as short as possible while still allowing for adequate knot security and hemostasis.
- Tissues should be handled as gently as possible with atraumatic instruments so as to avoid crush injury or loss of vascular supply. Forceps, retractors, and clamps should not be placed on structures not intended for dissection, reducing serosal denudation and vascular trauma. During surgical procedures the peritoneum is susceptible to crush, thermal, electrical, laser, mechanical, hypoxic, and strangulation injury, resulting in denudation of the superficial mesothelial layer. Disrupting the underlying connective tissue

Table 15.2: Recommended measures for preventing postoperative adhesion formation

Minimize tissue injury
- Constant irrigation to moisten tissues
- Avoid clamping and coagulating
- Limit abdominal packing
- Tapered needles
- Magnification

Decrease Inflammation
- Fine caliber non-reactive sutures
- Prophylactic antibiotics
- Minimizing suturing

Prevent raw surface apposition and fibrin deposition
- Intraperitoneal deposition
- Oxidised cellulose
- Heparinized ringer lactate irrigation

Extirpation of existing adhesions

and associated microvasculature elicits the inflammatory response, depresses fibrinolytic activity, and promotes adhesion formation.

- Maintaining proper line of dissection ideally in a vascular plane remains important
- Clamping, cutting and ligating which involves blood vessels should be done with strict attention to vascular supply since tissue ischemia resulting from devitalization has been implicated as a major cause in formation of adhesions.
- Careful approximation during suturing without undue tension on tissue surfaces caused by oversuturing.
- Thorough irrigation of pelvic cavity for removal of blood clots, lint and talc.
- Reperitonealization to be done only if it can be accomplished without undue tension upon peritoneal surfaces. If not possible peritoneal defects should be left to heal with secondary reperitonealization. There is evidence that peritoneal suturing increases adhesion formation.[6] Grafting or suturing of peritoneal defects increases ischemia, devascularization, and necrosis, predisposing the site to decreased fibrinolytic activity and increased adhesion formation. The presence of suture material and tightening the sutures to the point of ischemia potentiate adhesion formation. The practice of omitting the closure of the peritoneum is well supported in the literature.[7] Omental or peritoneal grafts should be avoided altogether.
- Microsurgical techniques are preferred.

2. *Cautery vs excision:* Lysis with cautery instead of sharp excision reduces adhesion formation. It may be due to improved hemostasis with decreased fibroblast proliferation into the region or due to tissue ischemia.

3. *Laparoscopic surgery:* Laparoscopic surgery is less adhesiogenic than laparotomy because of several reasons
   1. Trauma is minimized due to use of extremely precise energy sources such as the CO_2 laser, ultrasonic scalpel or high frequency electrosurgical needle.[8]

2. Infection is much less likely following laparoscopic surgery than laparotomy

3. Ischemia produced by surgical knots, which is a potent initiator of adhesion formation, can largely be avoided.

4. Laparoscopic surgery embraces the principles of microsurgery, with careful tissue handling, magnification provided by the laparoscope when held close to the tissue, copious irrigation to avoid tissue desiccation and strict attention to haemostasis with the use of microbipolar diathermy to coagulate individual bleeding vessels.

Although the results in terms of tubal patency were very similar, the subsequent fertility rate was much higher in the laparoscopy group and second-look laparoscopy showed much less adhesion formation in the women treated by laparoscopic salpingotomy.[9,10]

Endoscopy reduces *de novo* adhesions because of reduced peritoneal injury secondary to abrasion and reduced opportunity to create large areas of ischemic tissue. Adhesion reformation can occur with laparoscopy, and it has not been shown that laparoscopy is superior to microsurgical adhesiolysis in terms of subsequent pregnancy rates

4. *Selection of suture material*: All sutures elicit an acute inflammatory response resulting from trauma of suture placement. The most intense tissue reaction is associated with plain catgut followed by chromic catgut. Both these sutures cause more reaction than the synthetic sutures because both are absorbed by the process of cellular phagocytosis. A catgut suture, though rapidly absorbed, leads to greater tissue reaction, whereas polyglycolic acid derivatives and monofilament synthetics are less reactive. The synthetic absorbable sutures are absorbed by enzymatic hydrolysis and thus elicit less inflammatory response. Braided versus monofilament sutures contain microscopic pores that can harbor bacteria and lead to infection. The initial tensile strength and retention of tensile strength of

synthetic absorbable sutures are clearly superior to those of natural material. This characteristic allows use of smaller caliber suture if synthetic absorbable material is used, further reducing the amount of tissue inflammation and foreign body reaction. Non-absorbable sutures such as nylon and propylene cause even less acute reaction but they may lead to a foreign body granuloma formation. Hence for infertility surgery Dexon or Vicryl are superior. Catgut should be avoided.

5. *Irrigation solution*: Irrigating solution like Ringer lactate containing hydrocortisone 1000 mg and Heparin 5000 U in one liter have been used.

6. *Adjunctive procedures*:
   i. Suspension of adnexa
   ii. Uterine suspension: It is done by shortening of round ligament by triplication or fixation to the fascia. It prevents adhesions from forming in the pouch of Douglas. It may induce chronic pelvic pain.
   iii. Uterosacral plication: Sutures are placed through both uterosacral ligaments beginning towards the cervix and are tied in a fashion which buries the knot. The sutures are placed approximately 0.5 cm apart until ligaments are approximated providing coverage of raw or denuded peritoneal surface. It also provides a bunching effect which shortens the uterosacral ligament and produces a shelf on which the adenexa rests.

7. *Intraperitoneal agents:*
   A. *Drugs*
      1. *Corticosteroids:* Hydrocortisone 200 mg may be instilled intraperitoeally before closure.[11]
      2. *Heparin:* Acts by inhibition of thrombus formation in the vessels thus minimizing ischemia.[12] But this use of heparin was asso-ciated with hemorrhage and delayed wound healing. Low-dose intraperitoneal heparin irrigation (2,500/5,000 U/l) showed no benefit in adhesion reduction.

However, it was seen that anti-inflammatory agents and peritoneal instillates have no demonstrable benefit.[13]

B. *Mechanical barriers - Adjuvant barrier therapy*

Antiadhesion barriers basically fall under two main categories: macromolecular solutions and mechani-cal devices. In recent years both kinds of barriers have demonstrated real progress in adhesion prevention. The ideal barrier, besides being safe and effective, should be noninflammatory, nonimmunogenic, persisting during the critical remesothelialization phase. It should stay in place without sutures or staples, remain active in the presence of blood and be completely biodegradable without interfering with healing or promoting infection (Table 15.3).

Barrier Solutions

1. *Crystalloids:* The postsurgical peritoneal cavity is acidic, and consideration should be given to the irrigation solution used in surgery. Ringer's lactate is safe, inexpensive, readily available, and has a better buffering capacity than normal saline.

Intraperitoneal instillation of lactated Ringer's solution in animal models decreases adhesion formation and reformation.[14] The mechanism of action is unclear. The presence of a great volume of Ringer's lactate in the abdominal cavity separates raw peritoneal surfaces and prevents adhesion formation. It is also possible that Ringer's lactate cleanses the newly formed fibrin exudate that can serve as a matrix for fibroblast and capillary formation. This initial fibrin, if not removed by fibrinolysis or absorption, produces an inflammatory response, fibroblast proliferation, and adhesion formation.

The risks of leaving large volumes of fluid in the peritoneal cavity after surgery may reduce the ability of the host to eliminate infection by retarding the clearance

Table 15.3: Classes of surgical adjuvants used to minimize postoperative adhesions

Fibrinolytic agents
- Fibrinolysin
- Papain
- Strptokinase
- Urokinase
- Hyaluronidase
- Chymotrypsin
- Trypsin
- Pepsin

Anticoagulants
- Heparin
- Citrates
- Oxalates

Anti-inflammatory agents
- Corticosteroids
- Ibuprofen
- Antihistamines

Antibiotics
- Tetracyclines
- Cephalosporins

Mechanical separation (intrabdominal instills)
- Dextran
- Mineral oil silicone
- Povidone
- Petrolatum (Vaseline)
- Crystalloid solutions
- Carboxymethylcellulose

Barriers
Endogenous tissue
- Omental grafts
- Peritoneal grafts
- Bladder strips
- Fetal membrane

Exogenous tissue
- Oxidised cellulose fabric (Interceed)
- Oxidised regenerated cellulose
- Gelatin
- Rubber sheets
- Metal foils
- Plastic hoods
- Polytetrafluoroethylene (Gore- Tex)

of *E. coli* from the peritoneal cavity and its accumulation. It is thought to be because of dilution of opsonic proteins, and a decrease of the phagocyte-to-bacteria ratio because of an increased intraperitoneal volume.

2. *Hyaluronic acid combined with phosphate-buffered-saline (HA-PBS):* A macromolecular solution to prevent adhesion formation, called Sepracoat is applied intraoperatively, prior to dissection, to protect peritoneal surfaces from indirect surgical trauma (e.g. abrasion and desiccation). It significantly decreases incidence, extent, and severity of *de novo* adhesion in multiple sites following gynecologic pelvic surgery.

3. *Carboxymethylcellulose.* Carboxymethylcellulose is a derivative of cellulose. It is hydrophilic, negatively charged at physiological pH and freely soluble. It is a macromolecule with a similar mechanism of action as dextran. Carboxymethylcellulose works by separating raw surfaces and allowing independent healing of traumatized peritoneal surfaces

4. *Dextran:* It is antithrombotic solution and coats raw areas within the abdomen. It retards clot adherence and prevents surface approximation by drawing fluid into the peritoneal cavity. It has three predominant effect in reducing adhesions.

• Mechanical separation of traumatized tissue—the hydrofloatation effect. This effect is potentiated by the osmotic gradient created by large macromolecules which tend to draw more fluid into the cavity.

• Through dilution, dextran diminishes local fibrin concentration, preserves local plasminogen activators, and interferes with polymorphonuclear neutrophil expression of adhesion molecules.

• It coats and lubricates the tissues—The siliconizing effect.

• Alters clotting mechanism by decreasing the circulating levels of factors V, VIII and IX and reducing platelet adhesion. Several studies have suggested that 32% Dextran 70 is effective in reducing postoperative adhesions.[15] Although instillation of high-molecular-weight dextran (32% dextran 70) was popular, the results have been inconsistent.[16]

Side Effects
1. Transient weight gain
2. Labial edema
3. Ascitis
4. Allergic reaction including anaphylaxis.
5. Impairment of macrophage phagocytosis and host defence mechanism.
6. Fever
7. Ileus
8. Wound complications.

5. *Hyaluronic acid (HA):* HA is a naturally occurring glycosaminoglycan and a major component of the extracellular matrix, including connective tissue, skin, cartilage, vitreous and synovial fluids. HA is biocompatible, nonimmunogenic, nontoxic, and naturally bioabsorbable. Like carboxymethylcellulose, it is negatively charged at physiological pH and freely soluble. HA coats serosal surfaces and provides a certain degree of protection from serosal desiccation and other types of injury. However, its use after tissue injury is ineffective.

6. *Povidone:* It is a synthetic polymer marketed initially as a plasma substitute. It results in mechanical separation and lubrication of tissue which reduces the likelihood of peritoneal surfaces coming in contact with each other. It is not used as it has been shown to be retained indefinitely in the reticuloendothelium system.

Solid Barriers

A great number of natural and synthetic graft materials have been employed in an effort to reduce adhesion formation on traumatized surfaces. Natural materials have included peritoneum, omentum, HA, fat, amnion, as well as amnion and chorion. Synthetic materials like Gelfilm, Gelfoam, Silastic, meshes of polytetrafluorethylene (PTFE), Gore-Tex, Interceed - oxidized regenerated cellulose and Seprafilm - bioresorbable membrane chemically derived from sodium hyaluronate and carboxymethylcellulose (HA-CMC; Genzyme)

Natural Solid Barriers

1. *Autologous peritoneal transplants:* Experimental studies have demonstrated that covering lesions of the parietal peritoneum with microsurgically applied autologous peritoneal transplants can completely prevent severe adhesion formation. More significant was the decrease of visceral peritoneal adhesions with the use of autologous peritoneal transplants, i.e. injuries to the serosa of the uterine horn.

Synthetic Solid Barriers

1. *Interceed (TC 7)* Absorbable fabric composed of oxidized regenerated cellulose. It was seen that pelvic sidewalls covered with this substance showed a 90% improvement over controls with regard to adhesion formation.[17] The material forms a gel after becoming wet in 8 hours and is completely absorbed within 2 weeks of application. It can be applied easily by laparoscopy, follows the contour of the organ, and does not need suturing. It is not intended as a topical hemostat. Its effectiveness is lost if it becomes saturated with blood. The need for meticulous hemostasis and the fact that it should not be employed in the presence of infection are major limitations. The presence of blood significantly reduces its ability to minimise subsequent adhesion formation. Unfortunately, in situations where an adhesion barrier is desperately needed, like over a myomectomy incision, it is virtually impossible to achieve complete hemostasis.

   It reduces both raw surface area and the occurrence of adhesion formation-reformation by a margin of 20%.[18]

2. *Polytetrafluroethylene* (Gore-Tex surgical membrane) is a permanent non-porous nonreactive peritoneal substitute with small pores that inhibit cellular transmigration and tissue adherence. Its drawback is that it needs to be sutured in place and that it must be removed laparoscopically at a later date after reconstructive surgery. The very act of removal involves some degree of surgical trauma which might lead to adhesion formation. The use of PTFE in laparoscopy is cumbersome and not easy to handle. It has a distinct advantage that it may be safely and effectively employed at sites with less than perfect hemostasis. A PTFE barrier prevents adhesion formation and reformation regardless of the type of tissue injury or whether hemostasis is achieved.

3. *Seprafilm.* HA-CMC is a nontoxic, nonimmunogenic, material which is composed of modified hyaluronic acid and carboxymethylcellulose. It is effective in reducing incidence of severe postoperative adhesions. It turns to a hydrophilic gel approximately 24 hour after placement and provides a protective coat around traumatized tissue for up to 7 days during remesothelialization. It reduced the incidence of postoperative adhesions to the incision line by greater than 50%, and the mean adhesion rate was 40% less when compared to controls undergoing laparotomy. However, the sheets are rather firm and noncompliant and difficult to place at the required site during laparoscopic surgery.[19]

Adhesion formation is a complex process involving biochemical and biomechanical factors. The cascade leading to adhesion formation is the result of the body's response to an injury. A multifactorial approach to prevent adhesions includes minimizing tissue injury with meticulous surgical technique, appropriate prophylactic antibiotic usage to reduce infectious morbidity, and usage of biochemical agents with or without biomechanical barriers.

Severity and extent of adhesion have been scored by the American Fertility Society (Table 15.4).

Table 15.4: (A) The American Fertility Society Adhesion Scoring Method and (B) The More Comprehensive Adhesion Scoring Method (MCASM)[20]

A	Adhesions	<1/3 enclosed	<1/3 - 2/3 enclosed	> 2/3 enclosed
Ovary	Rt. Flimsy	1	2	4
	Rt. Dense	4	8	16
	Lt. Flimsy	1	2	4
	Lt. Dense	4	8	16
Tube	Rt. Flimsy	1	2	4
	Rt. Dense	4	8	16
	Lt. Flimsy	1	2	4
	Lt. Dense	4	8	16

B Location

Ant. abdominal wall 1-4
1. Lt. side to
2. Rt. side to
3. Incision line to
4. Above incision line to
   Ant. Cul-de-sac 5 – 8
5. Over uterus to
6. over bladder to
7. Rt. side to
8. Lt. side to
9. Post. uterus to
10. Post cul-de-sac to
11. Pelvic side wall left to
12. Pelvic side wall right to
13. Post broad ligament left to
14. Post broad ligament right to
15. Round ligament to tube left to
16. Round ligament to tube right to
17. Ovary left to
18. Ovary right to
19. Tube left to
20. Tube right to
21. Small bowel to
22. Large bowel to
23. Omentum to

Severity

0. No adhesions
1. Flimsy, avascular
2. Some vascularity and/or dense
3a. Cohesive, falls apart on touch
3b. Cohesive, visibly dissectable planes and can be dissected with minimal dissection
3c. Cohesive, no visibly dissectable planes and requires extensive dissection for separation

Extent

0. No adhesions
1. Mild – covering < 25 % of total area / length
2. Moderate – covering 25 - 50 % of total area / length
3. Severe – covering > 50 % of total area/length

Pelvic adhesions not only reduce the effectiveness of major surgery for infertility but in some cases may further impair fertility. The surgeon should be careful to minimize adhesions. Constant attention should be directed at avoiding serosal insults known to elicit inflammatory reactions. Such insults include tissue trauma, ischemia, hemorrhage, infection, foreign body reaction and exposure of raw material. It is essential that the infertility surgeon be aware of the medical and surgical modalities used to prevent or minimize adhesion occurence and their rationale, effectiveness and safety.

REFERENCES

1. Operative Laparoscopy Study Group: Postoperative adhesion development after operative laparoscopy: Evaluation at early second-look procedures. Fertil Steril 1991;55:700-4.
2. di Zerega GS: Contemporary adhesion prevention. Fertil Steril 1994;61:219-35.
3. Luijendijk RW, de Lange DCD, Wauters CCAP, et al: Foreign material in postoperative adhesions. Ann Surg 1996;223:242-8.
4. Levrant SG, Bieber EJ, Barnes RB: Anterior abdominal wall adhesions after laparotomy or laparoscopy. J Am Assoc Gynecol Laparosc 1997;4:353-6.
5. Pfeffer LH The effect of dexamethasone and promethazine administration on adhesion formation, tubal function and ultrastructure following microsurgical anastomosis of rabbit oviducts. Fertil Steril 1980;34:162.
6. Duffy DM, di Zerega GS: Is peritoneal closure necessary? Obstet Gynecol Surv 1994;49:817-22.
7. Malinak LR, Young AE: Peritoneal closure: When and why. Contemp Obstet Gynecol 1997;42:102-12.
8. Swank DJ, Swank-Bordewizk SC, Hop WCJ, van Erp WF, Janssen IM, Bonjer HJ, et al. Laparoscopic adhesiolysis in patients with chronic abdominal pain: a blinded randomised controlled multicentre trial. Lancet 2003;361:1247-51.
9. Lundorff B, Hahlin M, Kiallfelt B, Thornburn J, Lindblom B. Adhesion formation after laparoscopic surgery in tubal pregnancy: a randomized trial versus laparotomy. Fertil Steril 1991;55:911-5.
10. Gutt CN, Oniu T, Schemmer P, Mehrabi A, Buchler MW. Fewer adhesions induced by laparoscopic surgery? Surg Endosc. 2006; 20(6):999.

11. Cohen BM,Heyman T, Mast D. Use of intraperitoneal solutions for preventing pelvic adhesions in the rat . J Reprod Med 1983; 28: 649-53.

12. Al - Chalabi HA Otubo JAM. Value of a single intraperitoneal dose of heparin in prevention of adhesion formation: an experimental evaluation in rat. Int J Fertil 1987;32:332-25.

13. The Practice Committee of the American Society for Reproductive Medicine. Control and prevention of peritoneal adhesions in gynecologic surgery. Fertil Steril. 2006; 86 Suppl 5:S1-5.

14. Sahakian V, Rodgers R, Halme J, et al: Effects of carbon dioxide saturated normal saline and Ringer's lactate on postsurgical adhesion formation in the rabbit. Obstet Gynecol 1993;82:851-3.

15. Holtz G, Baker E,Tsai C. Effect of 32% dextran 70 on peritoneal adhesion formation after lysis 1980; 33:660.

16. Tulandi T: Intraperitoneal instillates. Infertil Reprod Med Clin North Am 1994;5:479-83.

17. Adhesion Barrier study group: Prevention of postsurgical adhesions by Interceed (TC 7), an absorbable adhesion barrier: postoperative randomized multicenter clinical study. Fertil Steril 1989; 51:933-8.

18. Larsson B: Efficacy of Interceed in adhesion prevention in gynecologic surgery: A review of 13 clinical studies. J Reprod Med 1996;41:27-34.

19. Burns JW, Skinner K, Colt MJ, Burgess L, Rose R, Diamond MP. A hyaluronate based gel for the prevention of post-surgical adhesions, evaluation in two animal species. Fertil Steril 1996;66: 814-21.

20. Adheron Scoring Group. Improvement of interobserver reproductivity of adhesions scoring system. Fertil Steril 1994;62: 984-98.

CHAPTER 16

IVF and Tubo-uterine Factors in Infertility

Shweta Mittal

Reproductive outcome in IVF depends on multiple factors. Embryo implantation remains the rate-limiting step in assisted conception programs. Factors affecting the interactions between blastocyst and endometrium are subjects of current research. This chapter aims to present uterine and tubal factors affecting endometrial receptivity during and around the implantation window in an IVF cycle.

Uterine Factors affecting Implantation

Uterine Fibroids

Different types of fibroids may affect reproductive outcome to different extent, with submucosal, intramural and subserosal fibroids (in decreasing order) being a cause of infertility and pregnancy wastage. It has been postulated that uterine fibroids may alter the uterine artery blood flow and may have an impact on implantation. Recent studies have also evaluated alterations in gene expression and local cytokine release, which may also play a role in implantation. Leiomyomas and polyps produce significant plasma glycodelin levels. Elevated glycodelin levels in the follicular and peri-ovulatory period may impair fertilization and implantation.[1]

Fibroids are associated with a lower rate of spontaneous pregnancies, and about 40% pregnancy rate can be expected after their removal.[2] The important questions are whether fibroids cause infertility and whether their removal increases one's chances to achieve a successful pregnancy during ART. There is clear evidence on the association between lower pregnancy (RR: 0.3 [95% CI: 0.1-0.7]) and higher miscarriage rates when fibroids with submucous components that distort the cavity are present. Removal of submucosal fibroids increases pregnancy rates (RR: 1.7 [95% CI: 1.1-2.5]).[3] It also seems evident that subserosal fibroids, regardless of their size, do not affect pregnancy rates. The effect of intramural fibroids is less clear. Most studies that have evaluated implantation and pregnancy rates reported controversial results with intramural fibroids that do not distort the cavity. These studies usually do not include women with myomas more than 6 cm in diameter.

Treatment of myoma before ART

- Submucosal myomas should be removed regardless of their size before ART.
- Subserosal myomas need not be removed unless they are symptomatic.
- Intramural fibroids should be removed if their diameter is more 6 cm. Intramural fibroids less 6 cm should be removed if they distort the cavity; otherwise, their removal does not appear to improve reproductive outcome, based on the currently available evidence.

Age: The age of the woman is a factor to consider. Younger woman with an intramural fibroid measuring less 6 cm should try IVF 2 to 3 times if necessary before proceeding with surgery. Older women under the same conditions should attempt IVF only once; but if the initial cycle fails, they should undergo a myomectomy.[3]

Uterine Polyps

There is still no consensus regarding the management of patients diagnosed with endometrial polyp in IVF cycles. Cycle cancellation cryopreservation and embryo transfer at a subsequent cycle preceding polypectomy is the current management of choice. However, small endometrial polyps discovered during ovarian stimulation do not negatively affect pregnancy and implantation outcomes of IVF cycles. Polyps less than 2 cm diameter do not require removal before IVF and do not affect the outcome of the subsequent pregnancy.[4]

Congenital Anomalies of Uterus

Congenital anomalies of the reproductive tract can be diagnosed in 1 to 2% of women. A uterine septum is the most common anomaly. It is associated with recurrent pregnancy loss. When a septum is diagnosed in a woman with recurrent pregnancy loss, an 85 to 90% miscarriage rate can be expected during a subsequent pregnancy if the septum is not surgically removed. Following surgical resection the loss rate is reduced to about 15%. There is no question about the benefit of septum resection in women with recurrent loss. It is less obvious whether a septum needs to be removed when it is diagnosed during infertility evaluation. However with the availability of operative hysteroscopy, the removal of a septum is a relatively simple and very safe procedure. One should not wait for a pregnancy to be lost, especially when a complex, expensive procedure like IVF is required to achieve the pregnancy. When a septum is found during the work-up, it should be removed hysteroscopically.[5]

Intrauterine Synechiae

In vitro fertilization (IVF) and embryo transfer offers the only realistic chance of conception in women with infertility due to genital tuberculosis. Although the medical treatment is successful in eradicating the infection, fibrotic sequelae of the disease may prevent the occurrence of an intrauterine pregnancy. Endometrial involvement may be noted in over half of the affected cases and the uterine cavity may be partially or totally obliterated with intrauterine synechiae.[6] Hysteroscopic lysis of intrauterine synechiae is indicated in such patients, affected by genital tuberculosis, to restore the uterine cavity before they are subjected to IVF and embryo transfer. Patients undergoing synechiolysis are put on cyclical estrogen therapy to build up estrogen receptors and endometrial growth. However in presence of severe adhesions prognosis is poor and patients may be advised surrogacy.

Unexplained Poor Endometrium

Aspirin, sildenafil (25 mg vaginal suppository QID), and L-arginine have all been evaluated in patients undergoing IVF with poor endometrial development.

Aspirin: Aspirin increases the level of the vasodilatory prostacyclin and therefore could improve uterine blood flow. However systematic review of 10 randomized controlled trials failed to find an improvement of pregnancy rates with aspirin.

L- arginine: The use of L-arginine, the precursor of nitric oxide, has not been found beneficial in the management of poor endometrial development.

Sildenafil: Sildenafil prevents the breakdown of cGMP and increases nitric oxide levels. It was shown to improve uterine blood flow in one study. This report was followed by a large case series that reported improved endometrial development and pregnancy rates with the use of vaginal sildenafil during ovarian stimulation.[7] The conclusions that can be drawn, however, are limited by the lack of a control group. A placebo-controlled, randomized, cross-over trial, however, reported no improvement with sildenafil. Further well-designed studies should evaluate these and other possible "adjuvant" treatments that are believed to improve IVF outcome.[8]

Tubal Factor Affecting Implantation

Hydrosalpinx

Patients with severe tubal damage have a poor prognosis with IVF- ET. Studies have shown that patients with hydrosalpinges seem to have lower implantation and pregnancy rates than patients suffering from other types of tubal damage. Different theories have evolved to explain the association of hydrosalpinx with poor pregnancy outcome which are as follows:

- Reflux of hydrosalpinx fluid into the uterine cavity diminishes embryonic endometrial aposition.
- Hydrosalpinx fluid is cosidered to be embryotoxic by releasing cytokines, prostaglandins and other inflammatory compounds.
- Association of hydrosalpinx with altered endometrial histology and lack of endometrial integrin (adhesion molecule) expression.

Prophylactic Salpingectomy

Two meta-analysis have estimated that hydrosalpinges diminished implantation rate by 35%.[9] Dechaud et al reported an improved implantation rate (10.4%) in the group with salpingectomy as compared to group without salpingectomy.[10] Prospective randomised multicenter trial of salpingectomy prior to IVF showed a significant difference in favor of salpingectomy in patients with bilateral hydrosalpinges and in patients with ultrasound visible hydrosalpinges. The clinical efficacy of prophylactic salpingectomy in presence of either unilateral hydrosalpinges or hydrosalpinges that are not visible on USG require further study. However, salpingectomy prior to IVF may impair the ovarian response as removal of fallopian tubes may have a detrimental effect on ovarian arterial supply. Bilateral tubal clipping can be performed laparoscopically in presence of dense pelvic adhesions where salpingectomy may not be possible.

Uterine and tubal pathologies do play an important role in the success of IVF. Since all pathologies do not need to be treated a thorough evaluation should be done before taking the patient for IVF to identify those which need therapy before IVF.

REFERENCES

1. Spencer S. Richlin, Ramchandran S, Shanti A, Ana A, Murphy, Parthasarathy S. Glycodelin levels in uterine flushings and in plasma of patients with leiomyomas and polyps: Implications for Implantation. Hum Reprod 2002; 17(10):2742-7.
2. Arici A. Fibroid and IVF Presented at the 7th World Congress on Controversies in Obstetrics and Gynecology and Infertility; Athens, Greece 2005; 14-17.
3. Rackow BW, Arici A. Fibroids and in-vitro fertilization: which comes first? Curr Opin Obstet Gynecol 2005;17:225-31.
4. Shokeir TA, Shalan HM, El-Shafei MM, Significance of endometrial polyps detected hysteroscopically in eumenorrheic infertile women. J Obstet Gynaecol Res. 2004; 30(2):84-9.
5. Donnez J. Resection of a uterine septum of IVF Presented at the 7th World Congress on Controversies in Obstetrics and Gynecology and Infertility; Athens, Greece 2005;14-17.

6. Sher G, Fisch JD. Effect of vaginal sildenafil on the outcome of in vitro Fertilization (IVF) after Multiple IVF failures attributed to poor endometrial development. Fertility and Sterility. 2002; 78(5):1073-6.

7. Varma TR. Genital tuberculosis and subsequent fertility. Int. J. Gynaecol Obstet 1991; 35:1-11.

8. Daya S. The use of aspirin and adjuvant therapy in IVF. Presented at the 7th World Congress on Controversies in Obstetrics and Gynecology and Infertility; Athens, Greece 2005;14-17.

9. Zeynelogu HB, Airci A, Olive DL. Adverse effects of hydrosalpinx on pregnancy rates after in vitro fertilization embryo transfer. Fertil Steril 1998; 70:492-9.

10. Dechaud H, Daures JP, Arnal F, Humeau C, hedon B. Does previous salpingectomy improve implantation and pregnancy rates in patients with tubal factor infertility who are undergoing in vitro fertilization? A pilot randomized controlled study. Fertil Steril 1998; 69:1020-5.

CHAPTER 17

Imaging Techniques in Tubo-uterine Pathology

Reeti Sahni

With advancements in imaging techniques diagnosing causes of infertility and guiding the gynecologist to the right medical or surgical treatment has become easier The most common female-related causes of infertility are tubal disease, pelvic adhesions, fibroids and ovulatory dysfunction. This chapter discusses multimode imaging of tubo-uterine pathologies in infertility.

UTERINE PATHOLOGY

Normal

3D Ultrasound: 3D Ultrasound of a normal uterus in the coronal plane. The endometrial cavity has a smooth triangular shape and cervix is at the bottom of the image (Fig. 17.1).

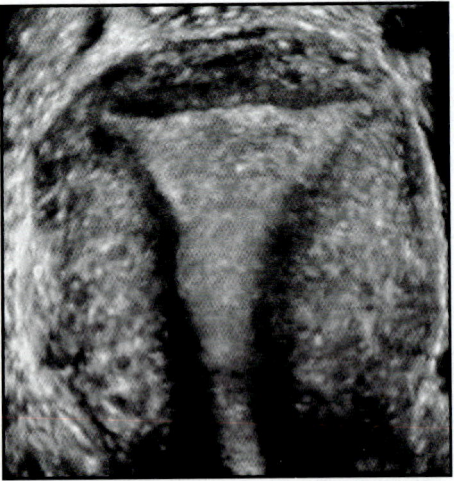

Fig. 17.1: 3D Ultrasound of a normal uterus

MRI: Sagittal T2-weighted image of the uterus shows the endometrium, junctional zone, and myometrium It also shows the epithelium, fibrous stroma, and peripheral myometrium of the cervix (Fig. 17. 2).

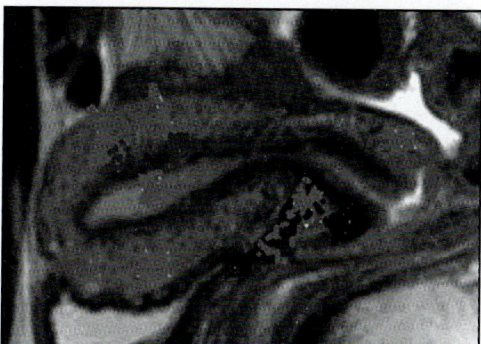

Fig. 17.2: MRI of a normal uterus

Uterine Malformations

Class I: Hypoplasia or agenesis: Failure of normal development of the müllerian ducts causes uterine agenesis or hypoplasia. (Mayer-Rokitansky Küster-Hauser syndrome). The uterus and upper two-thirds of the vagina are absent on MRI (Fig. 17.3).[1,2]

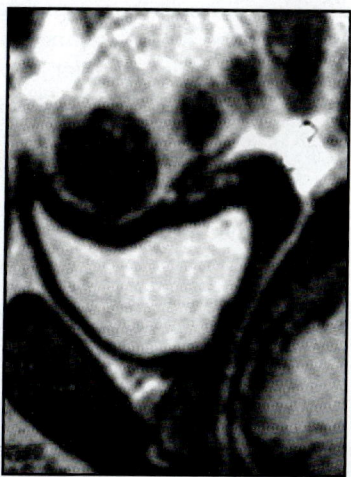

Fig. 17.3: Absent uterus and upper two thirds of vagina on MRI

Class II: Unicornuate uterus: It results from complete or incomplete arrest of development of one Müllerian duct. MRI image is seen in Figure 17.4. The uterus is banana shaped and the other horn (rudimentary) could be absent in 35% of cases.[3,4]

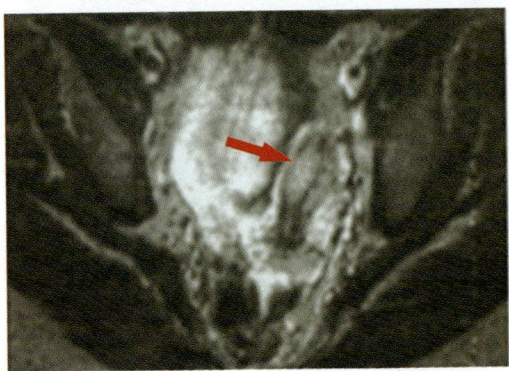

Fig. 17.4 MRI of unicornuate uterus

Class III: Uterus didelphus: It results from complete nonfusion of both Müllerian ducts resulting in two uterine bodies and two cervices[5] (Figs 17.5 and 17.6) (See Chapter 5).

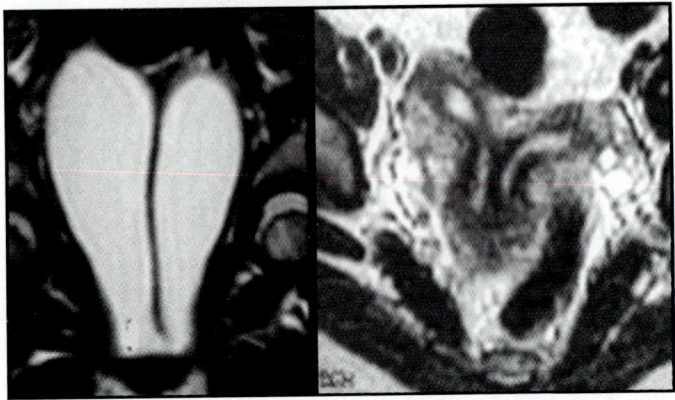

Figs 17.5 and 17.6: MRI of uterus didelphus

Class IV: Bicornuate: It results from partial nonfusion of the Müllerian ducts with double uterine bodies and a single cervix being present.[7,8] An arcuate uterus is considered a milder form of bicornuate uterus. MRI and 3D ultrasonography can accurately diagnose it (Figs 17.7 and 17.8).

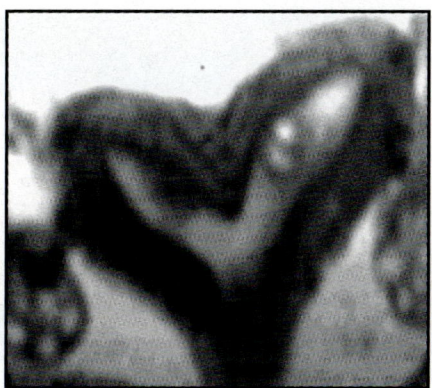

Fig. 17.7: MRI of bicornuate uterus

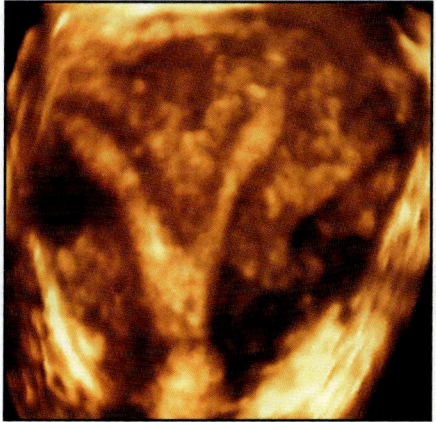

Fig. 17.8: 3D USG of bicornuate uterus

Class V: Septate uterus: It results from complete fusion of the Müllerian ducts with failure of resorption of the central septum. The septum may be partial or complete, and fibrous or muscular. (Figs 17.9 to 17.13). It can be differentiated from an arcuate uterus as the fundal contour is maintained.

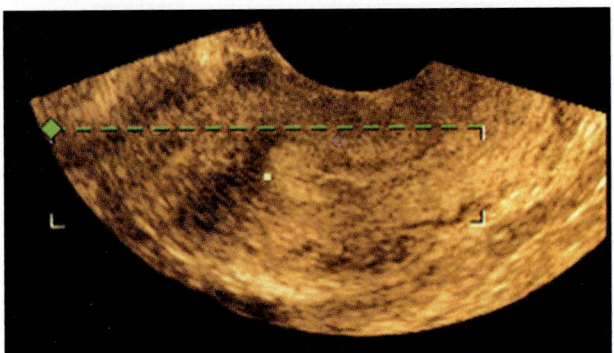

Fig. 17.9: USG of septate uterus

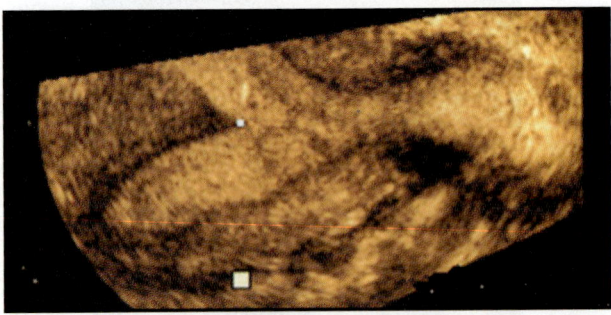

Fig. 17.10: 3D USG of septate uterus

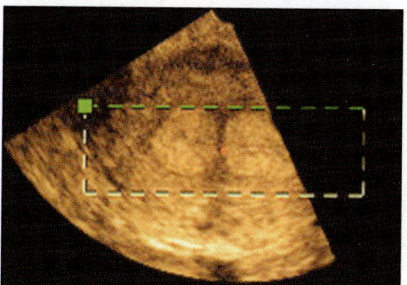

Fig. 17.11: USG of septate uterus

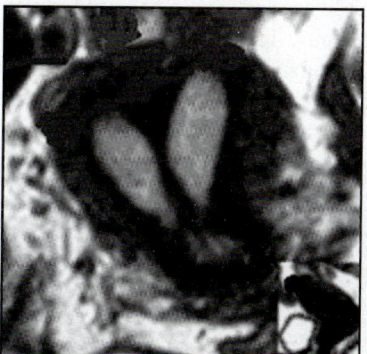

Fig. 17.12: MRI of septate uterus

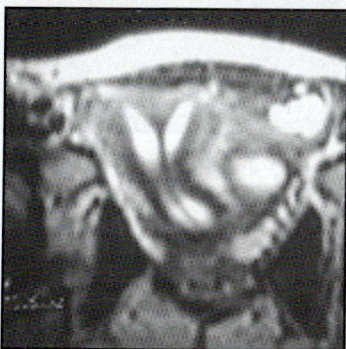

Fig. 17.13: MRI of septate uterus

Class VI: Arcuate: Arcuate uterus should be considered a normal variant, with a small indentation of the fundal endometrial canal and a normal external contour.

Class VII: Diethylstilbestrol related: Exposure to DES causes abnormal myometrial hypertrophy and results in uterine anomalies including T-shaped uterus, irregular constrictions, and hypoplasia.

Fibroids and Polyps

Uterine fibroids are the most common non-cancerous tumors in women of childbearing age and could cause infertility and recurrent pregnancy loss.[6,7] USG and MRI can accurately diagnose size , number and position of fibroid (Figs 17.14 and 17.15). Encroachment on cavity can be assessed also by HSG and saline infusion sonography (Figs 17.16 and 17.17).

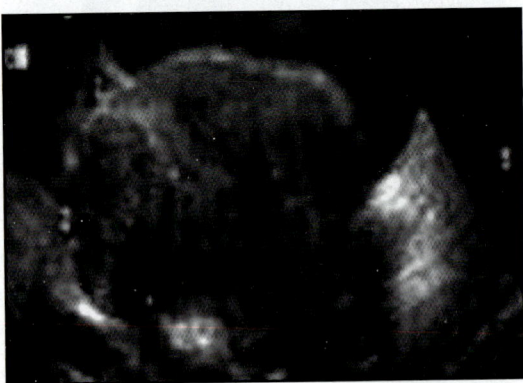

Fig. 17.14: USG showing fibroid

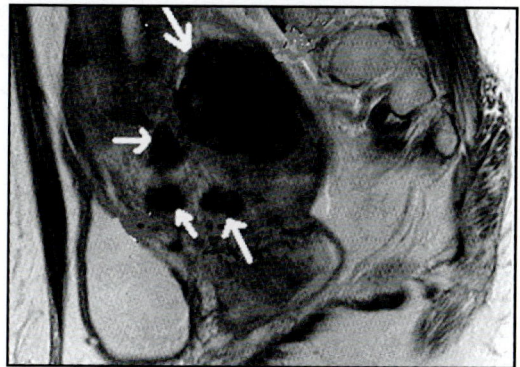

Fig. 17.15: Multiple fibroids on MRI

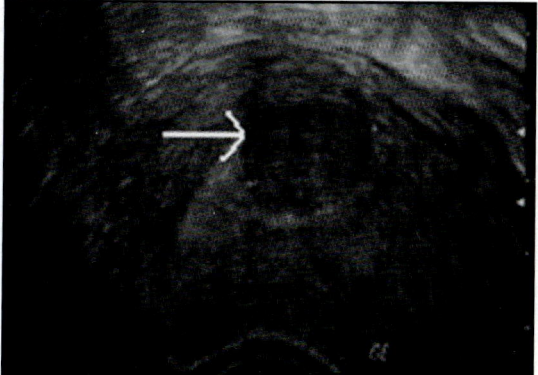

Fig. 17.16: Submucosal fibroids on USG

Adenomyosis

Adenomyosis is not a common cause of infertility. The exact reasons for infertility in patients with adenomyosis remain unclear, although an enlarged uterus may be associated with reduced uterine or endometrial receptivity.[8]

Both transvaginal ultrasound and MR imaging allow accurate, noninvasive diagnosis of adenomyosis.[9]

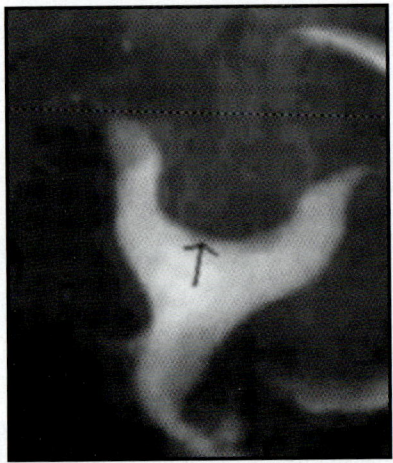

Fig. 17.17: Submucosal fibroids on HSG

The relevant diagnostic USG findings are:

(a) Thickening and asymmetry of the anterior or posterior uterine walls (Fig. 17.18).

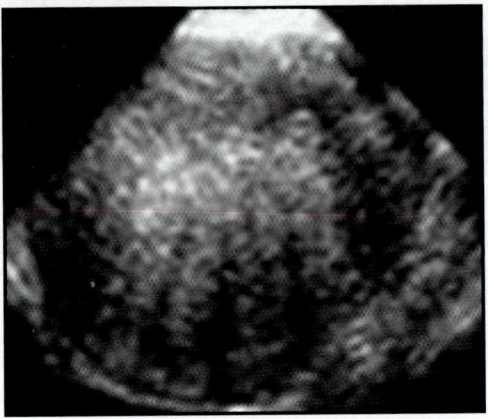

Fig. 17.18: Adenomyosis on USG showing thickened posterior wall

(b) A poorly defined area of decreased or increased echogenicity,

(c) Heterogeneous echotexture (Fig. 17.19)

(d) Myometrial cyst (Fig. 17.20).

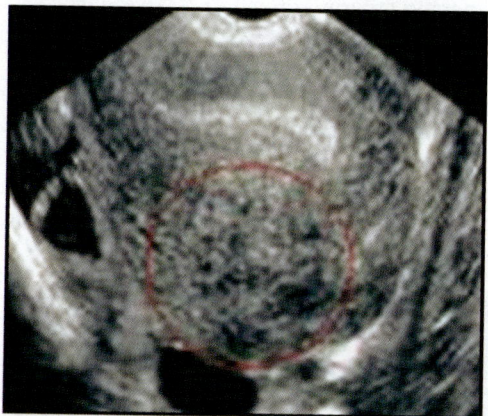

Fig. 17.19: Adenomyosis showing heterogeneous echotexture of the myometrium

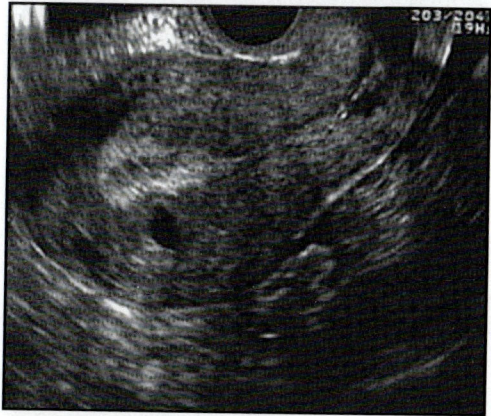

Fig. 17.20: Adenomyosis with myometrial cyst

MRI scan from the side showing a uterus with extensive adenomyosis (Fig. 17.21, black arrow), which appears as a darker shade of gray on this scan when compared to the normal portions of the uterine wall (Fig. 17.21, white arrow).

The MR Imaging criteria are:

(a) A myometrial mass of low signal intensity with indistinct margins on both T1- and T2-weighted images.

(b) Diffuse or focal widening of the junctional zone on T2-weighted images. A junctional zone thickness of 12 mm or more optimizes the accuracy of MR imaging for this diagnosis.

(c) Punctate high-signal-intensity foci, which correspond to ectopic endometrium, are often demonstrated on T2-weighted images (Fig. 17.22).

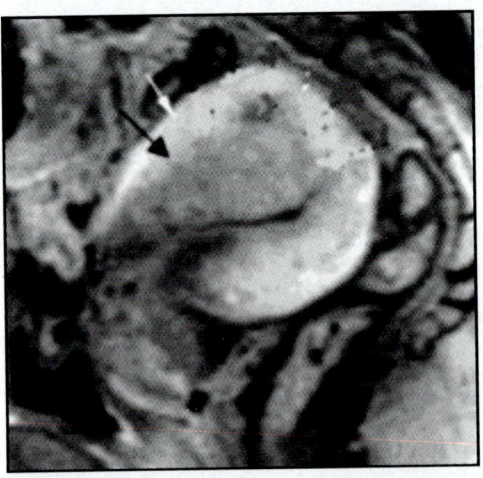

Fig. 17.21: Adenomyosis on MRI (Normal portion of myometrium—white arrow, Adenomyosis—black arrow)

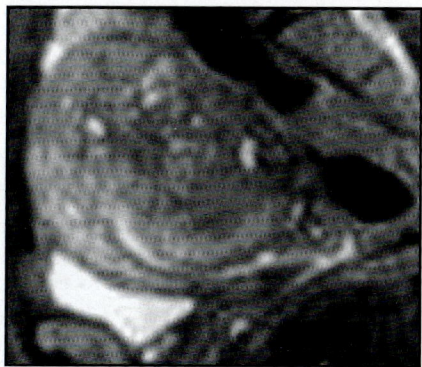

Fig. 17.22: MRI scan showing adenomyosis with thickened posterior wall and high signal intensity foci corresponding to ectopic endometrium

Lesions within the Endometrial Cavity

Intrauterine Adhesions (Asherman's Syndrome)

Menstrual disorders and infertility are the most common presenting symptoms in women with intrauterine adhesions other symptoms include recurrent pregnancy loss and placenta accreta. They can be diagnosed by hysterosalpingography and USG (Fig. 17.23).

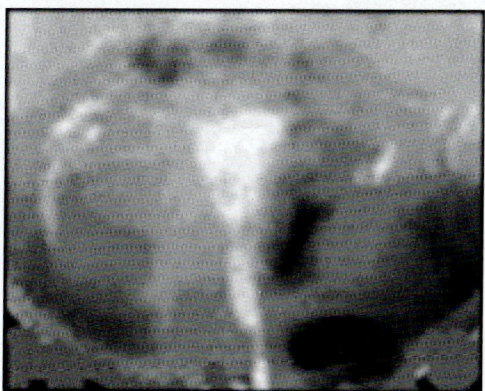

Fig. 17.23: HSG image of Asherman's syndrome

Polyps

Polyps and submucous fibroids can cause infertility. They can be accurately visualized by sonosalpingography and blood flow to them also can be demonstrated (Figs 17. 24 and 17.25).

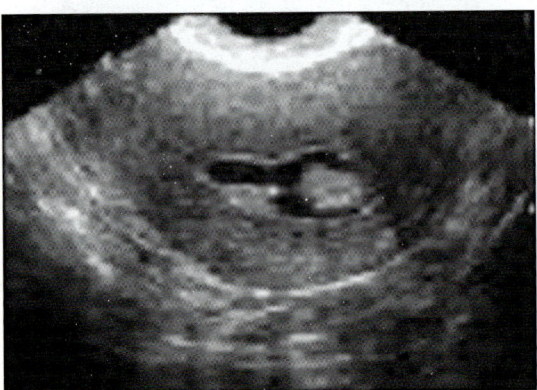

Fig. 17.24: Polyp seen on sonosalpingography

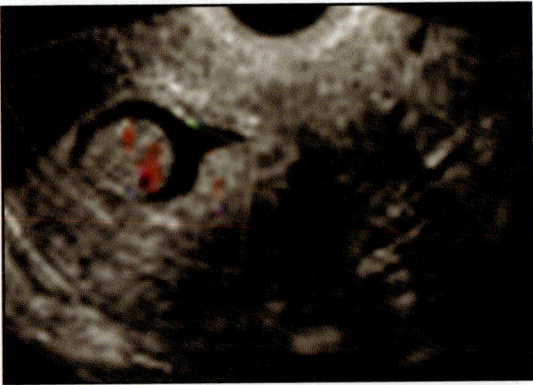

Fig. 17.25: Polyps with Doppler showing vascularity

Three-dimensional saline infusion contrast sonography:
A three-dimensional ultrasonography can be done with saline infusion. Advantage is decreased overall time of of examination, reduced quantity of saline required and higher accuracy. A large submucosal leiomyoma with a broad base is seen originating from the left posterior aspect of the uterus that almost entirely occupied the cavity (Fig. 17.26). HSG may be helpful in diagnosing myomas because of distortion of cavity (Fig. 17.27).

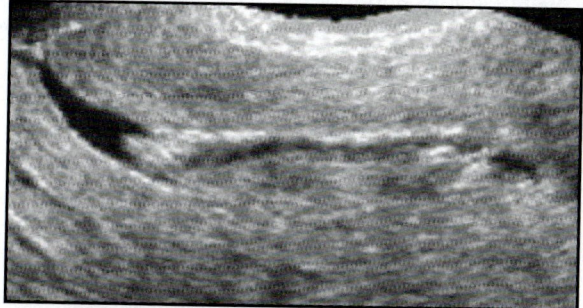

Fig. 17.26: Three-dimensional saline infusion contrast sonography showing large submucous myoma with a large base

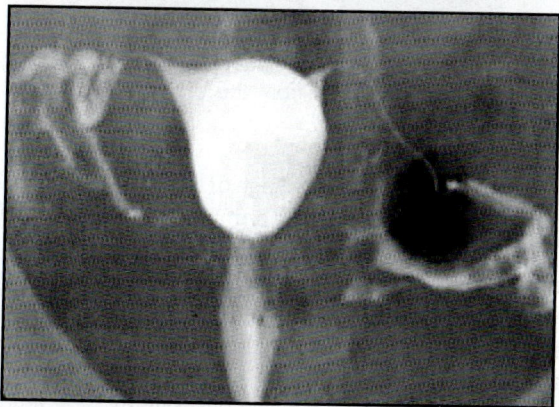

Fig. 17.27: HSG showing distortion of cavity due to myoma

Tubal Pathology

Tubal factor infertility accounts for about 20-25% of all cases of infertility. Tubal factor infertility is usually caused by either pelvic infection, such as pelvic inflammatory disease, pelvic surgery or endometriosis. The main imaging technique for the fallopian tubes is the conventional hysterosalpingography and now used in some centers sono-hysterosalpingography which delineates intracavitary lesions and tubes with greater clarity (Fig. 17.28). Both these procedures are real time. Tumors of the fallopian tubes are well visualized on MRI.

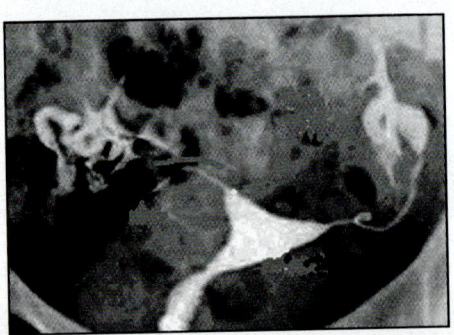

Fig. 17.28: Normal hysterosalpingogram. A smooth triangular uterine cavity and spill from the ends of both tubes

Hydrosalpinx/Pyosalpinx

Hydrosalpinx is caused by blockage of the fallopian tube usually resulting from infection and can be diagnosed on USG. (Figs 17.29 and 17.30). This reduces the chance of pregnancy because the fluid in the tubes is toxic to embryos and may leak into the uterine cavity during IVF and hinder embryo implantation rates. Infection of the long-standing fluid in the tubes can lead to pyosalpinx.

MRI accurately diagnoses an hydrosalpinx as a fluid filled tortuous mass (Fig. 17. 31).

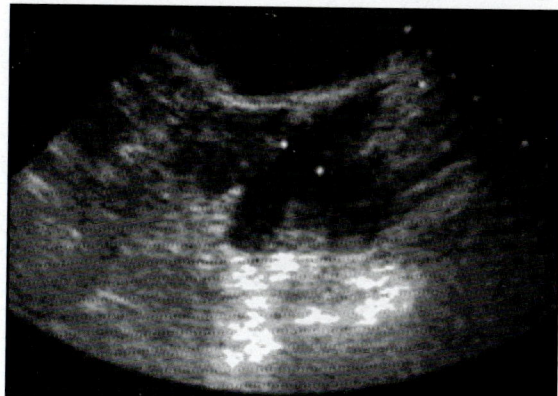

Fig. 17.29: Hydrosalpinx on USG

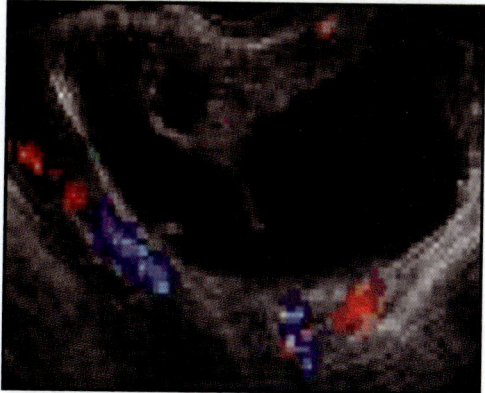

Fig. 17.30: Hydrosalpinx with Doppler showing blood flow

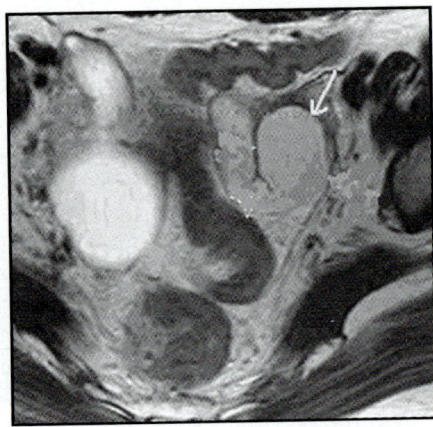

Fig. 17.31: MRI showing hydrosalpinx as a cystic mass of the left adnexa (arrow)

Tubo-ovarian Abscess

This can be seen clearly on an MRI (Fig. 17.32).

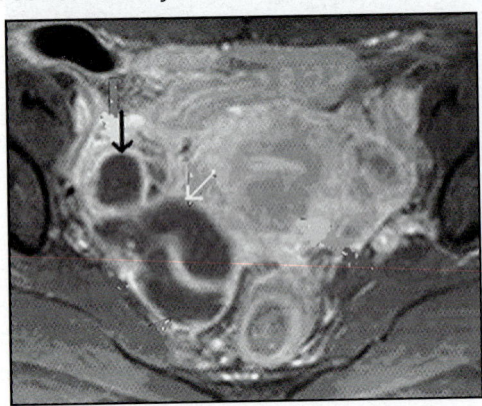

Fig. 17.32: Tubo-ovarian abscess. Axial T2-weighted (a) and contrast-enhanced fat-suppressed T1-weighted (b) images show a tortuous mass of the right adnexa. The mass consists of an ovarian abscess (black arrow) and hydrosalpinx (white arrow)

Ectopic Pregnancy

Ectopic pregnancy is the implantation and growth of products of conception outside the normal uterine cavity. It is a significant cause of morbidity and mortality. Ectopic pregnancies are most often located within the fallopian tube, but other potential sites include interstitial (cornual), ovarian, cervical, and fimbrial.[10]

Imaging: Transvaginal ultrasound should be used in the evaluation of patients at risk, especially for those in whom there has been no identification of an intrauterine pregnancy with transabdominal ultrasound. With ectopic pregnancy, the uterus is usually normal, but may contain a pseudosac, which fills the endometrial canal symmetrically as opposed to a gestational sac, which is usually asymmetric. If an intrauterine fluid collection is identified, but no fetal pole or yolk sac is seen, then the differentials include:

1. Ectopic pregnancy with pseudosac,
2. Intrauterine pregnancy too early to identify the yolk sac,
3. Abnormal intrauterine pregnancy.

Adnexal findings associated with ectopic pregnancy include: tubal ring sign, complex adnexal mass, simple adnexal cyst, and free fluid in the cul-de-sac (Figs 17.33 and 17.34). It is important to note that a normal transvaginal ultrasound exam does not exclude the presence of an ectopic pregnancy.

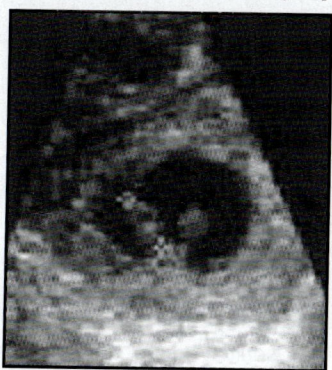

Fig. 17.33: Ectopic pregnancy in adnexa

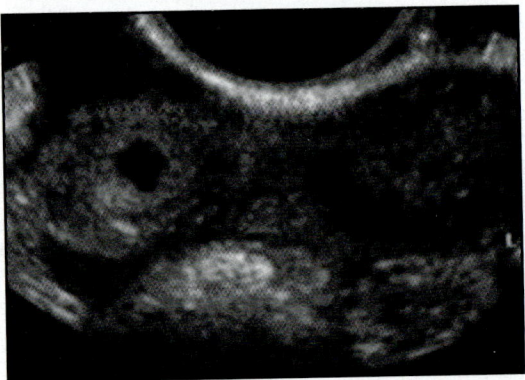

Fig. 17.34: Ectopic with fluid filled sac in adnexa

Cervical Pregnancy

The fundus will be empty, and gestational sac with embryo may be seen in the cervical canal. With inevitable abortion, the embryo will not be alive with the gestational sac in this position (Fig. 17.35). Color Doppler was also useful in this case to show perfusion of the placenta by the cervical tissue.[11]

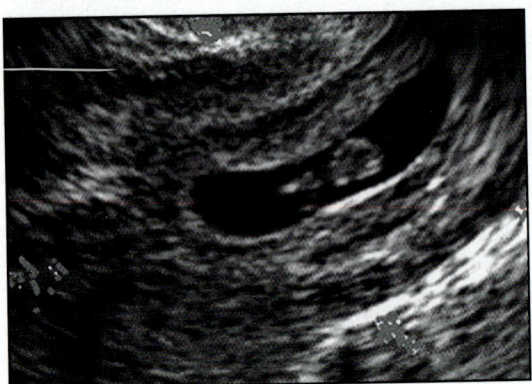

Fig. 17.35: This sagittal image shows a cervical ectopic pregnancy – The fundus is empty. The cervical canal shows a live embryo in the gestational sac

Cornual Ectopic Pregnancy

The ectopic pregnancy is found in the cornua and can be diagnosed on USG (Fig. 17.36).

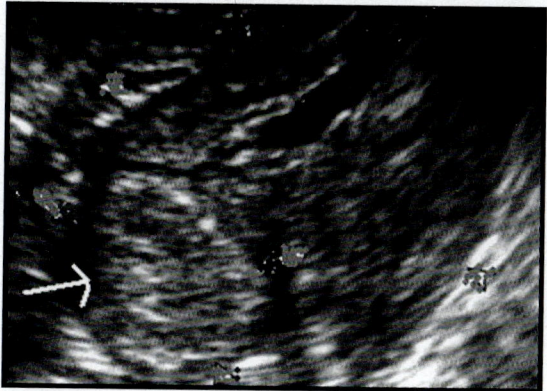

Fig. 17.36: Transverse image of a cornual ectopic pregnancy outlined by arrow. There is a small pseudo gestational sac in the endometrial cavity

Tubal Tumors

Primary malignant tumor of the fallopian tube is one of the rarest malignancies of the female genital tract. The most common histological type is the sdenocarcinoma. However, adenocarcinomas are only 0.3% of all gynecological cancers.[12] They can be diagnosed on USG and MRI (Figs 17.37 and 17.38).

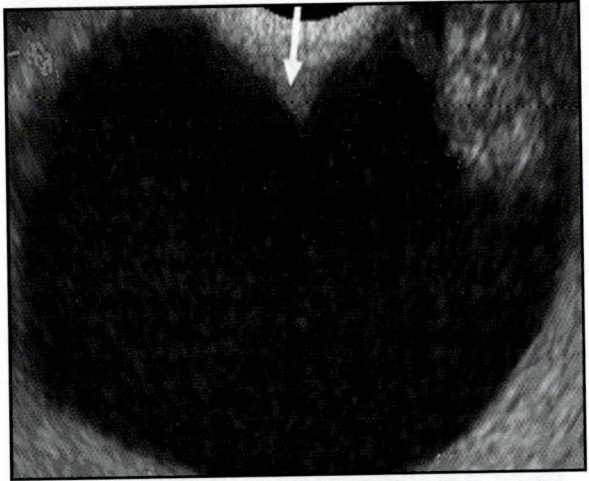

Fig. 17.37: USG image of fallopian tube mass

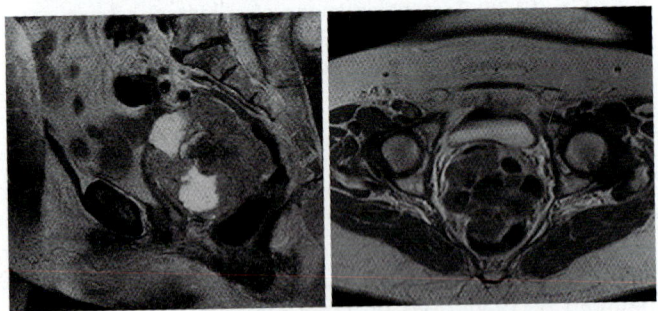

Fig. 17.38: MRI images of fallopian tube mass

Imaging by ultrasonography, sonohysterosalpingography, Hysterosalpingography and MRI are important for diagnosing uterine and tubal pathologies responsible for infertility and their subsequent management. MRI is most accurate in detecting uterine anomalies, fibroids and tubal pathologies. The 3D ultrasonography, a relatively new advancement detects uterine malformations without need for invasive techniques like hysteroscopy.

REFERENCES

1. Buttram VC, jr. Mullerian anomalies and their management. Fertil Steril 1983; 40:159-63.
2. Rock JA. Surgery for anomalies of the müllerian ducts. In Thompson JD, Rock JA (Eds): TeLinde's Operative Gynecology. 8th ed. Philadelphia: Lippincott-Raven, 1997; 687-729.
3. Brody JM, Koelliker SL, Frishman GN. Unicornuate uterus: imaging appearance, associated anomalies and clinical implications. Am J Roentgenol 1998; 171:1341-7.
4. Nahum GG. Uterine anomalies: how common are they, and what is their distribution among subtypes? J Reprod Med 1998; 43:877-87.
5. Minto CL, Hollings N, Hall-Craggs M, Creighton S. Magnetic resonance imaging in the assessment of complex Müllerian anomalies. BJOG 2001; 108:791-7.
6. Propst AM, Hill JA, 3rd. Anatomic factors associated with recurrent pregnancy loss. Semin Reprod Med 2000; 18:341- 50.
7. Casini ML, Rossi F, Agostini R, Unfer V. Effects of the position of fibroids on fertility. Gynecol Endocrinol. 2006 Feb;22(2):106-9.
8. C. Benecke, T.F. Kruger, T.I. Siebert, J.P. Van der Merwe, D.W. Steyn Effect of Fibroids on Fertility in Patients Undergoing Assisted Reproduction A Structured Literature Review Gynecol Obstet Invest 2005; 59:225-30
9. The Practice Committee of the American Society for Reproductive Medicine. Endometriosis and infertility. Fertil Steril 2006; 86(5): 156-60.
10. Braffman BH. Emergency department screening for ectopic pregnancy: A prospective Study. Radiology 1994; 190:797-802.
11. Frates M. Cervical ectopic pregnancy: results of conservative treatment. Radiology 1994; 191:773-5.
12. Sdaskalakis N, de Bree E, Giannikaki E, Tsousis S, Tsiftsis DD. Synchronous granulosa cell tumour of the ovary and fallopian tube adenocarcinoma: Two rare gynaecological malignancies. ANZJOG 2006; 46(6):558-9.

A

Absence of cervix 162
Advantages of laparoscopic
    surgery 229
Ampullary-ampullary
    anastomosis 252
Ampullary-infundibular
    anastomosis 253

C

Causes of tubal blockage 226
Complications of hysteroscopy
    217

E

Ectopic pregnancy 270, 369
    clinical presentation 371
    diagnostic aids 371
    etiology 370
    incidence 370
    treatment 375
        expectant 375
        medical 376
        surgical 381
Endometrial receptivity 200
    causes 201
    tests 201
    treatment 201
        change of drug 201
        estrogens 201
        immunosuppression 202
        luteal phase support 203

    reducing uterine
        contractility 202
    surgical treatment 204
Endometriosis 321
    classification 329
    clinical features 322
    investigations 325
        imaging studies 326
        lab studies 325
    physical findings 325
    procedures 326
    treatment 330
        expectant 330
        medical 331
        surgery 335
Endoscopic management of
    fibroid 101
Endoscopic microsurgical
    principles 277

F

Fibroid 53
    classification 54
        intramural 54
        pedunculated 54
        submucous 54
        subserous 54
    investigations 57
        CT scan 58
        diagnostic hysteroscopy
            59
        diagnostic laparoscopy 60
        hysterosalpingography 58

intravenous pyelogram
and barium enema 60
MRI 59
saline infusion sonography
58
ultrasonography 57
management 62
expectant management 63
medical therapy 63
prevalence 54
symptoms 54
abdominal mass 55
abnormal bleeding 54
pain 55
pressure symptoms 55
Fibroids and polyps 442
Fimbrioplasty 236, 282
Fluoroscopic fallopian tube
catheterization 264
contraindications 265
results 265
technique 264

G

Genital tuberculosis 314
clinical presentation 315
diagnosis 316
etiopathogenesis 315
treatment 318

H

Hematometra and cyclical pain
222
Hysterosalpingography 31
complications 31
limitations 31
Hysterosalpingosonography 36
accuracy 37
complications 37
technique 37

Hysteroscopic infertility surgery
207
Hysteroscopic tubal cannulation
for proximal tubal block 262
complications 263
technique 262

I

Interstitial pregnancy 396
diagnosis 396
treatment 397
medical 397
surgical 397
Intramural ampullary anastomosis
256
Intramural-isthmic anastomosis
254
steps 254
chromotubation to esta-
blish patency of
proximal segment 255
dissection of intramural
portion of tube 254
infiltration with vasopressin
254
inspection of both ends of
the tube 256
maintenance of hemostasis
255
myometrial sutures 256
preparation of distal stump
of tube 256
suturing of serosa and
mesosalpinx 256
transection of proximal
segment 254
Intrauterine adhesions 187
investigation 191
hysterosalpingography
191

hysteroscopy 193
magnetic resonance
  imaging 193
ultrasonography 191
signs 190
symptoms 190
treatment 193
Intrauterine septa 214
follow-up 216
hysteroscopic septal excision
  215
postoperative care 216
technique 215
Isthmic ampullary anastomosis
  250
Isthmic-Isthmic anastomosis 248
steps 248
    anastomosis of muscular
      layer 248
    application of serosal
      sutures 249
    approximation of
      mesosalpinx 249
    chromotubation 249
    excision of fibrous tissue
      248
    transection of distal stump
      of tube 248
    transection of proximal
      stump of tube 248

L

Laparoscopic myomectomy 104
anesthesia and positioning of
  patient 104
instruments 104
laparoscopic assisted
  myomectomy (LAM) 124
port placement 105
postoperative care 121

risk of laparoscopic
  myomectomy 121
Laparoscopic reconstructive
  surgery for tubal disease 277
Laparoscopic salpingo-ovariolysis
  278
technique 278
    lysis of abdominal wall
      adhesions 278
    salpingo-ovariolysis 278
Laparoscopic salpingostomy vs.
  medical management 387
Laparoscopic surgery for tubal
  and peritubal pathology in
  infertility 269
Laparoscopic tubal anastomosis
  288
Laparoscopy 38
advantages 38
disadvantages 40
Laparotomy vs laparoscopy 396
Lesions within the endometrial
  cavity 447

M

Management of endometriotic
  cysts associated with infertility
  345
impact on fertility 346
incidence 346
treatment 346
    expectant 346
    hormonal suppression 347
    IVF 349
    surgical treatment 348
    ultrasound guided cyst
      aspiration 347
Management of fibroid in the
  infertile patient 97

Management of infertile patient
following surgery 349
 controlled ovarian stimulation
  and intrauterine insemination 351
 factors affecting 350
  cul de sac obliteration 351
  early stage endometriosis
   350
  invasive adhesive
   endometriosis 350
  rectovaginal nodules 351
 impact of ART on endo-
  metriosis 354
 impact of endometriosis on
  IVF 352
 ovarian suppression prior to
  IVF 354
 post surgical medical treatment
  351
 presurgery ovarian
  suppression 351
Metroplasty 174
 Jones metroplasty 179
 Straussman's metroplasty 176
 Tomkins metroplasty 180
  advantages 182
  result 182
  treatment 183
Microsurgical approach to
 fallopian tube 230

N

Neosalpingostomy 239

O

Ovarian endometriosis 361
 large endometriomas 363
 moderate endometriomas
  363
 recurrent ovarian
  endometrioma 367
 superficial small ovarian
  endometrioma 363
 technique 363
  adhesiolysis 363
  control of bleeding 366
  decompression of the cyst
   363
  stripping the cyst wall 364

P

Pelvic inflammatory disease 303
 clinical characteristics 306
 diagnosis 307
  clinical diagnosis 307
  laboratory diagnosis 309
 etiology and pathogenesis
  304
 grading 310
 management 311
 risk factors 305
Peritoneal platform 243
Persistent ectopic pregnancy 273
Persistent tubal ectopic gestation
 387
Prefimbrial phimosis 237, 287
Prevention of postoperative
 adhesions 405
 barrier solutions 417
 etiology 406
 mechanism of infertility 406
 pathophysiology 407
 solid barriers 420
  natural 421
  synthetic 421
 types 410
  medical approach 410
  surgical approach 413
Proximal tubal cannulation 289

R

Recurrent endometriosis 345

S

Salpingectomy 242, 274
Salpingolysis 232
Salpingoplasty 236
Salpingostomy (salpingo-
　　neostomy) 287
Steps of adhesiolysis 233
Submucous myoma and polyp
　　217

T

Tests for assessing uterine cavity
　　and structural abnormalities 2
　　endometrial biopsy 22
　　hysterosalpingography 2
　　hysteroscopy 14
　　hysterosonography 11
　　magnetic resonance hystero-
　　　　graphy 14
　　MRI 22
　　ultrasound 22
Tests for evaluation of tubal
　　structure and function 29
Tests to assess uterine receptivity
　　22
　　markers of the embryo-
　　　　endometrial dialogue 25
　　tests that assess endometrial
　　　　changes 22
　　　　endometrial histology 22
　　　　hormonal levels 25
　　　　ultrasound and Doppler 23
Tubal anastomosis 291
　　indications 292
　　operative procedure 293
　　postoperative care 300

preoperative preparation 292
　　results 300
　　types 292
Tubal endoscopy 40
　　basic procedures 40
　　　　falloposcopy 41
　　　　salpingoscopy 41
　　complications 44
　　steps of the procedure 41
　　　　step I: gaining access to the
　　　　　　uterotubal ostium 41
　　　　step II: tubal catheterization
　　　　　　42
Tubal implantation 259
　　complications 262
　　procedures 260
　　　　cornual implantation 260
　　　　posterior wall implantation
　　　　　　260
　　steps 260
　　　　implantation 260
　　　　preparation of the proximal
　　　　　　portion of the distal
　　　　　　segment 260
　　　　preparation of the uterine
　　　　　　wall 260
Tubal pathology 450
　　cervical pregnancy 454
　　cornual ectopic pregnancy
　　　　455
　　ectopic pregnancy 453
　　hydrosalpinx/pyosalpinx 450
　　tubo-ovarian abscess 452
Tubal reanastomosis 246
Tubal reconstructive surgery 225
Tubal surgery vs ART 265
Tubal tumors 455
Tubo-cornual anastomosis for
　　proximal disease 253

Tubo-uterine factors in infertility
427
  tubal factor affecting
      implantation 431
  uterine factors affecting
      implantation 428
  uterine fibroids 428
  uterine polyps 429
  congenital anomalies of
      uterus 429
  intrauterine synechiae 430
  unexplained poor
      endometrium 430

U

Uterine anomalies 135
  classification 137
  development 136
  diagnosis 143
      hysterosalpingography
          143
      hysteroscopy 144
      intravenous pylography
          (IVP) 145
      laparoscopy 144
      magnetic resonance
          imaging 145
      transvaginal ultrasound
          144
  etiology 137

impact on fertility 142
incidence 136
management 148
symptoms 137
  gynecologic 137
  obstetric 137
Uterine cavity and endometrium
  1
Uterine malformations 437
  arcuate 442
  bicornuate 439
  diethylstilbestrol related 442
  hypoplasia or agenesis 437
  septate uterus 440
  unicornuate uterus 438
  uterus didelphus 438
Uterine pathology 436
Uterine-sparing treatment of
  fibroids 95

V

Vaginal atresia 150

W

William's vulvovaginoplasty 159
  advantages 161
  disadvantages 161
  indications 159
  technique 160